Cardiovascular
Nursing
SECRETS

Cardiovascular Nursing SECRETS

LESLIE DAVIS, MSN, RN, CS, ANP
Clinical Assistant Professor
School of Nursing
University of North Carolina at Chapel Hill
Chapel Hill, North Carolina

SERIES EDITOR

LINDA SCHEETZ, EdD, APRN, BC, CEN
Assistant Professor
College of Nursing
Rutgers, The State University of New Jersey
Rutgers, New Jersey

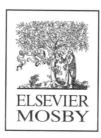

ELSEVIER
MOSBY

ELSEVIER
MOSBY

11830 Westline Industrial Drive
St. Louis, Missouri 63146

NOTICE

Cardiac Nursing is an ever-changing field. Standard safety precautions must be followed, but as new research and clinical experience broaden our knowledge, changes in treatment and drug therapy may become necessary or appropriate. Readers are advised to check the most current product information provided by the manufacturer of each drug to be administered to verify the recommended dose, the method and duration of administration, and contraindications. It is the responsibility of the licensed health care provider, relying on experience and knowledge of the patient, to determine dosages and the best treatment for each individual patient. Neither the publisher nor the author assumes any liability for any injury and/or damage to persons or property arising from this publication.

International Standard Book Number 0-323-03143-9

Acquisitions Editor: Sandra Clark Brown
Senior Developmental Editor: Cindi Anderson
Publishing Services Manager: Deborah L. Vogel
Senior Project Manager: Ann E. Rogers
Designer: Amy Buxton

Printed in the United States of America.

Last digit is the print number: 9 8 7 6 5 4 3 2 1

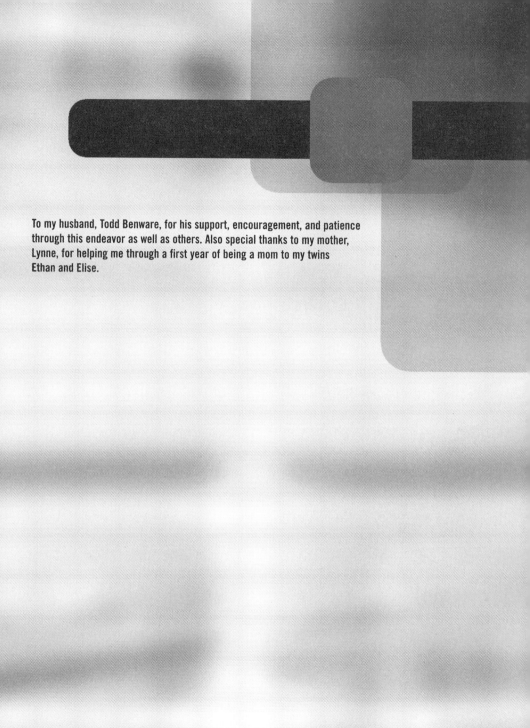

To my husband, Todd Benware, for his support, encouragement, and patience through this endeavor as well as others. Also special thanks to my mother, Lynne, for helping me through a first year of being a mom to my twins Ethan and Elise.

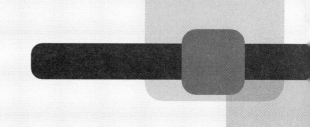

Contributors

MARGARET T. BOWERS, MSN, RN, CS, FNP
Assistant Clinical Professor
Duke University School of Nursing
Durham, North Carolina
    11, Heart Failure
    30, Diuretics and Nitrates

SHARON M. CASTINA, MSN, RN, WHCNP
Clinical Research Coordinator
School of Medicine
Department of Medicine, Division of Cardiology
University of North Carolina at Chapel Hill
Chapel Hill, North Carolina
    6, Selected Nuclear Cardiovascular Testing

KARI L. CRAWFORD, MS, RN-CS, PNP
Pediatric Nurse Practitioner
Cardiothoracic Surgery/Inpatient Cardiology
Brenner Children's Hospital/Wake Forest University Baptist Medical Center
Winston-Salem, North Carolina
    16, Congenital Heart Disease

PENELOPE ANN CRISP, ANP-C, MSN
Vascular Surgery Nurse Practitioner
Department of General Surgery
Wake Forest University School of Medicine
Winston-Salem, North Carolina
    15, Deep Vein Thrombosis and Pulmonary Embolism
    17, Peripheral Vascular Disease

LINDA K. DALEY, PHD, RN
Assistant Professor, Clinical and Assistant Dean for Pre-Licensure Programs
The Ohio State University College of Nursing
Columbus, Ohio
    8, Hypertension

LESLIE DAVIS, MSN, RN, CS, ANP
Clinical Assistant Professor
Adult Nurse Practitioner
School of Nursing
School of Medicine, Department of Medicine
Division of Cardiology
University of North Carolina at Chapel Hill
Chapel Hill, North Carolina

PAUL DUNN, MSN, FNP, CDE
Clinical Associate Professor
Department of Family Medicine
University of North Carolina at Chapel Hill
Chapel Hill, North Carolina

SUSAN K. FRAZIER, PhD, RN
Associate Professor
The Ohio State University College of Nursing
Columbus, Ohio

REBECCA GARY, RN, PhD
Assistant Professor
School of Nursing
Medical College of Georgia
Augusta, Georgia

PAULINE A. GEARING, RN, BSN, CCRC
Cardiac Research Manager
Research Department
University Community Hospital
Tampa, Florida

JANA M. GLOTZER, RN, MSN, CCRN, ACNP, ANP
Heart Failure Nurse Practitioner
Department of Medicine, Division of Cardiology
University of North Carolina at Chapel Hill
Chapel Hill, North Carolina
    33, Digoxin and Other Inotropic Agents

MARY JO GOOLSBY, EdD, MSN, ANP-C, FAANP
Director of Research and Education Department
American Academy of Nurse Practitioners
Austin, Texas
    29, Chronic Anticoagulation

CHRISTINE GREENWOOD, RN, BSN
Nurse Education Clinician
Department of Cardiology
University of North Carolina at Chapel Hill
Chapel Hill, North Carolina
    5, Noninvasive Cardiovascular Testing

JASON BARNES HARRELL, RN, MSN, ANP-C
Nurse Practitioner
Cardiology Department
Cardiology Specialists of North Carolina
Winston-Salem, North Carolina
    38, Cardiac Rehabilitation

WINNIE HENNESSY, RN, MSN, PhD(c)
Clinical Nurse Specialist: Palliative and Supportive Care
Medical and Surgical Oncology
Medical University of South Carolina
Charleston, South Carolina
    45, End-of-Life Care

KENDRA HENNINGS, AAS, RT(R) (CV) (ARRT)
Program Director, Clinical Instructor, Cardiovascular Specialist
Cardiac Catheterization Laboratory and Interventional Radiology
Wake Forest University Baptist Medical Center
Winston-Salem, North Carolina
    7, Invasive Cardiovascular Testing (Angiography and Electrophysiology Studies)

MARGARET C. HERBST, RN, MSN
Clinical Instructor of Medicine
Department of Medicine
University of North Carolina at Chapel Hill
Chapel Hill, North Carolina

CLAUDIA A. IRMIERE, RN, MS, CCRN
Clinical Nurse Specialist, Electrophysiology
Department of Electrophysiology
St. Joseph Regional Medical Center
Paterson, New Jersey

PENNY KAY KALPIN, MS, CNS, RN
Certified Clinical Nurse Specialist
Department of Nursing
Mayo Clinic, Saint Mary's Hospital
Rochester, Minnesota

JANE S. KAUFMAN, MS, RN, CS, ANP
Clinical Assistant Professor
School of Nursing
Adult Nurse Practitioner
Pulmonary Division
University of North Carolina at Chapel Hill
Chapel Hill, North Carolina

LISA A. KIGER, RN, MSN, APRN-BC, CCRN, FACCN
Cardiothoracic Nurse Practitioner
Cardiothoracic Surgery
Wake Forest University Baptist Medical Center
Winston-Salem, North Carolina

SCOTT KOWALCZYK, RN, BSN, CCTC
Cardiac Transplantation Coordinator
University of North Carolina Heart Center
Chapel Hill, North Carolina

VALERIE H. LUNSFORD, RN, MSN
Teaching Fellow and Doctoral Student
School of Nursing
University of North Carolina at Chapel Hill
Chapel Hill, North Carolina
   39, Psychosocial Considerations
   40, Cardiovascular Disease and Women

CORINNE M. MILLER, RN, BSN
Staff Nurse, Clinical Nurse IV
Cardiac Care Unit
Duke University Hospital
Durham, North Carolina
   9, Acute Coronary Syndromes

SARA PAUL, RN, MSN, FNP
Director, Heart Function Clinic
Hickory Cardiology Associates
Hickory, North Carolina
   1, History Taking for the Cardiovascular Patient
   2, Physical Examination of the Cardiovascular Patient
   31, Beta-Blockers and Calcium Channel Blockers
   32, Angiotensin-Converting Enzyme Inhibitors and Angiotensin-Receptor Blockers

KAREN PATTERSON PULIDO, RN, MSN
Acute Care Nurse Practitioner
Department of Medicine
Division of Cardiology
University of North Carolina at Chapel Hill
Chapel Hill, North Carolina
   4, Selected Laboratory Procedures

JULIE T. RUCH, MSN, ACNP
Nurse Practitioner, Clinical Instructor
University of North Carolina School of Medicine
Department of Medicine, Division of Cardiology
University of North Carolina at Chapel Hill
Chapel Hill, North Carolina
   36, Lipid-Lowering Strategies

SHARRON RUSHTON, RN, MS, MSN
Nurse Manager
Department of Nursing, Surgery Service
University of North Carolina Hospitals
Chapel Hill, North Carolina
   21, Cardiovascular Surgery

DEBORAH D. SMITH, BSN, RN
Research Coordinator, Cardiology
Department of Electrophysiology
Duke University Medical Center
Durham, North Carolina
   10, Myocardial Infarction
   27, Thrombolytic Therapy
   28, Antiplatelet and Antithrombotic Agents

JOHN STOVER, MSN, RN, FNP
Family Nurse Practitioner
Department of Anesthesia, Preoperative Screening
Duke University Medical Center
Durham, North Carolina
   14, Valvular Heart Disease

VICKIE STRANG, RN, BS, CCRN
Clinical Nurse III
Coronary Care Unit
University of North Carolina Hospitals
Chapel Hill, North Carolina
   22, Temporary Pacing, Cardioversion, and Defibrillation
   23, Ventricular Assist Devices and Intraaortic Balloon Pump

CINDI A. SULLIVAN, MS, RN
Director of Research
Department of Research
University Community Hospital
Tampa, Florida
   41, Cardiovascular Disease and the Elderly

BONNIE TAYLOR, RN, BSN
Certified Emergency Nurse
Emergency Department
Duke University Hospital
Durham, North Carolina
   44, Family Presence

BRENDA S. THOMPSON, RN, MS, CCRN, CNS
Advanced Practice Nurse
Program Director, Heart Failure Program
Cardiovascular Institute
St. Paul University Hospital at Southwestern Medical Center
Dallas, Texas
   42, Cardiovascular Disease and Ethnicity

RACHEL TUNSTALL, MSN, RN, CS, FNP
Clinical Research Coordinator
School of Medicine
Department of Medicine, Division of Cardiology
University of North Carolina at Chapel Hill
Chapel Hill, North Carolina
        5, Noninvasive Cardiovascular Testing
    12, Presyncope and Syncope

MARCIA VAN RIPER, RN, PHD
Associate Professor
School of Nursing/Carolina Center for Genome Sciences
University of North Carolina at Chapel Hill
Chapel Hill, North Carolina
    46, Genetics

KIMBERLY VITALE-SHELDON, RN, MS(C)
Clinical Field Specialist
ELA Medical, Inc.
Mission Viejo, California
    13, Arrhythmias

MONTY YODER, PHARMD, BCPS
Pharmaceutical Care Coordinator, Cardiology
Pharmacy Department
Wake Forest University Baptist Medical Center
Winston-Salem, North Carolina
    20, Percutaneous Coronary Interventions

Preface

The field of cardiology is growing rapidly in both hospital and outpatient settings. *Cardiovascular Nursing Secrets* is written by nurses for nurses in busy clinical practices; this book is intended to supplement basic knowledge in cardiovascular nursing. Common questions asked by new or experienced nurses in clinical practice are answered in this book, and topics are presented in a question-and-answer format for quick reference. "Pearls" of the trade are offered by expert clinicians, many of whom are advanced practice nurses. The book lends direction to the future of cardiovascular nursing by offering current clinical controversies and information on future directions at the end of most chapters.

The book is divided into eight sections. **Section I** provides a guide to assessment skills such as history taking and conducting a physical examination. Hemodynamic monitoring, both invasive and noninvasive, is also covered in the first section. **Section II** addresses various types of diagnostic testing pertinent to the cardiovascular patient population, including indications for each and tips for interpreting results. Patient preparation instructions and guidelines for patient and family education are also included. **Section III** covers symptoms and disease states for the most common cardiovascular conditions. Common etiologies of symptoms, differential diagnoses, the most common treatments, and controversies in the field are discussed. **Section IV** includes therapeutic treatment options—some invasive while others less so. **Section V** covers some of the major categories of pharmacologic treatment options for cardiovascular conditions, including indications for use, potential side effects, patient education, and any current controversies surrounding each treatment option. **Section VI** discusses areas of cardiovascular risk reduction that nurses commonly address when doing assessments, educating for primary and secondary prevention of cardiovascular events, and completing discharge planning. Common strategies are provided to optimize patient adherence. **Section VII** addresses special patient populations that are commonly seen in cardiovascular practice. Unique characteristics of each subpopulation in relation to cardiovascular disease are discussed. **Section VIII** covers special topics such as family presence, end of life, and genetics. These are topics not included in many general nursing educational programs yet commonly encountered in nursing practice.

References at the end of each chapter have been published primarily within the past five years, except for those which offer historical perspective for the topic presented.

In addition, special end-of-chapter features unique to the book include Internet Resources and a Key Points summary.

Finally, the Top Secrets for cardiovascular nursing are compiled as a reminder that clinicians should share "secrets" of the field to improve care for all of our clients.

Acknowledgments

I want to acknowledge my gratitude to the contributors for each of the chapters. They gave their time to share their expertise with nurses of today and of the future. I also am grateful to the thoughtful reviewers, Denise Buonocore and Jennifer Hebra, who offered suggestions to improve the book. I also would like to acknowledge Mary Jo Goolsby, whose support and encouragement to edit this book was incredible. I am also grateful to Linda Scheetz for her guidance in her role as the Nursing Secrets Series editor. Lastly, I would like to thank my mentors in the field of cardiology for the past two decades of my career—Carla Sueta, Magnus Ohman, Alan Hinderliter, Chris Granger, and Robert Califf.

Contents

VIII   CURRENT TOPICS IN CARDIOLOGY, 487

TOP SECRETS

1. **Top secret: *Listen to your patient.*** Even if the patient's objective signs don't correlate with the subjective symptoms, it is very important to listen carefully to the chief complaint. The history is the most important *diagnostic test* on which to base treatment decisions.
2. When taking a history, there is nothing more valuable than having patients express their symptoms in their own words. To that end, when asking follow-up questions, use the words (adjectives) that the patient uses. Don't call chest discomfort "pain" if the patient calls it "pressure."
3. Palpating a difficult-to-feel PMI: have the patient roll to the left side and lighten the fingertips of the hand you are using to assess the point of maximum impulse (PMI).
4. Auscultating difficult-to-hear heart sounds: place the patient in the left lateral recumbent position or have him or her sit up and lean forward. If still having difficulty hearing a sound, close your eyes to enhance concentration and block out extraneous sensory input.
5. Never auscultate through the patient's gown or other clothing. These items may interfere with accuracy of heart or lung sounds.
6. An incorrect blood pressure (BP) cuff size produces invalid BP readings: a cuff too large yields a falsely low measurement; a cuff too small yields a falsely high measurement.
7. Automated BP measurements will yield invalid results for patients with tachycardia, cardiac dysrhythmias (especially atrial fibrillation), shock, and/or vascular disease.
8. Common reasons for invalid pulse oximetry readings may be patient factors such as inadequate arterial pulsatile blood flow (i.e., hypothermia or hypotension), elevated venous pressure, and anemia, as well as system factors such as motion artifact, electrical interference, and interference with strong ambient light (heat lamps or surgical lights).
9. Treadmill testing should not be used for patients who have resting electrocardiogram (ECG) abnormalities, (e.g., 100% paced rhythm, atrial fibrillation, atrial flutter, or left bundle branch block) because these rhythms interfere with the interpretation of ST segment changes associated with ischemia. Likewise, patients who are receiving digoxin, have left ventricular hypertrophy (LVH), and/or are women have been associated with false-positive stress tests.
10. A 12-lead ECG provides a 10-second "snap shot" of the cardiac cycle. Therefore patients having dynamic ischemia (i.e., acute coronary syndromes) may have completely normal ECGs; hence the importance of serial ECGs for patients with ongoing or recurrent symptoms suggestive of cardiac ischemia. Similarly, ECGs performed at rest in the absence of stress or ongoing chest pain typically do not reveal ischemic changes.
11. The initial 12-lead ECG is diagnostic of an acute myocardial infarction (AMI) in only about 50%-60% of patients. Serial ECGs in this AMI population may reveal an additional 10%.
12. Suspect posterior wall MI in patients with signs and symptoms of AMI with ST depression in V_1-V_2 on the 12-lead ECG.
13. Suspect right ventricular (RV) infarct in inferior MI patients with markedly decreased BP;

check right-sided chest leads (V_{4R}) in these patients. Hypotension will occur with the use of nitroglycerin, magnesium sulfate, and diuretics with clear lung fields. IV fluid challenges, inotrope use, or balloon pump support may be required.

14. New left bundle branch block on a 12-lead ECG in a patient with ischemic symptoms is presumed to be an AMI until proven otherwise.

15. A tall-peaked and symmetrical T wave on the ECG often is the first change seen in patients with hyperkalemia.

16. Troponins are the "gold standard" for cardiac enzyme marker testing to rule out an AMI.

17. Ascertainment of serum troponin levels are very useful for patients who delay seeking treatment for symptoms associated with acute MI, as troponin levels remain elevated for up to 5 to 21 days post AMI (depending on which troponin test is done—troponin I versus T).

18. Target serum digoxin levels between 0.5 and 0.9 ng/dL should be used because additional efficacy is not attained with higher levels; yet side effects and toxicity risks are dose related.

19. Serum digoxin levels should be drawn at a minimum of 6 hours after dosing. Levels drawn sooner will be inaccurate.

20. Cardiac catheterization with selective coronary arteriography is the most reliable test for the diagnosis and quantification of coronary artery disease (CAD).

21. Post-PVC measurements of left ventricular ejection fraction (LVEF) done during a left ventriculogram may reveal a falsely elevated LVEF.

22. Chest pain worsened by respiration is typically non-ischemic.

23. For patients who complain of chest discomfort lasting hours at a time for several months with nondiagnositic ECGs of previous MI, the likelihood the pain is ischemic in origin is very low.

24. Prompt reperfusion is essential in treating AMI patients. However the longest delay in time to treatment for AMI patients continues to be the time of symptom onset to hospital presentation, which averages about $2\frac{1}{2}$ hours in the United States.

25. Recurrent chest pain in an AMI patient who has undergone successful reperfusion therapy (via percutaneous coronary intervention [PCI] or fibrinolytics) is worrisome and considered abrupt reocclusion or incomplete reperfusion until proven otherwise. Alternatively, recurrent chest pain days after an MI may reflect pericarditis.

26. Ventricular tachycardia is the most likely dysrhythmia to occur 7 to 9 hours after thrombolysis.

27. Diabetics, women, and the elderly are more likely to present with atypical signs of cardiac ischemia. In fact, approximately 20%-30% of AMI patients are completely asymptomatic at the time of coronary artery occlusion; many have diabetes and hypertension.

28. Assume that a diabetic patient has CAD until proven otherwise. Two thirds of patients with diabetes have CAD, with only about half of those having been previously diagnosed.

29. Coronary artery disease is the most common cause of heart failure in whites; hypertension is the most common cause for blacks.

30. One of the most common presenting symptoms of a patient with heart failure is decreased exercise tolerance. Fatigue and early satiety are also signs of cardiac decompensation.

31. Digoxin use in heart failure patients improves symptoms but not mortality.

32. Asymptomatic heart failure patients with low LVEF still benefit from angiotensin-converting inhibitors (ACE inhibitors) and beta-blockade.

33. The use of digoxin is not recommended for heart failure patients with preserved LVEF (also referred to as diastolic dysfunction).

34. Syncope in a patient with heart failure and low LVEF should be assumed to be due to ventricular tachycardia until proven otherwise.

35. Atrial fibrillation is the most common cardiac dysrhythmia to precipitate an episode of heart failure.

36. Suspect fluid overload in heart failure patients with a cough. Use of ACE inhibitors is often implicated as a cause of cough in HF patients, when in fact it may be more likely related to fluid overload.

37. Pulmonary congestion may or may not be present in patients with heart failure, as evidenced by the fact that 80% of patients with chronic heart failure who are hospitalized do not have rales.
38. Baseline resting tachycardia, hyponatremia, and hyperuricemia are poor prognostic indicators for patients with heart failure.
39. A wide complex tachycardia is assumed to be ventricular tachycardia until proven otherwise.
40. Suspect 2:1 atrial flutter in patients who have a supraventricular tachycardia at a rate of 150 beats per minute.
41. Patients who have undergone heart transplantation may have two distinct atrial P waves on the ECG; one from the preserved sinus node of the native heart and the second from the donor atria. The donor atrium controls the overall heart rate.
42. Chest pain, shortness of breath, and hypotension in patients with unstable cardiac dysrhythmias are typically associated with the cardiac dysrhythmia itself. Once the dysrhythmia resolves, the associated symptoms should dissipate.
43. Coronary artery disease is the most common cause of sudden death. Survivors of sudden death have a high recurrence of cardiac arrest. Thus an implantable cardioverter defibrillator (ICD) is often indicated for prevention of sudden death in these patients.
44. Survival rates after cardiac arrest from ventricular fibrillation decrease approximately 7%-10% for each minute that defibrillation is delayed.
45. Patients with permanent pacemakers may use cell phones, although they should use them on the opposite ear and should refrain from carrying the phone in the shirt pocket over the pulse generator.
46. The incidence of atrial fibrillation doubles with each advancing age of decade, from 0.5% at age 50 to 59 years and 10% at age 80 to 89 years.
47. The rate of stroke is 10 times higher in elders with atrial fibrillation, compared with younger patients.
48. Patient history and physical examination yield the cause of syncope in 45% of cases. A witness to the syncopal event is key; however, the etiology of approximately 50% of syncopal episodes is unknown.
49. Most patients with hypertension will need to be treated with at least two medications.
50. Individuals who are normotensive at 55 years of age have a 90% lifetime risk for developing hypertension.
51. Systolic BP of >140 mm Hg is a more important cardiovascular disease risk factor than diastolic BP.
52. Ninety percent of pulmonary emboli (PE) originate from deep vein thrombosis (DVT) of the legs. DVT from the thigh is more likely to cause a pulmonary embolus (PE) than is thrombosis of the veins in the calves. Thus a patient with a DVT has a high index of suspicion for PE.
53. A positive Homans sign (calf pain on dorsiflexion of the foot) is not a sensitive or specific test for DVT; results are positive in 50% of the patients with DVT and in 40% of those without DVT.
54. Presumed to be classic signs/symptoms of pulmonary emboli, hemoptysis, dyspnea, and chest pain occur in fewer than 20% of those diagnosed with PE. Of those who die of a massive PE, 60% have dyspnea, 17% have chest pain, and 3% have hemoptysis.
55. Aortic stenosis may cause angina in the absence of CAD.
56. The prognosis for patients with symptomatic aortic stenosis is poor, with the average survival being less than 3 years. For those patients with asymptomatic aortic stenosis, sudden death is rare.
57. Patients with severe mitral regurgitation (MR) may have a falsely elevated LVEF if measured by a left ventriculogram during cardiac catheterization. An echocardiogram should be done to evaluate LVEF in patients with severe MR.
58. More than 80% of patients with congenital heart disease are estimated to reach adulthood.

59. Doppler echocardiography is the most important diagnostic tool for evaluating congenital heart disease, often preventing the need for cardiac catheterization.

60. For those patients undergoing CABG, the internal mammary artery (IMA) is the conduit of choice, with patency rates (at 10 years) of approximately 83%, as compared to 41% for saphenous vein grafts.

61. Approximately 30% of patients undergoing open heart surgery are estimated to develop postoperative atrial fibrillation, most commonly on the second or third postoperative day.

62. Transdermal nitrate patches should be applied for a 12-hour to 14-hour period and then removed for 10 to 12 hours before the next patch is applied in order to reduce tolerance to nitrates. Sometimes this interval when the patient is free of topical nitrates is referred to as a "nitrate holiday."

63. Actually giving aspirin (ASA) to a post-MI patient is more important than the specific dose.

64. Combined studies in more than 100,000 patients have shown a 29% reduction in MI incidence in patients treated early with ASA.

65. A common adverse effect of milrinone is atrial fibrillation.

66. Even a half pack of cigarettes per day may increase the risk of development of peripheral vascular disease (PVD) by 30%-50%.

67. After 15 smoke-free years, the risk of a new MI or death from CHD is similar to that of those who never smoked.

68. Passive smoking (or second-hand smoke) increases the relative risk of CHD in men by 22% and in women by 24%.

69. An accurate lipid panel can be assessed only after 12 hours of fasting. If the patient doesn't fast, only a total cholesterol (TC) and a high-density lipoprotein cholesterol (HDL-C) should be obtained.

70. For patients with hyperlipidemia, treatment should focus on lowering the low-density lipoprotein (LDL) cholesterol.

71. Common causes of elevated triglyceride (TG) levels are uncontrolled diabetes, alcohol use, and estrogen or steroid use; all of which should be addressed before treating the hypertriglyceridemia.

72. Women have smaller diameter coronary arteries and have less developed collateral circulation than men, which may explain their atypical symptoms of ischemia.

73. During the first year after the diagnosis of CHD, women have a greater risk of both death and reinfarction as compared with men.

74. Depression has been associated with twice the risk of developing CHD.

75. **And the final secret is: *Listen to your patient.*** This is the most important secret, thus it is listed first and last. Care begins and ends with the patient—and that is best understood by listening to him or her!

Section I

Assessment

Chapter 1

History Taking for the Cardiovascular Patient

Sara Paul

1. When assessing a patient with a cardiovascular (CV) condition, what pertinent questions should a nurse ask?

The nurse questioning a patient with a CV disease should allow the patient to express his or her chief complaint in his or her own words. This gives the nurse some insight into the patient's understanding of the illness. Furthermore, patients may use their own adjectives to describe symptoms, such as referring to chest pain as "pressure," "tightness," or "burning" rather than calling it "pain." This may be an accurate description of the sensation in the patient's chest, or it may be a denial mechanism for the patient to avoid admitting that he or she could have a cardiac problem.

2. What are some specific CV questions to ask patients about symptoms?

There are a number of cardinal symptoms of heart disease, but the major ones include difficulty breathing, cough, chest pain or discomfort, palpitations, syncope, edema, and cyanosis. It is important to differentiate a pulmonary versus a cardiac origin when assessing difficulty breathing and cough. Chest pain has many different sources, and cardiac origin must be ruled out before any other cause. Other abnormalities may cause palpitations and syncope, but cardiac causes are most common and must be ruled out. Although edema is not a life-threatening symptom, it can arise from hepatic origin, renal disease, or serious CV illness such as heart failure. Cyanosis is a bluish discoloration of the skin and mucous membranes and is both a symptom and a physical sign of decreased oxygenation. It may be central, as in congenital heart disease, or peripheral, as in cutaneous vasoconstriction. Other minor symptoms that are broader in etiology include fatigue and hemoptysis. The table below outlines the pertinent questions surrounding each of these topics.

Questions to ask about symptoms of heart disease

Symptom	Questions
Difficulty breathing/cough	1. Did your difficulty breathing begin abruptly or come on gradually?
	2. Does your difficulty primarily occur with inspiration, expiration, or both?
	3. Do you find it difficult to breathe at rest or only with activity?

Questions to ask about symptoms of heart disease   *continued*

Symptom	Questions
Difficulty breathing/cough	4. Does your breathing cause any pain?
	5. Is your difficulty breathing associated with anxiety or hyperventilation?
	6. Do you hear yourself wheezing when it is difficult to breathe?
	7. Is it difficult to breathe lying flat? If so, how many pillows must you prop yourself up with to breathe comfortably?
	8. Does a change in position make your breathing easier?
	9. Do you ever wake up from your sleep with difficulty breathing and have to sit up in bed to breathe easier?
	10. Do you experience any other symptoms when it is difficult to breathe?
	11. Is your cough dry or wet? If wet, what do the secretions look like?
	12. Do you cough more at any particular time, such as early morning, only when lying down, during the night, or anytime?
	13. How long have you had this cough?
	14. Is your cough associated with sinus congestion, sore throat, runny nose, or fever?
	15. Do you smoke?
Chest pain or discomfort	1. Describe the location, radiation, and character of the discomfort.
	2. What causes it and what relieves it?
	3. What is the frequency of recurrence?
	4. In what setting does the discomfort occur?
	5. Are there other symptoms associated with the chest discomfort?
	6. When did it begin? How long ago did it start?
	7. How long does the discomfort last?
	8. Does the discomfort have maximal intensity from its onset, or is there a build-up for several seconds?
	9. Is there a family history of coronary artery disease?
Palpitations or syncope	1. Do you have episodes of your heart skipping beats or racing?
	2. When did it first begin, and how frequently does it happen?
	3. How long does it last?
	4. Does it occur with rest or activity or both?
	5. Does it occur after ingesting large quantities of caffeine or cigarettes?
	6. Are there associated symptoms with these palpitations?
	7. Have you ever counted your pulse during an episode of palpitations? If so, what was your heart rate?
	8. Have you ever passed out or felt like you were near to passing out (black vision or floaters in front of your eyes)?
	9. If you have passed out, what exactly happened before and after you lost consciousness?
	10. Is there a family history of syncope, arrhythmia, or sudden death?
Edema	1. Where is the swelling?
	2. Does it occur on both the right and left side, or is it unilateral?

Questions to ask about symptoms of heart disease   *continued*

Symptom	Questions
Edema	3. Is the swelling worse in the evenings and better in the mornings? 4. Are there any other symptoms associated with the swelling? 5. Does the swelling occur only after long periods of sitting or standing? 6. Do you take any medications that may cause swelling (nonsteroidal antiinflammatory agents, minoxidil, hydralazine, clonidine, calcium channel blockers, steroid hormones, or cyclosporine)?
Cyanosis	1. Have you noticed a bluish coloring to your skin on any part of your body? 2. Where do you notice the discoloration? 3. Does it only occur in cold weather? 4. How long have you had this discoloration? Did you have it as a child?
Others Hemoptysis	1. Have you ever coughed up blood? 2. Was your sputum blood streaked or tinged or frank blood? 3. Is it associated with coughing? 4. Is it associated with difficulty breathing or chest pain? 5. How long has this been happening?
Fatigue	1. How long have you felt fatigued? 2. How far can you walk without having to stop and rest? 3. How many steps can you climb? 4. What specific activities make you fatigued, and what level of activity can you perform?
Nocturia	1. Do you get up to urinate during the night? How many times? 2. How long have you been doing this?
Anorexia	1. Have you lost weight recently? How much? 2. Do you feel abdominal fullness or right upper quadrant discomfort? 3. Do you have any appetite? Do you get full quickly? 4. Have you had any nausea or vomiting lately?
Visual changes	1. Have you had any visual changes recently?

3. What are other questions to ask patients about their chief complaint?

Once the patient has voiced the complaint, the nurse must query the patient on issues surrounding the specific symptom, such as the following:

- When did the symptom begin?
- Has it happened before?
- How did it begin? (abrupt versus gradual onset)
- What were you doing at the time? (rest versus activity)
- How long does it last?
- How often does it occur?
- What brings on the symptom? (precipitating events)

- What relieves the symptom? (medication, rest, change of position)
- If there is pain, specify where the pain is felt and describe the pain.
- How severe is the pain or symptom? (usually measured on a scale from 1 to 10, with 1 being the least and 10 being the most severe)
- What other symptoms are associated with the complaint?

4. What essential questions should nurses ask CV patients when assessing past medical history?

Start with a query of the patient's general state of health, and then ask about any CV or non-CV illnesses. Special attention should be given to diseases that have a direct impact on the CV system, such as diabetes, hypertension, coronary artery disease/chest pain, past cardiac illnesses (e.g., myocardial infarction, heart failure, arrhythmias), peripheral vascular disease, and elevated lipid concentrations. Numerous illnesses, including, but not limited to, the neurological, endocrine, gastrointestinal, rheumatic, pulmonary, and hematological/oncology systems, have important effects on the CV system or mimic CV symptoms, and it is vital to assess for the presence of these and any other conditions. Examples of these include stroke, thyroid disorders, rheumatic disease, anemia, chronic obstructive pulmonary disease, and gastric reflux. Women should be queried about their menstrual status and if they have experienced menopause. Inquire about any childhood illnesses, especially streptococcal infections. The patient should be asked if he or she has any allergies to food, medications, or anything else. Ask the patient about any accidents or injuries he or she has had in the past, as well as any hospitalizations or procedures.

5. What are pertinent questions to ask about the patient's use of medications?

It is crucial to obtain a current list of all medications the patient is taking, including prescription drugs, over-the-counter medicines, and herbal remedies. The best way to do this is to have the patient's medications in front of you and go over them one by one, opening the bottles and actually looking at the pills. Ask the patient specifically how each one is taken. Do not rely on what the prescription on the bottle says. Many times, health care providers change dosages without giving the patient a new prescription. Opening the bottle and looking at the pills may provide interesting insights, such as pills that the patient has split in half or mixed together or that the number of pills in the bottle does not correspond with the date the prescription was filled. This may indicate that the patient has been taking the wrong dosage. Too many pills in the bottle may indicate that the patient has not been taking enough pills each day, and too few pills in the bottle may indicate that the patient has been taking a higher dose of the medicine than prescribed. Occasionally, the dosage of the pills in the bottle may differ from the dosage that was prescribed. This may come about by human error when the pharmacist filled the prescription. It is important to check these things because lay people are often less knowledgeable about prescription medications. Over-the-counter medications should be specifically discussed because they may interact with prescription drugs or may contain ingredients that the patient should not be taking. Examples include pseudo-ephedrine, which may cause tachycardia and should not be taken by cardiac patients, or nonsteroidal antiinflammatory drugs, such as ibuprofen or naproxen, which may increase the risk of bleeding in patients taking warfarin or cause swelling in heart failure patients. Herbal remedies are notorious for interacting with prescription drugs by increasing or decreasing the potency of many medications. Also ask about any recent medication changes.

6. **What essential questions should nurses ask CV patients when assessing past surgical history?**

Particular attention should be paid to a history of CV surgery, such as coronary artery bypass grafting, valve repair or replacement, pericardectomy, pacemaker or defibrillator implantation, ventricular resection, or congenital heart defect repair. The nurse should specifically ask about procedures that the patient has undergone because the patient might not consider a procedure to be surgical in nature and therefore will not volunteer the information, particularly if the procedure was not performed in an operating room. Examples of CV procedures include percutaneous coronary angioplasty, stent placement, pacemaker or implantable defibrillator insertion, cardiac catheterization, and ablation therapy. The patient should also be asked about any noncardiac surgery or procedures he or she might have undergone in the past. Examples include, but are certainly not limited to, gynecological surgery, dental surgery, and gastrointestinal, genitourinary, oncologic, and orthopedic procedures.

7. **What information in the patient's family history is pertinent when evaluating a CV patient?**

Some forms of CV disease are hereditary and may be passed on from parents to offspring. When asking about the patient's family history, specify that you want to know about the patient's immediate family members: father, mother, sisters, brothers, and their offspring. Distant relatives with CV disease (grandparents, aunts, uncles, cousins) do not increase the patient's risk of CV disease. Inquire about the health status of immediate family members, and determine those who are living and those who are deceased. Identify the cause of death and the age at which the family member died. If the patient's mother or father died of a myocardial infarction at age 40, this increases the patient's risk of experiencing a coronary event. However, if the patient's relative died at an advanced age (e.g., 80 years) from a myocardial infarction or is not a first-degree relative, the risk of the patient experiencing a coronary event is not increased.

8. **What essential questions should a nurse ask when assessing a CV patient's social history?**

Inquire about the patient's marital status, living situation, children, and any other support people who may help the patient during his or her illness. Job situation, education level, military service, and travel should be identified. The patient should be asked about personal habits such as exercise, cigarette smoking, alcohol intake, and use of drugs, illicit and otherwise. Inquire about previous charges of driving while intoxicated. The patient should be given information regarding complications of and remedies for unhealthful social practices to minimize future risk, such as smoking cessation information.

9. Where do CV risk factors fit into history taking?

A risk factor is a feature that is present early in life and is associated with an increased risk of developing future disease. It may be a behavior (smoking), an inherited trait (family history), or a laboratory measurement (elevated cholesterol). Particular attention should be paid to questions about factors that put the patient at increased risk for CV disease, as follows:

- Cigarette smoking—How many packs does the patient smoke daily? How long has the patient smoked? Has the patient ever tried to quit?
- Hypertension—How long has the patient had high blood pressure? What medicines and dosages is the patient taking for it? Who is the health care provider who manages the patient's hypertension? Does the patient have home blood pressure monitoring?
- Hyperlipidemia—When was the last time the patient's lipids were checked? What were the results? Is the patient on medicine to lower cholesterol? Who is the health care provider who manages the patient's hypercholesterolemia? Has the patient ever talked with a dietician about a low-cholesterol diet? What kind of diet is the patient on?
- Diabetes—How long has the patient had diabetes? Does the patient take oral agents, insulin, or both? What is the patient's average blood sugar value? Does the patient monitor his or her blood sugar at home? Who manages the patient's diabetes? Has the patient ever seen a diabetes educator? Is the patient compliant with a diabetic diet?
- Obesity—Has the patient always been obese? Was the patient also obese as a child, or did the obesity develop during adulthood?
- Sedentary lifestyle—Does the patient perform any type of regular exercise? If so, what type and how often? Does the patient have any physical limitations that prevent exercise?
- Mental stress—Is the patient under a great deal of mental stress? What are some major stresses in the patient's life? How does the patient deal with stress? What methods does the patient use (if any) to relieve stress?
- Hormone status (in women)—Is the patient premenopausal or postmenopausal? Does the patient take birth control pills? Is the patient on hormone therapy?
- Excessive alcohol intake—How many alcoholic drinks does the patient have each day or week? What are the type and specific amount of alcohol consumed? Does the patient have any history of alcohol abuse?
- Family history of CV disease—Does the patient have any immediate relatives who have had heart disease or a heart attack? If so, at what age were they diagnosed? Are they living or deceased?

10. Are there any special tips for obtaining a CV history?

Cardiologist Henry Marriott said, "A health care provider who cannot take a good history and a patient who cannot give one are in danger of giving and receiving bad treatment." That is particularly true for the CV patient. Much of the CV assessment information is obtained during the history, and adequate time must be spent obtaining this information. The nurse should have a routine system for questioning patients and consistently use this same routine each time he or she obtains a CV history. This way, no questions are forgotten or left out of the interview. Unfortunately, most health care institutions give new patients a standardized form to fill out with their entire history, and very few health care providers actually spend time obtaining the health history of their patients in a face-to-face manner. Much more data are obtained in a face-to-face interview, beyond simply the health history. The nurse is able to observe the patient and note the patient's understanding of his or her body and illness. Unspoken body gestures, facial grimacing, ability to make eye contact, mental status, speech patterns, intellectual capacity, family interaction, and fine motor movements are a few of the observations one can make while interviewing a patient.

11. Are there any special tips for interviewing patients?

The nurse should allow the patient to speak in his or her own words, but it is sometimes necessary to keep the patient on track and guide the patient to remain focused on the topic. Otherwise, the patient may ramble in his or her conversation or offer vague answers to questions that require specific information. Often, it is helpful to have a spouse or other family member in the room to offer a different perspective on the patient's description of the symptoms or to share information about the patient's compliance with medical advice. It is important to ask one question at a time, rather than piling up a series of questions for the patient to answer. The nurse must be concise in questioning and clear about the information he or she is attempting to obtain. This brings to mind the patient who, when asked to show her teeth to the medical resident (in a test for cranial nerve function), turned to her husband and said, "George, go out to the truck and fetch my teeth!" Clearly, she did not understand that the resident did not want to examine her false teeth but rather wanted to see if all of the patient's cranial nerves were intact. Clear communication is imperative when obtaining a history from patients.

 Key Points

- The nurse questioning a CV patient should allow the patient to express the chief complaint in his or her own words.
- There are a number of cardinal symptoms of heart disease, but the major ones include difficulty breathing/cough, chest pain or discomfort, palpitation or syncope, edema, and cyanosis.
- It is crucial to obtain a current list of all medications the patient is taking, including prescription drugs, over-the-counter medicines, and herbal remedies.
- The nurse should have a routine system for questioning patients and consistently use this same routine each time he or she obtains a CV history.

Internet Resources

Explore Health With Sentara, Incorporated:
http://explorehealth.sentara.com/library/healthguide/IllnessConditions/topic.asp?
HWID=ps1507

**University of California San Diego: A Practical Guide to Clinical Medicine, Exam of the
Heart:**
http://medicine.ucsd.edu/clinicalmed/heart.htm

**Beth Israel Deaconess Medical Center, Boston, Cardiac Services, Clinical Evaluation and
Testing:**
http://www.bidmc.harvard.edu/cardiac/eval_n_testing/default.asp

Bibliography

Bickley LS, Szilagyi PG: *Bates' guide to physical examination and history taking,* ed 8, Philadelphia, 2002,
Lippincott Williams & Wilkins, pp 1-42.

Braunwald E: The history. In Braunwald E, Zipes D, Libby P, editors: *Heart disease: a textbook of
cardiovascular medicine,* ed 6, Philadelphia, 2001, WB Saunders, pp 27-44.

Coulehan JL, Block MR: *The medical interview: mastering skills for clinical practice,* ed 4, Philadelphia, 2001,
FA Davis.

Marriott HJL: *Bedside cardiac diagnosis,* Philadelphia, 1992, JB Lippincott, pp 1-8.

Taylor GJ, Boyd GE: Physical examination. In Taylor JG, editor: *Primary care management of heart disease,*
St Louis, 2000, Mosby, pp 24-35.

Woods SL, Froelicher ES, Motzer SA, editors: *Cardiac nursing,* ed 4, Philadelphia, 1999, Lippincott Williams
& Wilkins, pp 226-258.

Chapter 2

Physical Examination of the Cardiovascular Patient

Sara Paul

1. **When performing a physical exam on a cardiovascular (CV) patient, what should be assessed during *inspection*?**

   Inspection of the CV system begins with a general inspection of the patient and careful assessment of the skin, mouth, and extremities. Certain findings may indicate CV disorders:
   - Flushed cheeks—mitral stenosis
   - Tall in stature and thin body features—Marfan syndrome
   - Pulsatile eyes and earlobes—tricuspid regurgitation
   - Bobbing of the head with each pulse—aortic regurgitation
   - Central cyanosis—right-to-left shunting (such as occurs with congenital heart disease)
   - Peripheral cyanosis—vascular disease
   - Clubbing of fingers and toes—congenital heart disease
   - Lipid deposit in the inner aspect of the eye (xanthoma)—hyperlipidemia

   Inspection of the anterior chest may reveal abnormal pulsations, bony deformities, abnormal respiratory patterns, skin lesions, or surgical scars. With the patient supine at about a 30-degree angle, inspect the patient's chest from the right side, particularly noting the areas illustrated in the figure on the next page.

2. **What is meant by a *normal carotid upstroke*?**

   The carotid arterial pulse is the most accurate reflection of aortic pulsation, except in patients with carotid bruits or carotid obstruction. Carotid pulsations are visible just medial to the sternomastoid muscles and should be palpated bilaterally, *one side at a time*. The normal upstroke of the carotid pulse is smooth and rapid, and immediately follows the first heart sound. Decreased carotid pulsations with a slow upstroke may represent decreased stroke volume, as occurs in heart failure, hypovolemia, and severe aortic stenosis or atherosclerotic narrowing of the carotid artery. A bounding carotid pulse may be caused by fever, anemia, hyperthyroidism, aortic regurgitation, bradycardia, or heart block.

3. **How is jugular venous distention assessed and measured?**

   The jugular venous pulse provides important information concerning body fluid volume; the presence of venous distention may indicate congestive heart

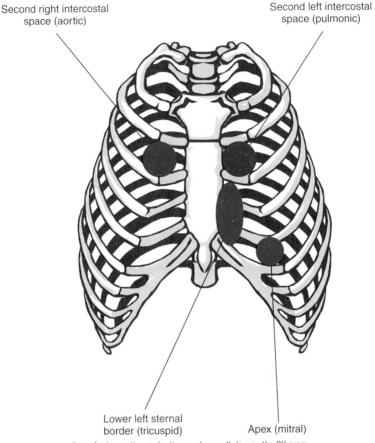

Second right intercostal space (aortic)

Second left intercostal space (pulmonic)

Lower left sternal border (tricuspid)

Apex (mitral)

Areas for inspection, palpation, and auscultation in the CV exam.

failure. It also can indicate abnormal right heart structure or function and may provide clues about cardiac arrhythmias when the venous pulse wave is abnormal. The internal jugular vein is usually assessed with the patient supine at about 30-45 degrees using a light shined tangentially across the right side of the patient's neck. Two assessments can be made of the venous pulse: the level of venous pressure and the venous wave pattern. It is difficult to assess the venous wave pattern; this is usually done by an experienced clinician. However, the venous pressure may be determined by measuring from the patient's sternal angle to the top of the distended jugular vein, per the following figure. This is done by identifying the highest point of the right internal jugular venous pulsation on the patient's neck and measuring the vertical distance at a right angle down to the sternal angle, using a ruler that shows centimeters. Because the right atrium is about 5 cm below the sternal angle, add 5 to the number of centimeters measured from the top of the venous pulsation. The normal jugular venous pressure should not exceed 9 cm.

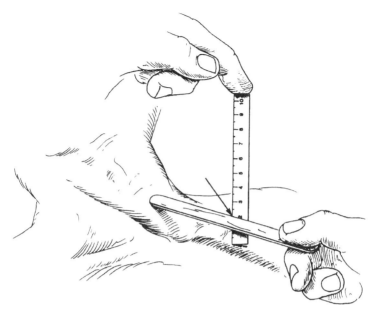

Measuring jugular venous pressure. *(From Adair O: Cardiology secrets, ed 2, Philadelphia, 2001, Hanley & Belfus.)*

4. What is a *point of maximum impulse* (PMI), and why is it useful to assess?

The PMI is caused by the lower anterior portion of the left ventricle striking the chest wall at the time of aortic valve opening. It is normally located at the midclavicular line in the fifth intercostal space. It is a pulsation that should be the size of a quarter and is tapping in quality. The PMI may be laterally displaced when the heart becomes volume overloaded or dilated, and it may be more forceful in left ventricular hypertrophy or dilated cardiomyopathy.

5. How does a nurse locate a patient's PMI, and what are tips for a nurse to use when having difficulty locating the PMI?

With the patient supine, the nurse should palpate the fifth intercostal space at the midclavicular line, using the fingerpads or fingertips with light pressure applied and moving the fingers laterally until the apical pulse is felt. The PMI may not be palpable in the supine position in as many as half of all patients over age 50. If it is difficult to find, have the patient partially roll onto the left side and raise the left arm over the head to make the heart fall laterally and increase palpability of the apical pulse. You may also ask the patient to fully exhale and stop breathing for a few seconds while you palpate for the PMI.

6. What does a *lift* mean, and how does a nurse assess for this?

Right ventricular pressure overload (as in pulmonary hypertension or pulmonic stenosis) and volume overload (as in right ventricular failure, atrial septal defect, or tricuspid regurgitation) can cause a palpable anterior systolic movement along the left parasternal border. This is also known as a *right ventricular heave*. Using your fingerpads with the patient supine, palpate along each of the areas shown in the figure in Question 1, feeling for an anterior systolic motion. You will know you have identified a lift (or heave) if your fingers are visibly lifted up and down on the patient's chest with each pulsation.

7. What is a *thrill*, and how does a nurse assess for this?

A thrill is a vibratory sensation that is a palpable manifestation of loud, harsh murmurs. It is best felt with the flat heel of the hand, while palpating each of the sites shown in the figure on page 12, and could be described as feeling like the throat of a purring cat.

8. When palpating pulses, what are the most essential things for a nurse to do?

Pulses must be palpated and compared bilaterally for symmetrical equality at the carotid, radial, brachial, femoral, popliteal, dorsalis pedis, and posterior tibial sites. Pulses that are not equal bilaterally may indicate reduced arterial blood flow on the side with the weaker pulse. It is important to remember that you should never palpate both sides of the carotid pulse at the same time.

9. What is the appropriate size of blood pressure (BP) cuff to use to provide the most accurate reading?

Many nurses do not think about the size of the BP cuff when they measure a patient's BP. The rubber bladder that is inside the cuff should be 80% of the circumference of the patient's limb, and the width of the cuff should be 40% of the patient's limb circumference. It is very important to use the correct size because a cuff that is too small gives an artificially high reading and a cuff that is too big gives an artificially low reading. Remember that antihypertensive medications are prescribed and dosages are adjusted on the basis of the BP readings obtained by nurses. A BP that is measured falsely high may result in unnecessary medication (or increase in medication), whereas a BP reading that is measured falsely low may result in less-than-adequate therapy. Medications are expensive and have considerable side effects; consequently, a correct BP reading is imperative!

10. What is *pulsus paradoxus*, and how is it measured?

Pulsus paradoxus is a weakening of the pulse during inspiration. Normally, during inspiration, the systolic BP does not drop more than 10 mm Hg. However, in pulsus paradoxus, the systolic BP drops more than 10 mm Hg. This may indicate diseases of the pericardium, pericardial effusion, or constrictive pericarditis. To check for pulsus paradoxus, the BP cuff should be inflated above the patient's usual systolic BP while the patient is supine. The cuff should be deflated so that the initial Korotkoff sounds are heard while the patient slowly exhales. Next, the peak systolic BP should be checked during inspiration. Differences of 10 mm Hg or more in the BPs indicate pulsus paradoxus.

11. **When assessing for edema in the extremities, what are essential points to remember?**

It is important to compare one extremity with the other when evaluating peripheral edema. When checking for pitting, press your thumb into the extremity firmly but gently for at least 5 seconds. The severity of edema is graded on a 4-point scale that ranges from slight, indicated as "+" to very marked, indicated as "++++". Causes of peripheral edema include deep venous thrombosis, chronic venous insufficiency (incompetence of venous valves), lymphedema, heart failure, and tumors that are obstructing venous return. The most common causes of generalized edema seen by the clinician include congestive heart failure, cirrhosis, nephrotic syndrome and other forms of renal disease, and premenstrual edema and pregnancy.

12. **What is the best method to use for auscultating lung sounds in a CV patient?**

Auscultate lung sounds with the patient sitting up at 90 degrees. The posterior and lateral chest should be auscultated bilaterally, beginning at the top and working your way down, alternately listening to the right and left sides. Have the patient breathe with the mouth open, somewhat more deeply than normal. Repeat this procedure on the anterior chest.

13. **What are tips for a nurse to use in patients whose lung sounds are hard to hear, and what does this mean?**

Clothing should be removed from the areas of auscultation because clothes, paper gowns, and even thick chest hair can create confusing sounds that interfere with auscultation. If the patient's chest hair interrupts the ability to clearly auscultate by creating a crackling sound, either press harder with the stethoscope or wet the chest hair. Breath sounds may be difficult to hear in obese patients or patients with restrictive airway disease.

14. **What are some other bedside methods to use to evaluate the lungs during the physical exam if an abnormality is suspected?**

Percussion may be used to determine whether lung tissue is fluid filled, air filled, or solid and should be performed in the same locations and manner as auscultation. If you suspect that air-filled lung tissue has been replaced by fluid-filled or solid lung tissue, you may test the patient's transmitted voice sounds to identify areas of lung that are no longer air filled. Ask the patient to say "99" while auscultating symmetrical areas over the chest wall. Normally, the words should sound muffled, but if the patient's voice transmits loudly (known as *bronchophony*), the lung tissue is no longer air filled. The same is true if the patient's whispered "99" sounds louder and clearer (known as *whispered pectoriloquy*). You can also have the patient say "eee" and listen for a normally muffled "eee" sound. If the patient's voice sounds like "aay" through your stethoscope on the chest (known as *egophony*), you are auscultating over an area of lung that is no longer air filled. It would be reasonable to contact the patient's physician and obtain a chest radiograph to evaluate the patient's pulmonary status.

15. What are the essential things for a nurse to assess when auscultating heart sounds?

Auscultation of the heart should be performed at each of the sites in the Question 1 figure, beginning at the apex and moving up the chest, while listening with the diaphragm and the bell at each site. It is reasonable to begin at the apex because the first heart sound is heard best here; once you have established the first and second heart sounds (S_1 and S_2, respectively), you can identify whether murmurs or extra heart sounds occur during systole or diastole. Sounds that are heard between S_1 and S_2 occur during systole, and sounds that occur after S_2 and before S_1 occur during diastole. There are characteristics of heart sounds that should be considered when auscultating, as follows:

- Timing—Whether the sound occurs during systole or diastole
- Location—Where the sound is heard the loudest on the chest
- Point and duration during the cardiac cycle—Whether the sound occurs in early, mid, or late systole or diastole or the sound lasts throughout systole or diastole *(holosystolic)*
- Pitch—Low pitch (heard best with the bell) or high pitch (heard best with the diaphragm)
- Intensity—Loudness of the sound
- Quality—Descriptive sound of a murmur, such as "blowing," "harsh," "rumbling," or "musical"
- Shape or configuration—Whether the sound starts soft and becomes louder *(crescendo)*, starts loud and becomes softer *(decrescendo)*, starts soft and becomes louder and then softer *(crescendo-decrescendo)*, or maintains the same intensity from the start of the murmur to the end *(pansystolic)*. Each murmur is known for its configuration. For example, mitral stenosis usually has a crescendo configuration, whereas aortic insufficiency is a decrescendo murmur.
- Radiation—When the sound radiates on the chest or body (e.g., mitral regurgitation is associated with radiation to the left axilla; aortic stenosis is associated with radiation to the right side of the neck above the clavicle)
- Changes—Changes in the sound affected by changes in respiration, body position, or medications

Placement of stethoscope for cardiac sounds

Cardiac Sound	Heard Best With	Location	Possible Findings	Causes
S_1	Diaphragm	Apex	Split S_1*	Right bundle branch block
S_2	Diaphragm	Upper left sternal border	Physiological splitting Fixed splitting throughout inspiration and expiration	Split only during inspiration (normal finding) Right bundle branch block, pulmonic stenosis, atrial septal defect, mitral regurgitation

*A split S_1 or S_2 sounds like one heart sound split into two halves of equal intensity and pitch.

Placement of stethoscope for cardiac sounds *continued*

Cardiac Sound	Heard Best With	Location	Possible Findings	Causes
S_3	Bell	Apex	Low-pitched early diastolic sound heard immediately after S_2	Normal in children In adults, decreased myocardial contractility, heart failure, ventricular volume overload
S_4	Bell	Apex	Low-pitched late diastolic sound heard immediately before S_1	Corresponds to atrial contraction (atrial "kick") with a stiff ventricle; caused by hypertension, coronary artery disease, aortic stenosis, cardiomyopathy; not heard in atrial fibrillation

16. If a heart murmur is heard, how can a nurse determine what kind of murmur the patient has?

You can differentiate between a systolic and a diastolic murmur by palpating the patient's carotid pulse while auscultating the chest. If the murmur is heard during a palpable carotid pulse (between S_1 and S_2), then the murmur is systolic, because a pulsation occurs during systole. If the murmur is heard between pulsations, then it is a diastolic murmur, occurring during ventricular filling. By auscultating at each of the sites designated in the Question 1 figure, you can determine the site at which the murmur is best heard. For instance, if a systolic murmur is heard the loudest at the mitral valve site, it is very likely mitral regurgitation. Diastolic murmurs are usually harder to hear and have more of an "echo" sound, rather than a direct sound.

Systolic and diastolic murmurs

Systolic Murmur	Diastolic Murmur
Mitral regurgitation*	Mitral stenosis
Tricuspid regurgitation	Tricuspid stenosis (extremely rare)
Aortic stenosis	Pulmonic insufficiency
Pulmonic stenosis	Aortic insufficiency

*The terms *regurgitation* and *insufficiency* may be used interchangeably.

17. Review the grading system for murmurs.

Cardiac murmurs are graded on a scale of 1 to 6, based on intensity. The grade is usually written in Roman numerals (I-VI) as a fraction. For example, I/VI indicates that a murmur is very quiet, a grade 1 (the softest sound) of 6 (the loudest). The murmur grading scale may be defined as follows:

Grade I—Very faint; may not be heard in all positions; may be intermittently heard; usually heard by more experienced listeners

Grade II—Quiet but heard consistently with each heartbeat

Grade III—Moderately loud

Grade IV—Loud

Grade V—Quite loud and clear

Grade VI—May be so loud that it is heard with the stethoscope off the chest

(Note: Grades IV-VI are usually associated with a thrill.)

18. If an extra heart sound is heard on the exam, how can a nurse determine what it is and whether it is a significant finding?

The first action is to determine at what point in the cardiac cycle the sound is best heard. If it occurs immediately after S_2, the sound is probably an S_3 extra-cardiac sound. It has a lower pitch than S_2 and is best heard with the bell of the stethoscope. If the sound occurs immediately before S_1, it is an S_4 extracardiac sound and, again, is heard best with the bell. One trick to use to determine whether the extra sound is an extracardiac sound is to lightly rest the bell of the stethoscope on the chest at the apex (where the sound is heard best). The extracardiac sound should be heard fairly well. By pressing the stethoscope harder onto the chest, the skin beneath the bell is stretched and effectively creates a diaphragm. Because low-pitched sounds are not heard well with a diaphragm, the extracardiac sound should be diminished. By releasing pressure on the stethoscope, it becomes a bell again and the extracardiac sound should return. Do this several times until you are convinced that what you are hearing is indeed an S_3 or an S_4.

19. Are there tips for hearing heart sounds better in patients who have distant heart sounds?

It is important to remove the patient's clothing to auscultate heart sounds, but the patient should be appropriately draped to maintain his or her dignity. Auscultate with the patient in the supine position initially, but if the heart tones are difficult to hear, you may have the patient roll partially onto the left side with the left arm above the head. You may also have the patient sit up and lean forward while you auscultate. Both of these maneuvers drop the heart forward, moving it closer to the chest wall and your stethoscope. In women who have large pendulous breasts, you may need to move the breast aside or lift it up and listen around it or under it to better hear heart sounds. In obese or large-breasted women, the sounds may be heard better at the sternal border.

20. **When should apical pulses be assessed instead of radial pulses when checking vital signs in CV patients?**

When the heart rhythm is irregular, the rate should be determined by apical assessment. A radial pulse assessment in the setting of an irregular heartbeat may underestimate the heart rate. If you are still in doubt as to the accuracy of the heart rate, obtain an electrocardiogram on the patient, especially if the irregular heart rhythm is a new finding. Chances are that you will find a dysrhythmia.

21. **When taking an apical radial pulse assessment, why are some apical beats not felt at the radial artery?**

Heartbeats in which the stroke volume is reduced may not be strong enough to create a palpable peripheral pulse. Examples of beats with reduced stroke volume include premature atrial or ventricular contractions and rapid heart rhythms.

22. **When should heart rate be counted over a full minute?**

If the heart rhythm is unusually fast or slow or if it is irregular, the rate should be counted for 1 full minute.

23. **When is it important for a nurse to auscultate for bruits, and what is the appropriate auscultation technique to hear one?**

A *bruit* is a low-pitched systolic sound like the purring of a cat that can be heard when the bell of the stethoscope is lightly placed over an artery. It represents about 50% obstruction to blood flow in an artery and could signify peripheral vascular disease. As the obstruction worsens, the bruit becomes high pitched and louder. The nurse should auscultate for bruits any time a cardiovascular exam is performed, particularly with elderly patients or if arterial stenosis or obstruction is suspected. Sites to auscultate for bruits include over the carotid arteries, the epigastrium, and in each upper quadrant of the abdomen. If poor arterial circulation to the legs is suspected, the nurse should auscultate over the aorta, the iliac arteries, and the femoral arteries.

24. **What is the best way for nurses to organize a head-to-toe assessment when examining CV patients?**

It is very important to develop a systematic way in which you approach every patient for a CV exam. If you are consistent and examine every patient in the same way, you will rarely forget to perform any segment of the CV exam and you will be far more likely to recognize abnormal findings when they occur (see following table). Begin by examining the patient from the right side with the patient sitting up at 90 degrees, noting the patient's mental status, viewing the skin color and turgor, and looking for any bony deformities. Palpate the carotid pulses bilaterally (not at the same time); then auscultate the lungs. Lay the patient down at about 30 degrees and evaluate the jugular venous pulse on the right side. Expose the chest and observe for any abnormalities before you palpate each of the sites designated in the Question 1 figure. First palpate with the fingerpads and then with the heel of the hand, feeling for any lift or thrill. Be sure to examine the point of maximum impulse. Auscultate each of the sites in the Question 1 figure with the diaphragm of your stethoscope, beginning with the mitral site, moving to the tricuspid and pulmonic sites, and ending with the aortic site. Repeat this step with the bell of the stethoscope. Palpate the arterial pulses, starting with the brachial and moving on to radial, femoral, popliteal, dorsalis pedis, and posterior tibial pulses, noting skin color and temperature while comparing bilaterally. Assess for peripheral edema.

Head-to-toe cardiovascular exam

Patient Position	Segment of Exam
Sitting up at 90 degrees	General inspection: mental status, skin color, obvious bony deformities
	Carotid pulses/carotid bruits
	Lung sounds (posterior and anterior)
Supine at 30 degrees	Inspect for jugular venous distention
	Inspect chest
	Palpate chest with finger pads and heel of hand
	Auscultate heart sounds
	Palpate arterial pulses bilaterally
	Assess for peripheral edema
	Assess abdomen for bruits, hepatomegaly, ascites

Key Points

- The cardiovascular exam requires careful observation of findings and "hands-on" palpation in a quiet room.
- Eight essential characteristics for a nurse to assess when auscultating heart sounds are timing; location, duration, and point during the cardiac cycle; pitch; intensity; quality; shape or configuration; radiation; and changes.
- When auscultating heart sounds, the nurse should stand on the patient's right side and listen at each of the auscultation points on the chest, first with the diaphragm of the stethoscope and then with the bell.

Internet Resources

University of California San Diego: A Practical Guide to Clinical Medicine, Exam of the Heart
http://medicine.ucsd.edu/clinicalmed/heart.htm

HeartSite.com, Physical Exam
http://www.heartsite.com/html/physical.html

Richard Rathe, MD, University of Florida, Cardiovascular Examination
http://www.medinfo.ufl.edu/year1/bcs/clist/cardio.html

Explore Health With Sentara, Incorporated
http://explorehealth.sentara.com/library/healthguide/IllnessConditions/topic.asp?HWID=ps1507

Heart Sounds and Murmurs, University of Washington School of Medicine
http://depts.washington.edu/~physdx/heart/demo.html

Beth Israel Deaconess Medical Center, cardiovascular exam websites
http://research.caregroup.org/clinicalSkills/clinSkills_List.asp?skillID=2

Bibliography

Bickley LS, Szilagyi PG: *Bates' guide to physical examination and history taking,* ed 8, Philadelphia, 2002, Lippincott Williams & Wilkins, pp 245-332.

Braunwald E: Physical examination of the heart and circulation. In Braunwald E, Zipes D, Libby P, editors: *Heart disease: a textbook of cardiovascular medicine,* ed 6, Philadelphia, 2001, WB Saunders, pp 45-81.

Perloff JK: *Physical examination of the heart and circulation,* ed 3, Philadelphia, 2000, WB Saunders.

Taylor GJ, Cope D: Physical examination. In Taylor JG, editor: *Primary care management of heart disease,* St Louis, 2000, Mosby, pp 36-53.

Weber JR: *Nurses' handbook of health assessment,* ed 4, Philadelphia, 2000, Lippincott Williams & Wilkins, pp 154-173.

Chapter 3

Hemodynamic Monitoring

Susan K. Frazier

1. What is the purpose of hemodynamic monitoring?

Hemodynamic monitoring is a means to evaluate the energy generated by the heart and the subsequent movement of blood through the cardiovascular circuit. Indirect and direct measures may be obtained to provide information to the clinician.

2. Describe a typical indirect hemodynamic measurement that is made at the bedside.

The most common indirect hemodynamic measurement is evaluation of blood pressure by the auscultation technique using a sphygmomanometer, an inflatable blood pressure cuff, and a stethoscope. This type of evaluation is dependent on blood flow. Although the technique for this measurement is not complex, a number of technical difficulties can produce significant measurement error. Common technical difficulties are given in the following table.

Common errors in auscultation technique	
Technique Error	**Result**
Incorrect cuff size	
Cuff that is too large	False low measurement
Cuff that is too small	False high measurement
Incorrect cuff placement	
Cuff that is applied too loosely	False high measurement
Cuff that is not centered over brachial artery	False high measurement
Incorrect arm placement	
Arm above heart level	False low measurement
Arm below heart level	False high measurement
Failure to accurately detect start of Korotkoff sounds	False low measurement

3. What is blood pressure?

Blood pressure is a measurement of the force exerted by the blood on blood vessel walls. It is a function of the pressure produced by cardiac ejection and the resistance of the arterial blood vessels to forward blood flow. Systolic blood pressure is associated with ventricular contraction and ejection (cardiac output). Diastolic blood pressure is associated with vascular resistance.

4. Are there other methods of indirectly measuring blood pressure in addition to the auscultation technique?

Yes. They are all dependent on blood flow and are described in the following table.

Indirect measurement of blood pressure

Technique	Procedure	Advantages/Disadvantages
Auscultation technique	With arm supported at heart level, blood pressure cuff is inflated until the brachial artery is compressed and blood flow ceases. Clinician auscultates brachial artery as cuff is deflated. Return of flow produces Korotkoff sounds (produced by turbulent blood flow) correlated to systolic and diastolic blood pressures.	Quiet environment and normal hearing acuity are required. Multiple sizes of cuffs must be available. Appropriate cuff size is critical. Valid, reliable measures may be difficult to obtain in hypotensive patients who have cool or clammy skin due to vasoconstriction
Palpation technique	This is performed through palpation of radial or brachial pulse, occlusion of blood flow by cuff, and detection of return of pulse. Pressure measurement obtained at point of pulsatile flow return is measure of systolic blood pressure.	This is a simple technique. Minimal equipment is usually readily available. Appropriate cuff size is critical. Technique is not dependent on hearing acuity. This provides a measure of only systolic blood pressure. With vasoconstriction and/or decreased cardiac output, systolic pressure is underestimated.
Doppler flow detector	Pulsatile blood flow is detected with hand-held Doppler device. Cuff is inflated until pulsatile flow is obliterated; then, inflation is gradually released. Point at which pulsatile blood flow detected is systolic blood pressure measure.	This is a simple technique. Appropriate cuff size is critical. Technique is not dependent on hearing acuity. This provides an estimate of only systolic blood pressure. Doppler device may not be readily available in all clinical areas.

Indirect measurement of blood pressure   *continued*

Technique	Procedure	Advantages/Disadvantages
Oscillatory technique	Cuff is inflated and then deflated as clinician observes mercury column or aneroid needle. Systolic blood pressure is detected when oscillations of mercury meniscus or aneroid needle begin. Point at which oscillations reach maximal strength and begin to decrease is estimate of mean arterial pressure.	This is a simple technique. Measurement is not dependent on hearing acuity. Appropriate cuff size is critical. The estimate of mean arterial pressure is subjective and may not be reliable. Estimates only are provided of systolic and mean arterial pressures. Hypotensive individuals may have weak to absent oscillations.
Automated blood pressure measurement	Place cuff of automated device over the brachial artery. Program an estimate of systolic blood pressure and frequency of desired measurement, and initiate measurement. Most devices provide an estimate of systolic, diastolic, and mean arterial pressures using one of four techniques: oscillometric detection, plethysmography, Doppler blood flow detection, or intrasonographic detection of Korotkoff sounds.	Reliable estimates of blood pressure may be obtained with hemodynamically stable individuals. Appropriate cuff size is critical. This technique should not be used in unstable, critically ill patients; invalid results are obtained in patients with tachycardia, cardiac dysrhythmias (e.g., atrial fibrillation), shock, and/or vascular disease. Automated measures depend on pulsatile blood flow; reduced accuracy occurs with hypothermia/cold extremities, hypotension, arm movement, tachycardia, measurements too frequently (1 measure every 3 minutes). Do not place cuff proximal to intravenous catheter. Remove cuff routinely to evaluate underlying skin surface. Nerve compression and nerve damage are potential complications. Patients often find routine cuff inflation to be an annoyance.

5. Is there a direct measure of blood pressure that can be obtained at the bedside?

Yes. Direct arterial blood pressure is evaluated by the placement of a fluid-filled catheter (arterial catheter [A-line]) directly into an arterial vessel. The catheter is connected to a transducer that converts the detected pressure into an electrical signal, which is received by a monitoring system. The signal is amplified and displayed as an arterial waveform, as shown in the following figure.

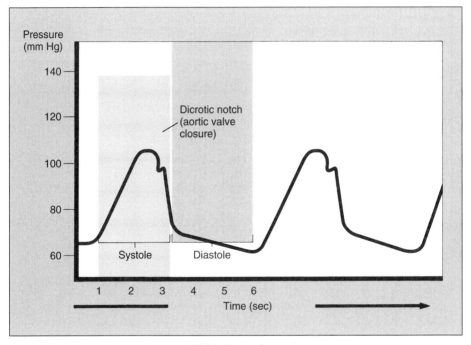

Arterial pulse waveform.

6. What are the indications for placement of an arterial catheter?

An arterial catheter is commonly placed for continuous, direct evaluation of arterial blood pressure, and successive arterial blood sampling. The information obtained with use of an arterial catheter is commonly used to continuously evaluate patient hemodynamic status and hemodynamic response to therapies like fluid administration or vasoactive medications.

7. Where and how are arterial catheters placed?

Arterial catheters are commonly placed in the radial artery. Other sites that may be used for catheter placement include the brachial, axillary, femoral, and dorsalis pedis arteries. Placement of the catheter is generally performed through percutaneous puncture using a catheter over a needle (Intracath), although the placement of a guide wire followed by a catheter (Seldinger technique) or surgical cutdown may also be used. Catheter placement in either the radial artery or dorsalis pedis artery requires evaluation of collateral circulation. An Allen's test may be performed by placing the arm and hand in a neutral position. The examiner should occlude both the radial and ulnar arteries, request that the patient gently move his or her fingers, and observe loss of color of the hand and fingers. When the fingers and hand exhibit pallor, the examiner should maintain compression of the radial artery but release the pressure on the ulnar artery. Return of normal color to the hand and fingers within 7 seconds is purported to be an indication of adequate ulnar circulation. Compression of both the dorsalis pedis and posterior tibial arteries in the foot permits evaluation of collateral circulation (adequate collateral flow indicated by color return within 10 seconds). The clinician *must* be aware that collateral circulation may be inadequate to the hand in a significant number (14%) of patients even when the Allen's test indicates adequate flow.

8. Is the directly measured arterial pressure the same in all arteries?

No. Blood pressure measurements differ as measurement is made more distal from the heart. For example, systolic blood pressure measured via a catheter in the dorsalis pedis artery is higher than that measured in the radial artery, whereas diastolic pressure is lower. This phenomenon is due to the transmission of the pulsatile pressure wave after ejection of blood from the left ventricle. The ejection of blood into the aorta initiates a forward moving, pulsatile pressure wave. This pressure wave is transmitted to increasingly smaller arterial branches as blood moves forward. In the smallest, distal arterioles, this initial rapid pulsatile wave is actually reflected back toward the heart and is superimposed on the next forward moving pulsatile wave. This produces a characteristic elevation in systolic pressure and a lowering of diastolic pressure in more distal arteries. This response is enhanced with vasoconstriction and reduced with vasodilation, common responses that may occur with drug therapy or underlying pathophysiological conditions like sepsis.

9. What is the best indication of tissue perfusion?

Mean arterial pressure (MAP), the average pressure of the arterial system during the cardiac cycle (systole and diastole), is the best indicator of tissue perfusion. This measure is ideal, because MAP is constant throughout the arterial circulation and does not vary by vessel location. Adequate tissue perfusion may be inferred with an MAP greater than 70 mm Hg. MAP may also be estimated using values obtained via indirect measurement methods. The MAP that is calculated is not a mathematical average value, because diastole is a longer portion of the cardiac cycle than systole. Thus, a time-weighted average value must be calculated. MAP may be estimated using the following formula: $MAP = DBP + (PP/3)$, where DBP is the diastolic blood pressure and PP is the pulse pressure or difference between systolic and diastolic blood pressures. For example, with a blood pressure of 120/60 mm Hg, the pulse pressure is 60 mm Hg. The MAP would then be $60 + (60)/3$, or 80 mm Hg. This formula is often an invalid measure because it assumes a resting heart rate of 60 bpm, but in individuals with a stable heart rate, it may be used to evaluate trends.

10. Should the indirect measurement of blood pressure be equivalent to measures obtained via a direct method like an arterial catheter?

No. Indirect blood pressure measurement is dependent on blood flow, whereas direct pressure measurement via an arterial catheter is an actual measure of pressure. Because two very different variables are measured, do not assume that these results will be the same.

11. What are potential complications of an arterial catheter?

A common complication is **acute hemorrhage**. Significant blood loss can occur with movement and/or dislodgment of an arterial catheter. Disconnection of any portion of the fluid-filled monitoring system can produce a rapid loss of blood. **Vascular insufficiency** due to partial or total occlusion of the cannulated vessel is another complication. Blood flow in the vessel may be reduced or obliterated by a cannula that is too large for the vessel, an embolus, or a thrombus and/or ruptured plaque. Injection of drugs into an arterial catheter can produce **severe arterial spasm** with subsequent vascular insufficiency. Arterial catheters should be clearly labeled to prevent intraarterial administration of medications. As with any vascular catheter, the likelihood of bacterial colonization and **infection** is associated with the length of time the cannula is in place. Although the longer the duration of catheter placement, the greater is the chance of infection, research investigations do not support routine replacement of arterial catheters. Rather, a catheter may remain in place until it is no longer necessary for patient evaluation and therapy, as long as there are no signs of local or systemic infection. For recommendations and further references, see http://www.cdc.gov/mmwr/preview/mmwrhtml/rr5110a1.htm.

12. What nursing assessments should be made during arterial monitoring and after the removal of an arterial catheter?

Regular neurovascular evaluation of the extremity distal to the site of an arterial cannula is mandatory. This is particularly true with a radial artery catheter, because immobilization of the site in other than a neutral position may produce neurovascular injury and loss of function. Insertion sites should be regularly evaluated for signs of occult bleeding or infection. During monitoring, high and low pressure alarms should be used to alert the clinician to abrupt change in pressure. This may indicate a change in patient condition or disconnection in the system that could produce significant blood loss.

13. What common difficulties occur during arterial pressure monitoring?

Some common problems and solutions are detailed in the following table. It goes without saying, of course, that the nurse should evaluate the patient first and then address equipment difficulties.

Troubleshooting common difficulties with arterial pressure monitoring

Common Difficulty	Cause	Solution
Absence of arterial waveform on the monitor	Arterial catheter displaced Loose connection or disconnection in fluid-filled monitoring system Obstruction in fluid-filled system: stopcock turned off to patient, kink in tubing	Ensure monitor is receiving power; evaluate catheter placement (aspirate blood); inspect monitoring system: tighten loose connections, ensure stopcocks turned in correct direction; assess zero reference point, recalibrate
Damped waveform: loss of much of pressure signal	Partial obstruction of catheter: may be due to blood or movement of catheter tip against vessel wall Presence of air bubbles in tubing or transducer dome Hypotension	Ensure air bubbles removed from fluid-filled system; evaluate catheter patency and placement
Arterial waveforms with artifact: false signals	Electrical interference from other equipment Excessive patient movement Movement of catheter within the artery: catheter whip	Remove equipment producing interference; evaluate patient need for pain medication or sedation or other comfort measures; assess catheter patency and position, redress and secure catheter to reduce movement within vessel Evaluate dynamic response (ability to measure pressure change) of monitor using square wave test
Inaccurate measurement of pressure (too high or too low)	Transducer not leveled or zeroed correctly Loss of system calibration Presence of air bubbles or kinks in fluid-filled system Partial occlusion of catheter with thrombus Automatic flush device providing flush at too high a rate (typically deliver 3 ml/hr)	Evaluate catheter patency; level transducer at the phlebostatic axis, zero system: remove effects of atmospheric and hydrostatic pressure; remove air bubbles from fluid-filled system, ensure fast flush system is functioning correctly: fill pressure bag with appropriate pressure for system

14. **What patient and family teaching is helpful for a patient with an arterial catheter?**

The patient and family should understand the reason for insertion of the arterial catheter, the procedure for insertion, and potential complications of this procedure prior to provision of informed consent. Once the catheter is in place, the patient and family should understand the importance of minimal catheter movement in the vessel. Although it may be difficult to immobilize the catheter insertion site and prevent catheter movement, the patient and family should receive information about the importance of catheter stability. The patient and family should also understand the reasons for frequent neurovascular assessments and signs and symptoms that would be associated with neuro-vascular insufficiency, and they should be informed about the clinical status of the patient and treatment decisions that are based on hemodynamic parameters.

15. What is a Swan-Ganz catheter?

The Swan-Ganz catheter is a pulmonary artery (PA) catheter. The name "Swan-Ganz" is derived from the names of two physicians who were instrumental in the development of the flow-directed PA catheter. A PA catheter is a flow-directed, multilumen catheter that is used to evaluate volume state and left ventricular function.

16. How are PA catheters placed?

A flow-directed technique is used to place these catheters. The catheter is advanced into a central venous vessel, most commonly via the internal or

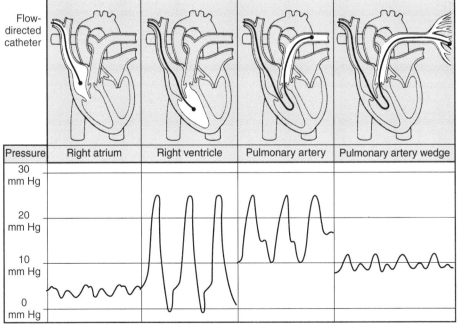

Insertion of pulmonary artery catheter and pressure waveform.

external jugular vein or subclavian vein. The balloon near the tip of the catheter is inflated. As the catheter is advanced, blood flow carries the inflated balloon through the right atrium, tricuspid valve, right ventricle, and pulmonic valve into the PA. Pressure waveforms are monitored and evaluated during insertion so that the clinicians can determine catheter location and intracardiac pressures. Typical waveform and pressure changes alert the clinicians to the movement of the catheter tip through the right heart chambers and into the wedged or occlusion position. The occlusion position indicates that the balloon has floated into a small branch of the pulmonary circuit where the inflated balloon diameter is greater than the diameter of the vessel lumen. The balloon is passively deflated and the typical PA waveform should return if the catheter is appropriately placed. See the figure on page 30.

17. What are the indications for insertion of a PA catheter?

PA catheters are placed primarily to assess cardiovascular function and response in critically ill and high-risk patients and to evaluate cardiovascular responses to therapy. The information from the PA catheter provides clinicians with information that can assist them in optimizing cardiovascular function by carefully guided titration of pharmacological agents that influence preload, afterload and contractility. Additionally, clinicians will be able to determine whether pulmonary edema is cardiogenic or noncardiogenic in origin and to implement appropriate therapy.

18. What useful information can be measured with a PA catheter?

Measures that may be obtained with a PA catheter are described in the following table. See also the figure to Question 16.

Measurements obtainable from PA catheters

Measurement	Normal Range for Adults
Right atrial pressure—Transducer connected to proximal infusion port, measure of central venous pressure	-1 to 8 mm Hg
Right ventricular pressure—Pressure obtained during insertion of catheter	15-25 mm Hg systolic pressure 0-8 mm Hg diastolic pressure
PA pressure—Continuous measure with transducer connected to distal catheter	15-25 mm Hg systolic pressure 8-15 mm Hg diastolic pressure

Measurements obtainable from PA catheters   *continued*

Measurement	Normal Range for Adults
PA occlusion pressure or wedge pressure—Obtained with balloon inflated; in presence of normal mitral valve, this pressure provides an indication of left heart function	6-12 mm Hg
Cardiac output—Obtained by either bolus or continuous thermodilution technique	4-8 L/min
Cardiac index—Cardiac output indexed to body surface area for the individual	2.5-4 L/min/m^2
Pulmonary vascular resistance—Calculated value that provides an estimated value reflecting pulmonary vascular tone and resistance to blood flow	<250 dynes•sec/cm^5
Systemic vascular resistance—Calculated value that provides an estimated value reflecting the vascular tone and resistance to blood flow exerted by the systemic vessels	800-1200 dynes•sec/cm^5
Right ventricular ejection fraction—Obtained with specialized PA catheter; measure of the proportion of blood in the right ventricle (end-diastolic volume) that is ejected into the PA	40-60%
Right ventricular end-diastolic volume—Measure of the volume of blood in the right ventricle at end-diastole; reflection of the preload of the heart	100-160 ml
Svo$_2$—Mixed venous oxygen saturation obtained continuously with specialized catheter	60-80%

19. What are potential complications related to PA catheters?

Cardiac dysrhythmias, in particular ventricular ectopy, are common. Dysrhythmias typically occur during insertion but can occur during monitoring or catheter removal. Right bundle branch block due to irritation and edema of the conduction system may develop after placement of a PA catheter. With preexisting left bundle branch block, complete heart block may develop and require a cardiac pacemaker. **Lack of clinician knowledge** about insertion of and evaluation of the values obtained with a PA catheter can result in inappropriate management strategies. Pulmonary complications include the development of a **pneumothorax,** usually during insertion of the catheter. **Pulmonary infarction** may occur if the catheter migrates to a wedged position and obstructs pulmonary blood flow for a prolonged period of time. **Damage to the PA** may range from minimal intimal damage to rupture of the artery and subsequent hemorrhage. **Local (insertion site)** or **systemic infection (sepsis)** may occur directly related to the placement of the PA catheter. **Balloon rupture** results in the introduction of a small volume of air (0.8-1.5 ml) into the pulmonary circulation, which is generally not a problem. Repeated injections of air into the ruptured balloon may produce a pulmonary air embolus. Rupture of the balloon may produce fragments of balloon that embolize and obstruct blood flow in distal branches of the pulmonary circulation. **Catheter knotting** is a rare complication in which, during insertion, the catheter is reflected backward, curls or twists, and forms a knot.

20. What nursing assessments should be made during PA monitoring and after removal of the catheter?

Continuous cardiac monitoring is necessary to observe for alterations in cardiac rhythm. Auscultation of breath sounds alerts the clinician to the presence of a significant pneumothorax. The clinician must also continuously observe and evaluate the PA waveform to ensure that the catheter does not float into a wedged position and obstruct blood flow to a portion of the pulmonary system. Evaluation of PA pressure, occlusion pressure, and cardiac output requires the clinician have a *comprehensive* understanding of physiology and technology. Misinformation and lack of knowledge can result in ineffective and/or deleterious therapeutic interventions that may increase morbidity and mortality.

21. Are there common difficulties that occur during PA monitoring? What interventions may be helpful for these difficulties?

These are detailed in the following table. It goes without saying that patient evaluation is the initial response to alterations in hemodynamic waveforms.

Troubleshooting common difficulties with PA pressure monitoring

Common Difficulty	Cause	Solution
Absence of PA waveform on the monitor	Catheter misplaced Catheter occluded by thrombus Loose connection in fluid-filled transducer system Stopcock turned off to patient, kink in tubing	Ensure monitor is receiving power; evaluate catheter placement (aspirate blood); inspect monitoring system— tighten loose connections, ensure stopcocks turned in correct direction; assess zero reference point, recalibrate.
Damped PA waveform (decreased amplitude of waveform)	Significant alteration in patient condition Air bubbles in tubing or transducer dome Thrombus formation in catheter Catheter tip against vessel wall Lack of calibration Forward migration of catheter to near-wedged position	Evaluate patient immediately for hemodynamic instability; ensure air bubbles removed from fluid-filled system; calibrate; evaluate catheter patency and placement; notify physician of need for catheter repositioning.

Troubleshooting common difficulties with PA pressure monitoring *continued*

Common Difficulty	Cause	Solution
Inability to obtain a PA occlusion pressure	Balloon rupture Movement of catheter to proximal PA or right ventricle	Evaluate catheter position, notify physician of the need for repositioning as necessary; if balloon rupture occurs, *ensure* that balloon is no longer used.
Inaccurate pressure measurement (too high or too low)	Transducer not leveled or zeroed correctly Loss of system calibration Presence of air bubbles or kinks in fluid-filled system Partial occlusion of catheter with thrombus Automatic flush device providing flush at too high a rate (>3 drops/min) Significant position change	Evaluate catheter patency; level transducer—one-half of anterior posterior chest diameter below angle of sternum; zero system—remove effects of atmospheric and hydrostatic pressure; remove air bubbles from fluid-filled system, ensure fast flush system is functioning correctly—pressure bag with appropriate pressure. Evaluate patient position for significant changes; relevel and rezero system as needed.

22. What patient and family teaching is helpful for a patient with a PA catheter?

The patient and family should understand the reason for insertion of the PA catheter, the procedure for insertion, and potential complications of this procedure before provision of informed consent. The patient and family should be informed about the clinical status of the patient and treatment decisions based on hemodynamic parameters obtained with the PA catheter.

23. How do you ensure that invasive pressure measurements are valid?

To ensure the electronics are functioning properly, the clinician must correctly prepare and maintain the fluid-filled system, level the air–fluid interface of the transducer system with the phlebostatic axis (for vascular pressures) and zero reference the system, perform a square wave test to evaluate the frequency response, and calibrate the equipment.

24. How is cardiac output measured with a PA catheter?

The PA catheter contains a thermistor or thermometer that continually measures blood temperature in the PA. A precise volume of solution with a known temperature (warm, room temperature, or cold solution may be used) is injected into the right atrium via the PA catheter. The thermistor detects changes in PA blood temperature as the solution is ejected from the right ventricle into the pulmonary circulation. Temperature changes are transmitted to the computer, and a curve that displays change in PA blood temperature over time is constructed. In patients with a low cardiac output, blood temperature requires a greater length of time to return to the baseline temperature and the area under the curve is greater. In those with a larger cardiac output, blood temperature returns to baseline much quicker and the area under the curve is less. Cardiac output is inversely proportional to the area under this curve. Thus, individuals with a low cardiac output will have a greater area under the curve, and those with a high cardiac output will have less area under the curve (see the following figure).

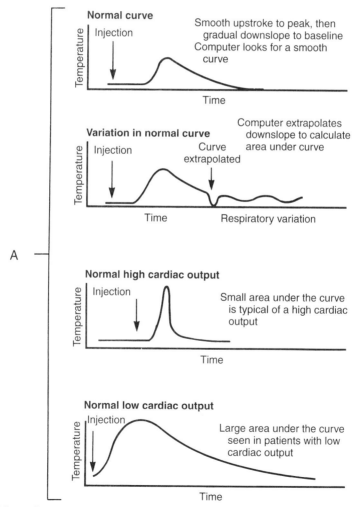

Thermodilution cardiac output curves. Individuals with a low cardiac output will have a greater area under the curve, and those with a high cardiac output will have less area under the curve.

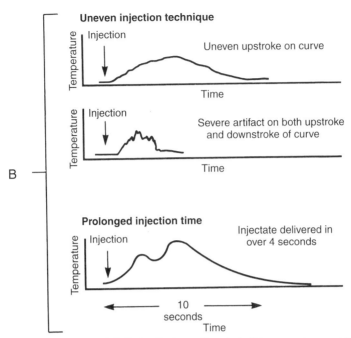

Thermodilution cardiac output curves. Individuals with a low cardiac output will have a greater area under the curve, and those with a high cardiac output will have less area under the curve.

25. Are there measures of cardiac output that do not require placement of a PA catheter?

Yes. There are technologies that provide noninvasive estimates of cardiac output.

- *Thoracic bioelectrical impedance* technique sends an electrical current through the chest between four pairs of electrodes. The impedance, or resistance, to electrical current flow is associated with changes in thoracic blood volume; as thoracic blood volume varies during the cardiac cycle, thoracic impedance changes. These electrode pairs not only deliver a harmless, low-voltage current but also receive and sense this current. This information is transmitted to a computer and processed to provide hemodynamic measures like cardiac output and stroke volume.
- The *noninvasive measurement of cardiac output* may also occur with analysis of changes in expired carbon dioxide. A disposable ventilatory circuit is interfaced with a patient's endotracheal tube and the cardiac output computer. With this technique, volumetric carbon dioxide ($\dot{V}CO_2$) is measured and used to calculate cardiac output by using a modified Fick equation. Baseline $\dot{V}CO_2$ is compared with the $\dot{V}CO_2$ obtained during a rebreathing cycle and used to calculate cardiac output.

26. Are there bedside measures that provide information about oxygenation status?

Oxygen is transported in two ways: it is bound to hemoglobin (98% of oxygen transport) or dissolved in the plasma (2% of oxygen transport). The partial pressure of oxygen (PaO_2) obtained with an arterial blood gas (ABG) measurement is a measure of the oxygen dissolved in the plasma. Oxygen saturation (SaO_2) obtained by an ABG measurement is a measure of the degree of oxygen binding to the hemoglobin molecules. Pulse oximetry provides a noninvasive estimate of arterial oxygen saturation (SpO_2).

27. Is there a difference in the measurement of oxygen saturation by pulse oximetry and an ABG?

Yes. The measurement of oxygen saturation by either method is based on hemoglobin absorption of different wavelengths of light. Hemoglobin molecules bound to oxygen, oxyhemoglobin (HbO_2), absorb a greater degree of infrared light. In contrast, deoxygenated or reduced hemoglobin absorbs more red light. With pulse oximetry (SpO_2), erythrocytes are exposed to *two* wavelengths of light (one red and one infrared). From this analysis, a *functional* measurement of hemoglobin saturation is obtained (ratio of oxygenated hemoglobin to deoxygenated hemoglobin). The oxygen saturation value obtained with an arterial blood gas (SaO_2) uses similar technology; but four or more wavelengths of light are used. The SaO_2 value obtained with this technique is a *fractional* measurement of oxygen saturation (the ratio of oxygenated hemoglobin to the *total* number of hemoglobin molecules, not just deoxygenated hemoglobin).

28. Which is a better measure?

The *fractional* measurement obtained with an ABG provides a more comprehensive evaluation of oxygen saturation. This can be extremely important for certain individuals (e.g., those with smoke inhalation or carbon monoxide poisoning). For example, a patient with an increased proportion of hemoglobin bound to carbon monoxide (carboxyhemoglobin) might present with a functional SpO_2 of 98%-100%. However, a fractional measure of SaO_2 would provide an accurate measure of oxygenated hemoglobin in relation to the total volume of hemoglobin. For this patient, perhaps only 50% of total hemoglobin is bound to oxygen and most of the remainder is bound to carbon monoxide. This critical situation would not be evident from the SpO_2 value.

29. What problems occur in the measurement of oxygen saturation by pulse oximetry?

Several factors can influence the precision and accuracy of SpO_2 values, as listed in the following box. There also is good evidence that the accuracy of SpO_2 values decreases as hypoxemia develops.

Reasons for inaccurate Spo₂ values

Patient Factors
- Inadequate arterial pulsatile blood flow—May be due to hypothermia or hypotension
- Venous pulsatile blood flow—Elevated venous pressure
- High proportion of hemoglobin unavailable for binding with oxygen—Carboxyhemoglobin or methemoglobin
- Anemia
- Hyperlipidemia or administration of lipid solutions
- Circulation of systemic dyes (indocyanine green, methylene blue)

System or Technical Factors
- Motion artifact
- Interference by strong ambient light (heat lamps, surgical lights)
- Optical shunt—Light wavelengths detected without passing through vascular bed
- Electrical interference from other equipment
- Optical cross-talk—Detection of red or infrared light from another piece of equipment

30. **Current controversy: Does hemodynamic monitoring with a PA catheter improve patient care?**

    The use of a PA catheter to manage the care of critically ill patients has become increasingly commonplace since its introduction in the early 1970s. However, there are no well-designed, controlled clinical trials that provide substantive evidence that the use of PA pressure monitoring to guide therapy improves patient outcomes. Until this evidence is available, the decision to insert a PA catheter should be individualized for each patient. Before the insertion of a PA catheter, the risk-benefit ratio should be evaluated to determine whether the potential benefits are greater than the potential risks.

 Key Points

- Hemodynamic monitoring is a means to evaluate the energy generated by the heart and the subsequent movement of blood through the cardiovascular circuit.
- An arterial catheter is commonly placed for continuous, direct evaluation of arterial blood pressure and for successive arterial blood sampling.
- MAP, the average pressure of the arterial system during the cardiac cycle (systole and diastole), is the best indicator of tissue perfusion.
- Regular neurovascular evaluation of the extremity distal to the site of an arterial cannula is mandatory.
- PA catheters are placed primarily to assess cardiovascular function and response in critically ill and high-risk patients and to evaluate cardiovascular responses to therapy.

Key Points *continued*

- The PA catheter contains a thermistor (or thermometer) that continually measures blood temperature in the PA.
- Intermittent thermodilution cardiac output measurements are computer calculated from PA blood temperature curves. The thermistor detects changes in PA blood temperature as a precise volume of solution with a known temperature is injected into the right atrium and then ejected from the right ventricle into the pulmonary circulation.

Internet Resources

ACP/ACC/AHA Task Force Statements. Introduction: Clinical Competence in Hemodynamic Monitoring: A Statement for Physicians From the ACP/ACC/AHA Task Force on Clinical Privileges in Cardiology:
http://www.acc.org/Clinical/competence/pdf/acp_690002.pdf

RnCeus.com: Interactive Online Continuing Education for Nurse Professionals. Hemodynamic Monitoring: An Introduction:
http://www.rnceus.com/course_frame.asp?exam_id=46&directory=hemo

Critical Care Nurse Hemodynamic Monitoring Course:
http://www.eonreality.com/demos/e-learning/ccn/index2.html

Philips Hemodynamics Monitoring Webcast:
http://www6.medical.philips.com/CMSMedia/hemo_1/

Bibliography

Baldwin IC, Heland M: Incidence of cardiac dysrhythmias in patients during pulmonary artery catheter removal after cardiac surgery, *Heart Lung* 29:155-160, 2000.

Brandstetter RD, Grant GR, Estilo M et al: Swan-Ganz catheter: misconceptions, pitfalls, and incomplete user knowledge—an identified trilogy in need of correction, *Heart Lung* 27:218-222, 1998.

Bridges EJ: Monitoring pulmonary artery pressures: just the facts, *Crit Care Nurs* 20:59-80, 2000.

Grap MJ, Pettrey L, Thornby D: Hemodynamic monitoring: a comparison of research and practice, *Am J Crit Care* 6:452-456, 1997.

Headley JM: Invasive hemodynamic monitoring: applying advanced technologies, *Crit Care Nurs Q* 21:73-84, 1998.

McGhee BH, Woods SL: Critical care nurses' knowledge of arterial pressure monitoring, *Am J Crit Care* 10:43-51, 2001.

Shoemaker WC, Belzberg H, Wo CCJ et al: Multicenter study of noninvasive monitoring systems as alternatives to invasive monitoring of acutely ill emergency patients, *Chest* 114:1643-1652, 1998.

Section II

Diagnostic Procedures

Selected Laboratory Procedures

Karen Patterson Pulido

1. **From a cardiovascular (CV) standpoint, what are the most important components of the complete blood cell count (CBC) for nurses to be aware of and what are normal values for these components?**

   Hemoglobin (Hgb) and platelets are the most important components of the CBC in regard to CV patients. Normal values are as follows:
   - Hgb (g/dl): male, 13.5-17.5; female, 12-16
   - Platelets ($\times 10^9$/L), 150-399

2. **With regard to CV patients, why is the CBC monitored?**

   In a patient who has angina, severe anemia can produce ischemia as a result of inadequate blood supply. The decreased oxygen-carrying capacity of the Hgb and the increased cardiac output demanded by anemia can precipitate cardiac failure. However, most patients who develop congestive heart failure (CHF) with anemia have underlying heart disease. Thrombocytopenia (platelets $<150,000 \times 10^9$/L) is a well-recognized complication of heparin therapy, usually occurring within 4-10 days after heparin treatment has started.

3. **What are the normal values for a basic chemistry panel?**

   Normal basic chemistry panel values

Sodium (Na)	137-147 mmol/L
Potassium (K)	3.4-5.3 mmol/L
Chloride (Cl)	99-108 mmol/L
CO_2 (carbon dioxide)	22-29 mmol/L
Blood urea nitrogen (BUN)	8-21 mg/dl
Creatinine (Cr)	0.5-1.3 mg/dl
Blood glucose, fasting	60-109 mg/dl

4. **What are the implications of abnormal values in the basic chemistry panel for a CV patient?**
   - **Hyponatremia** in patients with heart failure results from an inability to excrete ingested water; therefore the sodium is diluted in the excess fluid. This problem

is largely related to the associated fall in cardiac output and systemic blood pressure.

- **Hypokalemia** due to increased urinary potassium losses most often occurs in CHF with the use of loop or thiazide-type diuretics. Potassium depletion can increase the incidence of arrhythmias, particularly in patients who are also being treated with digoxin. As a result, maintaining the plasma potassium concentration above 4 mEQ/L is desirable in these patients. Hypokalemia can contribute to an increased incidence of sudden death in patients with hypertension and left ventricular hypertrophy. Potassium depletion may have two additional deleterious effects in patients with hypertension: it can raise the blood pressure by a mean of 5 to 7 mm Hg (probably due in part to sodium retention), and it can increase the incidence of stroke, independent of other CV risk factors.
- A tall-peaked and symmetrical T wave is the first change seen on the electrocardiogram (ECG) in a patient with **hyperkalemia.** Ultimately the QRS widens further due to a severe conduction delay and may eventually result in a flat line on the ECG with complete absence of electrical activity. Hyperkalemia in CHF is typically mild (plasma potassium concentration <5.5 mEQ/L) unless exacerbated by the concurrent use of potassium chloride supplements, a potassium-sparing diuretic, or an angiotensin-converting enzyme (ACE) inhibitor in CHF.

5. What are normal values for calcium, magnesium, and phosphorus?

Calcium (Ca)	8.7-10.7 mg/dl
Magnesium (Mg)	1.8-3.0 mg/dl
Phosphorus (P)	2.5-4.6 mg/dl

6. What are the implications of abnormal values of calcium, magnesium, and phosphorus?

- **Hypocalcemia:** Many patients have symptoms when their serum total calcium concentration is about 7 mg/dl. Patients with symptomatic hypocalcemia should be treated immediately. Severe, symptomatic hypocalcemia may result in CV collapse, hypotension unresponsive to fluids and vasopressors, and dysrhythmias. Prolongation of the QT interval in normal persons is due to inward potassium channels. Hypocalcemia can prolong the QT interval because calcium can modulate a potassium channel.
- **Hypercalcemia:** Long-standing hypercalcemia can lead to the deposition of calcium in heart valves, coronary arteries, and myocardial fibers. Hypercalcemia also directly shortens the myocardial action potential, which is reflected in a shortened QT interval.
- **Hypomagnesemia:** Hypotension, vasodilatation, bradycardia, heart block, and cardiac arrest can occur with hypermagnesemia. Hypomagnesemia may cause cardiac arrhythmias such as torsades de pointes. Hypomagnesemia can cause tachycardia, hypertension, cardiac dysrhythmias, and ventricular fibrillation. Magnesium regulates several cardiac ion channels. Arrhythmias can be due to concurrent hypokalemia, hypomagnesemia itself, or both.

- **Hypermagnesemia:** Intracellular magnesium blocks several cardiac potassium channels. These changes can combine to impair CV function. Hypermagnesemia can cause hypotension and heart block. It is difficult to replace potassium if hypomagnesemia or hypocalcemia is also present.
- **Hypophosphatemia:** The symptoms of hypophosphatemia are due to the consequences of intracellular phosphate depletion. Intracellular ATP levels fall with severe hypophosphatemia, and those cell functions dependent on phosphate begin to fail. When the plasma phosphate concentration falls to 1.0 mg/dl (0.32 mmol/L), the reduction in cardiac output may become clinically significant, leading to CHF.

7. What are the different types of cardiac enzymes used to rule out myocardial infarction (MI), and what are the current recommendations for testing?

For many years, the diagnosis of acute MI has relied on chest discomfort characteristic of ischemia, ECG manifestations, and typical elevations in serum markers of myocardial injury. Two of the three criteria were required for diagnosis. It is now clear, however, that substantial numbers of patients with acute MI have an ECG that reveals only nonspecific changes or may even be normal. Many patients have no recognizable symptoms. For these reasons, more reliance has been placed on the evaluation of biochemical markers of myocardial injury (see the following table).

Biochemical markers of myocardial injury

Test	Onset	Peak	Duration
Creatine kinase–MB	3-12 hr	18-24 hr	36-48 hr
Troponins	3-12 hr	18-24 hr	Up to 10 days
Myoglobin	1-4 hr	6-7 hr	24 hr
Lactate dehydrogenase	6-12 hr	24-48 hr	6-8 days

Cardiac troponin I (cTnI) and T (cTnT) are cardiac regulatory proteins that control the calcium-mediated interaction of actin and myosin. cTnI is somewhat smaller than cTnT. Troponins are the markers of choice and should be used instead of creatine kinase (CK)-MB. They are highly specific for myocardial injury, rise early at 3 to 6 hours, and remain elevated for up to 10 days. However, because of the long duration, it is difficult to estimate from an elevated serum troponin value alone whether infarction is acute or occurred in the days before admission.

The appropriate use of measures of these enzymes in patients with renal insufficiency is less clear, because elevations in serum troponins are commonly observed in patients with renal insufficiency who do not have clinical evidence of myocardial damage.

CK-MB may be helpful to determine the timing of events and should be used predominantly for that purpose. CK-MB rises early but remains elevated for only 36 to 48 hours. An elevated serum CK-MB level in the appropriate setting is indicative of a recent acute MI.

Total CK and lactate dehydrogenase (LDH) really no longer have a role. The use of percentage criteria of CK-MB relative to total CK can be misleading in a number of clinical settings, including myopathies or skeletal muscle injury, hypothyroidism, renal failure, and combined skeletal muscle and cardiac injury.

Myoglobin is a heme protein with a low molecular weight. Because of its small size, myoglobin is rapidly released from damaged tissue.

8. What are the various components of the liver function test (LFT), and what are their normal values?

Alanine aminotransferase (ALT or SGPT)	19-72 units/L for males
	15-48 units/L for females
Aspartate aminotransferase (AST or SGOT)	19-55 units/L for males
	14-38 units/L for females
Gamma-glutamyl-transferase/transpeptidase (GGT/GGTP)	13-68 units/L for males
	11-48 units/L for females
Alkaline phosphatase (ALP)	36-126 units/L
Total bilirubin	0.1-1.2 mg/dl

9. What are the implications of an abnormal LFT for a cardiology patient?

As a result of hepatic congestion, patients with right-sided heart failure frequently have elevated liver enzymes. Another cause of elevated AST or ALT values could be as an adverse effect of statin therapy for hyperlipidemia (see Chapter 36, Lipid-Lowering Strategies).

10. What new lab tests are being evaluated in cardiology?

Homocysteine is an amino acid. Increasing evidence suggests that moderate hyperhomocysteinemia is associated with an increased risk of coronary and cerebrovascular disease. The effect of lowering homocysteine levels on CV risk remains unknown. Currently the treatment of hyperhomocysteinemia is folic acid (1 mg/day), pyroxidine (10 mg/day), and vitamin B_{12} (0.4 mg/day). A clinical trial assessing the efficacy of supplementation in patients with normal serum homocysteine levels is ongoing.

C-reactive protein (CRP) is an acute-phase reactant that rises with most inflammatory disorders. Thus elevated values can be considered predictive only if there is no other apparent cause. The mechanisms responsible for the association between CRP and CV disease are not clear. CRP may be only a marker of inflammation and thrombotic risk, without any specific role in the degree of atherosclerosis. Before routine CRP measurement becomes an accepted practice, there are a number of issues that affect the use and cost-effectiveness of this test. There is as yet no targeted therapy to lower serum CRP and there is no direct evidence that lowering CRP alone results in a reduction in CV risk. The only current therapy that has been evaluated is the administration of a statin.

11. What are a PT/INR and aPTT?

PT stands for *prothrombin time*. This measurement is used to monitor anti-coagulation in patients who are taking warfarin for reasons such as atrial fibrillation and valve replacement. The normal range for a PT is 13.2-17 seconds, with some institutional variation. The level is usually maintained between 2 to 3 times control, or the "normal" value. In patients who have had a valve replacement, levels are kept between 2.5 and 3.5 times control (see Chapter 29, Chronic Anticoagulation).

aPTT stands for *partial thromboplastin time*. This measurement is used to monitor heparin therapy. The critical therapeutic level of heparin can be reached within 24 hours. The goal of maintenance heparin therapy is to maintain the aPTT in the range of 1.5-2.5 times the patient's aPTT baseline value (see Chapter 28, Antiplatelet and Antithrombotic Agents).

12. What is TSH, and what is its normal value?

TSH is *thyroid-stimulating hormone*, and the normal value is 2-7.3 microIU/ml.

13. What are the implications of an abnormal TSH for a cardiology patient?

The major CV changes that occur in **hypothyroidism** (often recognized by an elevated TSH level) include a decrease in cardiac contractility and mass, a reduction in heart rate, and an increase in peripheral vascular resistance. In addition to a slow pulse rate, hypothyroid patients may have ventricular premature beats and, rarely, ventricular tachycardia with a long QT interval (torsades de pointes).

Patients with **hyperthyroidism** (often recognized by a low TSH level) may display CV symptoms and signs such as tachycardia (at rest, during sleep, and during exercise), palpitations (due to both tachycardia and more forceful cardiac contraction), systolic hypertension with widened pulse pressure, and exertional dyspnea. Hyperthyroidism may cause atrial premature contractions, paroxysmal atrial tachycardia, atrial fibrillation, and atrial flutter. Among these arrhythmias, atrial fibrillation is the most common. Patients with angina may have chest pain more often when they become hyperthyroid, presumably because of the increase in cardiac oxygen consumption.

14. What does the creatinine clearance test measure?

The creatinine clearance test compares the level of creatinine in urine with the creatinine level in the blood, usually based on assessments of a 24-hour urine sample and a blood sample drawn at the end of the 24-hour period. Clearance is often measured as milliliters per minute. Because creatinine is found in stable plasma concentrations, is freely filtered and not reabsorbed, and is minimally secreted by the kidneys, creatinine clearance is used to estimate the glomerular filtration rate (GFR). The GFR in turn is the standard by which renal function is assessed. Creatinine clearance is a more precise measure of renal function than is serum creatinine alone.

15. How do you calculate a creatinine clearance?

The following formulas are used to calculate the patient's creatinine clearance:

$$\text{Creatinine clearance (male)} = \frac{(140 - \text{age in years}) \times \text{body weight (kg)}}{72 \times \text{serum creatinine (mg/dl)}}$$

$$\text{Creatinine clearance (female)} = \frac{(140 - \text{age in years}) \times \text{body weight (kg)} \times 0.85}{72 \times \text{serum creatinine (mg/dl)}}$$

 Key Points

- In a patient who is having anginal pain, evaluation of the CBC and a thyroid function study is important to assess for underlying anemia or thyroid disease as an etiology.
- A tall-peaked and symmetrical T wave on the ECG often is the first change seen in patients with hyperkalemia.
- Hypomagnesemia can lead to fatal arrhythmias.
- Troponins are the "gold standard" for cardiac enzyme marker testing to rule out an MI.

 Internet Resources

The Journal of the International Federation of Clinical Chemistry and Laboratory Medicine. 6. Evaluation of Risk Markers for Acute Myocardial Infarction and Heart Failure: Present and the Future:
http://www.ifcc.org/ejifcc/vol14no2/140206200307n.htm

The Doctors' Medical Library: CBC Interpretation:
http://www.medical-library.net/sites/_cbc_interpretation.html

MEDLINEplus Medical Encyclopedia: CHEM-2 (chemistry values of normal and abnormal results):
http://www.nlm.nih.gov/medlineplus/ency/article/003468.htm

What Is Homocysteine?
http://www.americanheart.org/presenter.jhtml?identifier=535

Bibliography

Alexander R, Schlant R: *The heart,* ed 9, New York, 1998, McGraw-Hill.

Braunwald E, Fauci A: *Harrison's manual of medicine,* ed 15, New York, 2002, McGraw-Hill.

Jaffe AS et al: It's time for a change to a troponin standard, *Circulation* 102:1216, 2000.

Leier CV, Dei Cas L, Metra M: Clinical relevance and management of the major electrolyte abnormalities in congestive heart failure: hyponatremia; hypokalemia, and hypomagnesemia, *Am Heart J* 128:564, 1994.

Missov E, Calzolari C, Pau B: Circulating cardiac troponin I in severe congestive heart failure, *Circulation* 96:2953, 1997.

Warkentin TE, Chong BH, Greinacher A: Heparin-induced thrombocytopenia: towards consensus, *Thromb Haemost* 79:1, 1998.

Noninvasive Cardiovascular Testing

Rachel Tunstall and Christine Greenwood

1. **What are the indications for performing a 12-lead electrocardiogram (ECG)?**

   A 12-lead ECG is the noninvasive method of choice for the diagnosis of arrhythmias, conduction disturbances, and acute ischemia. It may also be used to assess or diagnose cardiac hypertrophy, cardiomyopathy, pericarditis, electrolyte or metabolic imbalances, pacemaker function, and the effectiveness of cardiac drugs.

2. **What patient education is provided before patients undergo an ECG?**

   - Provide patient education regarding why the test is being performed.
   - Advise the patient that the test lasts no longer than 15 minutes.
   - Explain to the patient what the procedure entails. Explain that the test is painless and that he or she will be lying down for the procedure. Instruct the patient that any clothing (e.g., pantyhose, bra, socks, undershirt) that would impede skin contact with the electrode, which is necessary for a good signal, must be removed. The patient may undress and use a patient gown if necessary for completion of this test. State the number of electrodes being used and where they will be placed (i.e., chest, arms, and legs). Alcohol may be used to clean the areas where the electrodes will be placed. Any hair on the chest or legs where electrodes are placed is clipped to receive a good signal for the ECG.
   - Explain to the patient that he or she needs to remain as quiet and as still as possible while breathing normally. Also remind any family member in the room to not touch the patient. Any excess movement, talking, or touching of the patient interferes with the ECG and requires that the test be repeated.

3. **What is a Holter monitor test?**

   A Holter monitor test is a continuous recording of the electrical activity of the patient's heart over a period of time. This test allows for an examination of the heart's electrical activity during a routine day in the patient's life. For this test, a patient is asked to wear electrodes for either 24 or 48 hours. The patient is also asked to record in a diary all events (e.g., sleep, medications taken, exercise, symptoms) that occur while the patient is wearing the monitor. At the end of the test, the patient is asked to come to the physician's office or lab and to return the Holter device. The Holter monitor data and correlating diary are then examined by a cardiologist. The results are given to the health care provider so that a plan of care can be determined for the patient.

4. What are the indications for a Holter monitor test?

- Diagnose arrhythmias and any relationship to activity or chest pain
- Assess the effectiveness of cardiac medications or other therapy used to treat arrhythmias

5. Is an event recorder the same test as a Holter monitor test?

- An event recorder (also known as a *loop recorder*) is *not* the same test as a Holter monitor test. An event recorder records only at intermittent intervals, such as when an arrhythmia occurs (sometimes the recording is activated by the patient pressing a button), whereas a Holter monitor test is a continuous recording of the heart's electrical activity.
- Each test aims to provide crucial information at the time symptoms occur to provide a diagnosis—that is, to detect, document, and/or characterize abnormal cardiac electrical activity)—and to provide guidance in determining a plan of care for the patient.
- Event recorders are used with patients who experience infrequent symptoms and where a clinical correlation is being determined.
- Event recorders are used over a longer period of time, such as 4- to 6-week intervals, due to the infrequent periods of symptoms with this group of patients.
- The process and patient education for an event recorder and Holter monitor test are essentially the same. The one difference is that patients with event recorders need to learn how to place electrodes and use the equipment; this is a result of the longer observation period and because patients are allowed to shower or bathe.

6. What patient education is given for patients who are using either a Holter monitor or an event recorder?

1. Tell the patient that the test is painless.
2. Inform the patient how many electrodes are being used and where they are placed (i.e., the chest).
3. Explain that any clothing that would impede skin contact with the electrode needs to be removed.
4. Explain that the areas where the electrodes will be placed will be cleaned with alcohol and that any hair on the chest in those areas will be shaved so that a good signal can be received.
5. A patient diary is to be kept to record the times of any activity (e.g., exercise, sleep), physical symptoms, and medications taken.
6. Tell the patient that he or she cannot remove, change, or disconnect the electrodes while the recording is taking place. Therefore the patient is not able to shower while on the Holter monitor.
7. The patient must be instructed to avoid items that would interfere with the Holter monitor test or event recorder such as magnets or metal detectors.

7. Should a patient with a pacemaker and/or defibrillator wear a Holter monitor or an event recorder?

A patient with a pacemaker and/or implantable cardioverter-defibrillator (ICD) may wear a Holter monitor. Event recorders are less common in this population. Indications for the use of a Holter monitor in this population of patients include the following:

- Evaluation of the pacemaker or ICD function (i.e., failure of the device)
- Assessment of whether changes need to be made in the programming of the devices
- Assessment of pacemaker and/or ICD function with concomitant medication

8. What is an echocardiogram (echo), and what are its indications?

Echocardiography is a simple, painless, noninvasive procedure. It uses high-frequency sound waves to create an image of the cardiac anatomy (size, shape, and thickness) and to assess the movement of cardiac structures. Doppler analysis uses the sound waves to evaluate blood flow, thus permitting detection of valvular regurgitation, stenosis, and intracardiac shunts. Other indications include assessment of overall left ventricular function and prosthetic valve function and detection of endocarditis, thrombus, cardiac tamponade, pericardial diseases, cardiac tumors, ventricular aneurysms, cardiomyopathies, and congenital abnormalities.

9. What can the patient expect when undergoing echocardiography?

Initially, ECG leads are placed on the chest of the patient. An ECG is done during the echo because it helps in the timing of various cardiac events. Then the patient is usually asked to lie on the left side. This position allows the heart to move forward in the chest cavity for better visualization.* A transducer is placed on the chest wall with some gel placed in the midsternal and apical areas to find the acoustic windows (the areas where the heart can easily be visualized).* The patient may be asked to change positions, hold his or her breath, or exhale during the procedure. The transducer sends images to the computer for visualization. Patients will also hear a "swooshing" sound during the Doppler study, which assesses the blood flow through the heart valves.

10. What is transesophageal echocardiography (TEE)?

TEE is a specialized type of cardiac ultrasonography that is obtained by means of a transducer mounted on a flexible gastroscope and positioned behind the heart via the esophagus.

---

*Some factors that can limit the visualization of the heart are chronic obstructive pulmonary disease (excess air in the lungs decreases the transmission of the sound waves) and obesity.

11. What are the indications for TEE?

The major indications for TEE include the following:
- Detection of the source of an embolus in the left atrium and left atrial appendage before cardioversion
- Assessment of the severity of valvular disease, especially of prosthetic valves
- Assessment for aortic dissection
- Diagnostic procedure of choice to exclude vegetation and detect complications of infective endocarditis
- Provides more definitive information for patients with a suboptimal transthoracic echo result
- Used extensively in the operating room during cardiac surgery

12. What can the patient expect when undergoing TEE?

Consent is obtained from the patient after an explanation of the risks and benefits. An intravenous line is placed to administer sedation. The patient is mildly sedated via conscious sedation for this procedure (the combination of meperidine and midazolam is used most often). The patient must swallow the flexible tube. The scope is positioned in the esophagus, which lies directly behind the heart. Images are obtained by positioning of the probe and by changing its angle. The actual test takes approximately 10-20 minutes. A total of 2 hours is typically required for preparation and recovery time. Blood pressure, heart rate, and oxygen saturation are monitored every 5-10 minutes throughout the test and for approximately 30 minutes after the test. Patients are given oral lidocaine to decrease the gag reflex and therefore are not able to resume their diet for about 1 hour after the procedure. It is suggested that patients start with clear liquids, followed by soft foods, when resuming oral intake. Patients may experience minor throat soreness.

13. What are the preparations for TEE?

The patient must be NPO for 6 hours before the procedure and may take his or her medication with sips of water. The outpatient must have someone available to drive him or her home and be available to observe the patient for approximately 4-6 hours after the procedure.

14. What are the clinical indications for an exercise stress test?

- Assist in determining the etiology of chest pain stratified as low risk (see Chapter 9, Acute Coronary Syndromes)
- Identify dysrhythmias that may arise during exercise
- Assess the efficacy of drug therapy for dysrhythmias and angina

15. How do a "stress test," an "exercise tolerance test," and a "treadmill test" differ?

- These are synonymous terms for an exercise stress test; other terms are "exercise ECG" and "graded exercise test."

- Some centers may use a stationary bike and call the test a "bicycle ergometer test." In this situation, a bicycle is used instead of a treadmill and resistance to pedaling is gradually increased during the test.

16. What instructions should be given to a patient who is to undergo a stress test?

- Tell the patient that this noninvasive cardiovascular (CV) test takes about 30 minutes to complete.
- Explain that either a physician or nurse (and sometimes both) is present for the entire duration of the test.
- Instruct the patient to not eat, drink alcohol, or smoke for at least 3 hours before the exam; the patient may have sips of water before the procedure.
- Typically, beta-blockers are withheld before the exam because they blunt the response that occurs with exercise and prevent the test from being a true stress test for the heart.
- Other medications are continued per the discretion of the health care provider.
- Advise the patient to wear comfortable shoes and loose clothing for the test.
- If there are changes in the treadmill speed or incline, advise the patient that he or she will be informed of the changes before they are implemented during the exam.
- Advise the patient to report any chest pain, fatigue, or leg pain during the test. If any of these symptoms occur, the test is usually discontinued.
- Explain the number of electrodes that are applied to the patient and where they are placed. In addition, discuss that before electrode placement, the areas at which an electrode will be placed are cleaned with alcohol and chest hair on those areas is shaved for better electrode placement and to obtain a better signal.
- Explain to the patient that he or she is under continuous ECG monitoring during the test. Therefore heart rate and electrical conduction of the heart are monitored at all times. In addition, a blood pressure cuff is applied and measurements are taken periodically during the test.
- Tell the patient that the heart rate and blood pressure are monitored for about 15 minutes after the procedure as well.

17. Are there any complications (minor and major) for patients undergoing an exercise stress test? How would a nurse assess for these potential complications?

Potential Complications	Nursing Implications
Minor: Induced ischemia during the exam	Assess for chest pain, chest tightness, chest heaviness, arm pain, shortness of breath, dizziness, or fatigue.
Major: Myocardial infarction	To ensure the ischemia or myocardial infarction is accurately assessed, the patient is continuously monitored for the above and, via ECG, for changes (i.e., ST-segment depression or ST-segment elevation or T-wave inversion).

18. What is a treadmill stress echo?

This test uses a combination of the treadmill stress test and echocardiography. An echo is performed before the patient walks on the treadmill and immediately after. The indications and preparations are the same as for all stress tests.

19. What is a dobutamine stress echo?

Dobutamine stress echo is a stress test of the heart in which dobutamine is used to increase heart rate and contractility and echocardiography is used to evaluate changes in wall motion. A baseline echo is obtained to rule out contra-indications and to ensure good visualization of all of the walls of the heart. Dobutamine is infused in increasing doses every 3 minutes to increase heart rate and contractility. The heart rate is increased to 85% of the maximum predicted heart rate for the patient according to age. If dobutamine is not effective in increasing the heart rate, small doses of atropine (0.25 mg at a time, up to 1.0 mg total) are also given. The echo is assessed before dobutamine is given, after the low dose is given, at the peak dose, and about 10 minutes postinfusion.

20. What are the indications for a dobutamine stress echo?

The primary indication for a dobutamine stress echo is to rule out ischemia. It is most often used to risk stratify patients before noncardiac surgery or to evaluate patients presenting with symptoms suggestive of coronary artery disease. It may also be used to evaluate patients with known coronary artery disease. Myocardial viability can also be evaluated using lower doses of dobutamine.

21. What can the patient expect when undergoing a dobutamine stress echo?

Consent is obtained after an explanation of the risks and benefits. A baseline echo is obtained to detect the presence of good acoustic windows. The patient has an intravenous line inserted. A 12-lead ECG and blood pressure are monitored throughout the procedure. The test takes approximately 60-90 minutes, including preparation and recovery. The medication infuses for 15-20 minutes. Patients most often feel the heart beating stronger and faster; this can cause a feeling of anxiety or restlessness. Other common feelings during the infusion include nausea, tingling, headache, and chest pressure. These symptoms resolve shortly after the medication infusion is complete (most often within 5 minutes).

22. What are the preparations for a dobutamine stress echo?

- The patients may not eat, drink, or smoke for 4 hours before the test.
- Beta-blocker medication should be held for 48 hours before the test.
- The patient may take other medications with sips of water.

23. What is a "bubble study," or contrast study, and what is its purpose?

During an echo, a syringe of agitated saline solution is injected through the patient's intravenous line. The fine bubbly solution passes into the right atrium of the heart. No bubbles should be seen early in the left atrium during the first three to five heartbeats after the injection. The test is used to determine if the patient has an atrial septal defect or patent foramen ovale. It is most often used to determine the source of an embolus in a patient who has had a neurological event such as a transient ischemic attack or cerebrovascular accident.

Key Points

- Examples of noninvasive CV tests include ECG, Holter monitoring, echo, TEE, exercise stress test, and dobutamine stress echo.
- For each of the noninvasive CV tests listed in this chapter, there are three items to know: a description of the test, indications for each test, and patient education topics.
- The most common noninvasive CV test performed on any cardiac patient is a 12-lead EEG. It is the method of choice for the diagnosis of arrhythmias, conduction disturbances, and acute ischemia. In addition, it can be used to assess other cardiac issues, such as cardiomyopathy, pericarditis, pacemaker function, and effectiveness of cardiac drugs.
- There are four types of echocardiographic testing: a basic echo, TEE, a dobutamine stress echo, and a treadmill stress echo.
- A basic echo uses an ultrasound probe on the chest wall to evaluate valves and heart function. It requires no preparation.
- A TEE uses an ultrasound probe, which is passed into the esophagus to evaluate heart valves for abnormalities and endocarditis and the cardiac chambers for thrombi. A TEE allows for clearer views of the heart valves and chambers. This study requires conscious sedation in most cases, and the patient needs to be NPO for 6 hours before the procedure. The study requires an informed consent be obtained and an intravenous line.
- A dobutamine stress echo combines the basic echo with an infusion of dobutamine (beta-agonist), which increases the rate and contractility of the heart to evaluate for ischemia with stress. The preparation includes withholding beta-blockers before the procedure and having the patient NPO for 4 hours. The study requires an informed consent and an intravenous line.
- A treadmill stress echo combines the basic echo with a treadmill stress test to evaluate for ischemia with stress. This requires the same preparation as the dobutamine stress echo. The patient must be able to walk briskly. The study also requires an informed consent.

Internet Resources

Health-Nexus.com: Echocardiogram:
http://www.health-nexus.com/echocardiogram.htm

Noninvasive Cardiac Test Center: HeartCenterOnline for Patients:
http://www.heartcenteronline.com/The_Noninvasive_Cardiac_Test_center.html

St. Vincent's Hospital: Noninvasive Cardiac Testing:
http://www.angelfire.com/ab/cardiosv/echo.html

Bibliography

Allen MN: *Diagnostic medical sonography: a guide to clinical practice*, ed 2, Philadelphia, 1999, Lippincott Williams & Wilkins, pp 349-370.

Arnold SE: What you should know about cardiac stress testing: your patient has questions—here's how to answer them, *Nursing* 27(1):58-61, 1997.

Johnston K, Goth R: The use of ECGs to record heart activity, *Prof Nurse* 14(6):417-423, 1999.

Kadish AH et al: ACC/AHA clinical competence statement on electrocardiography and ambulatory electrocardiography, *Circulation* 104(25):3169-3178, 2001.

Mee CL, Possanza CP: How to record an accurate 12-lead ECG, *Nursing* 27(3):60-63, 1997.

McConnell EA: Applying cardiac monitor electrodes, *Nursing* 28(8):26, 1998.

Oh JK, Seward JB, Tajik JA: *The echo manual*, ed 2, Philadelphia, 1999, Lippincott Williams & Wilkins.

Pinner J: Patient teaching for x-ray and other diagnostics: stress test and thallium stress test, *RN* 54(3):32-36, 1991.

Reynolds T: *The echocardiographer's pocket reference*, ed 2, Phoenix, Arizona Heart Institute, 2000, pp. 188-234.

Teaching your patient about cardiovascular tests: help him prepare both physically and emotionally, *Nursing* 32(1):62-64, 2002.

Selected Nuclear Cardiovascular Testing

Sharon M. Castina

1. What is nuclear cardiology?

Nuclear cardiology is the use of chemical agents combined with imaging techniques to provide a noninvasive method of evaluating the heart. The two most common types of nuclear cardiology studies are *myocardial perfusion imaging* (MPI) and *dynamic studies*. These studies assess myocardial blood flow, evaluate pumping function, and visualize the area of a myocardial infarction (MI).

2. What is MPI?

MPI is used in conjunction with exercise stress testing to visually assess blood flow to the heart muscle. An imaging agent (thallium, sestamibi, or tetrofosmin) is injected into the bloodstream during exercise and at rest, after which a gamma camera is used to measure the uptake by the heart of the imaging material; this is usually referred to as a *treadmill-thallium* or *treadmill-MIBI* test. Decreased blood flow is detected in ischemic areas of the myocardium during exercise, indicating significant blockage of a coronary artery or scarring from an MI. Scanning can be performed using planar images from three primary views or with single-photon emission computed tomography (SPECT) imaging. In SPECT imaging, a series of planar views are collected as the camera rotates in an arc around the patient, allowing for three-dimensional pictures when reconstructed. The three-dimensional views of SPECT allow enhanced localization of perfusion abnormalities and better diagnostic sensitivity (85%) than the individual planar images obtained in traditional MPI.

3. What does the procedure involve?

The patient receives an initial intravenous dose of the radioactive agent (thallium, tetrofosmin, or sestamibi) during exercise or chemical stress. At the end of exercise (or chemical stress), a scanning device is used to assess coronary blood flow, which is proportional to myocardial uptake of the agent, thereby indicating defects in perfusion caused by coronary artery disease (CAD). Images are also taken at rest after a few hours. During these images at rest, comparison scans are used to determine if the perfusion defect is permanent (e.g., after an MI) or reversible (e.g., ischemia).

4. Compare thallium with ^{99m}Tc (sestamibi, tetrofosmin) tracers.

- Thallium is a potassium analog, and it was the first radiotracer used for clinical MPI. It provides rapid myocardial extraction and minimal uptake by abdominal organs during exercise, allows visualization of myocardial ischemia with one injection, and provides diagnostic and prognostic value from lung uptake. A distinct advantage of thallium is that it is an excellent marker of myocardial viability. However, it is limited by a long half-life (72 hours), extended imaging requirements due to slow redistribution, low energy emission, and off-site production that requires shipment.
- ^{99m}Tc tracers were developed to overcome the limitations of thallium. ^{99m}Tc tracers remain trapped in the myocytes, allowing imaging as soon as 15 minutes and after as long as 4 hours. Due to its higher energy emission than thallium, sestamibi is preferred for women or larger men to reduce artifact caused by obesity or breast tissue. ^{99m}Tc tracers have a half-life of 6 hours, allowing the administration of a higher dose and producing higher-quality images and a slightly higher specificity in detecting CAD than thallium. ^{99m}Tc agents are more readily available due to their on-site production, and they allow analysis methods that simultaneously evaluate myocardial perfusion and left ventricular function.

5. Why should MPI be performed instead of routine exercise stress testing?

Routine exercise stress testing (see Chapter 5, Noninvasive Cardiovascular Testing) is often indicated to establish the diagnosis of CAD. Information is obtained by assessing blood pressure changes, electrocardiographic (ECG) changes, and the production of symptoms during exercise. In comparison, MPI provides a visualization that is more accurate when the resting ECG is abnormal, has greater sensitivity, is able to localize and characterize the extent of ischemia, and provides direct measurement of ventricular function.

6. What are some contraindications for exercise stress testing?

Contraindications include amputation, musculoskeletal or other orthopedic problems, peripheral artery disease, aortic aneurysm, left bundle branch block, and lung disease.

7. What agents are used to chemically stress the heart?

Pharmacological vasodilators (dipyridamole [Persantine] and adenosine) or catecholamines (dobutamine) can be used to chemically stress the heart, achieving a comparable effect to the exercise stress test. Possible side effects include chest pain, ECG changes, palpitations, headache, and flushing. The antidote for dipyridamole is aminophylline, which rapidly (within minutes) reverses its effects.

8. **What instructions should be given to the patient before undergoing pharmacological stress testing?**

Patient instructions for pharmacological stress testing

Dipyridamole, Adenosine
- These are contraindicated in patients with a history of asthma.
- No caffeine is to be consumed 12 to 24 hours before test.
- The patient must fast overnight (for at least 8 hours).

Dobutamine
- This is contraindicated in patients with recent uncontrolled hypotension or hypertension, aortic outflow obstruction, myocardial infarction, glaucoma, or ventricular arrhythmias.
- Beta blockers are withheld on the day of the test.

---

9. **What are contraindications to stress testing?**
   - Uncontrolled hypertension
   - Uncontrolled ventricular arrhythmias
   - Acute MI (within 2 days)
   - Acute aortic dissection
   - Known left main coronary stenosis
   - Decompensated heart failure
   - Severe aortic stenosis
   - Acute myocarditis or pericarditis

10. **When is MPI indicated?**
    - Diagnosis
    - Initial evaluation for chest pain to determine the presence of CAD
    - Prognosis
    - Preoperative risk assessment, post-MI stratification, determination of therapeutic efficacy, evaluation of the functional significance of angiographically determined stenoses, and myocardial viability

11. **What does radionuclide ventriculography evaluate, and how does it do so?**

Radionuclide ventriculography (RNV)/radionuclide angiography (RNA) is a dynamic study that provides information about valvular function and cardiac chamber integrity. It can also be used to evaluate any damage to the myocardium caused by cardiotoxic drugs. In this study, a radioactive imaging agent (usually technetium or thallium) is injected into the bloodstream, thus tagging the red blood cells, which are then counted in the left ventricle by a gamma camera in systole and diastole. The fraction of counts lost from diastole to systole is the *left ventricular ejection fraction (LVEF)*. This study can be done at rest or as part of a rest/exercise study to determine if heart function is altered during and after exercise. This test is also called a multiple gated acquisition or *MUGA scan*.

12. What are some features of positron emission tomography (PET)?

- Higher sensitivity than achieved with conventional nuclear medicine cameras
- Higher spatial resolution
- Quantitative rather than qualitative data given regarding radiopharmaceutical distribution in the body

13. When is PET scanning used?

PET scans evaluate both blood flow and metabolic activity in the myocardium. The combination of perfusion agents (^{13}N ammonia or rubidium) and metabolic imaging with ^{18}fluorodeoxyglucose (^{18}FDG) is the gold standard for the evaluation of myocardial viability. PET-FDG imaging can delineate ischemic but still viable and potentially salvageable myocardium with greater sensitivity than thallium exercise or chemical stress scanning. It is useful in selecting patients who will benefit from revascularization procedures such as angioplasty or coronary artery bypass graft surgery.

14. What are some advantages and disadvantages of cardiac magnetic resonance imaging (MRI)?

Advantages and disadvantages of cardiac magnetic resonance imaging

Advantages
- MRI provides three-dimensional images of body structures.
- During stress, MRI assesses left ventricular contractility, myocardial perfusion, coronary artery blood flow, and myocardial metabolism.
- MRI is ideal for assessing congenital disease, pericardial abnormalities, aortic aneurysm or dissection, and trauma.

Disadvantages
- The patient is placed within an enclosed space.
- MRI has a high cost.
- MRI cannot be used to image unstable patients because monitoring capabilities are limited (ECG tracing is distorted).

15. Which patients cannot undergo cardiac magnetic resonance imaging (MRI)?

Patients who cannot undergo cardiac MRI are those with
- Implanted ferromagnetic plates
- Pacemakers

- Defibrillators
- Other metal devices

16. Can patients with a prosthetic heart valve undergo MRI?

Most can, but patients with a Starr-Edwards 1200 series ball-cage valve cannot. However, limited information is obtained in the area of the valve due to absorption of imaging agent by metallic structures within the heart.

17. How should the patient be prepared before a cardiac MRI?

The nurse should ask the patient to arrive 30 minutes before the appointed time to fill out a safety profile and to change into a hospital gown. The hospital gown should be worn with the opening in the front because ECG wires are placed on the chest throughout the exam. The nurse should also explain that the table and tube are somewhat enclosed. There is a knocking sound as the device takes pictures, but the patient is provided with headphones or videos to reduce the noise stimuli. The patient may be asked to hold his or her breath for 3-20 seconds at a time to reduce artifact.

Key Points

- Nuclear cardiology uses chemical agents combined with imaging techniques to provide a noninvasive method of assessing myocardial blood flow and pumping function.
- Myocardial perfusion imaging is used in conjunction with exercise stress testing to visually assess blood flow to the heart muscle.
- Routine exercise stress testing is often indicated to establish the diagnosis of CAD by evaluating blood pressure and ECG changes and symptom production during exercise, whereas MPI is more sensitive, evaluates the location and extent of ischemia, and directly measures ventricular function.
- RNV/RNA is dynamic study that provides information about valvular function and cardiac chamber integrity and can be used to evaluate left ventricular function.

Internet Resources

Thallium Stress Test (American Heart Association):
http://www.americanheart.org/presenter.jhtml?identifier=4743

Computer Imaging/Tomography (American Heart Association):
http://www.americanheart.org/presenter.jhtml?identifier=4554

American Society of Nuclear Cardiology (ASNC):
http://www.asnc.org/

Bibliography

Bhola R, Quaife RA: Nuclear cardiology, magnetic resonance imaging, and computed tomography. In Adair OV, editor: *Cardiology secrets*, ed 2, Philadelphia, 2001, Hanley & Belfus, pp 55-64.

Cerqueira MD, Lawrence A: Nuclear cardiology update, *Nuclear Cardiol Update* 39(5):931-946, 2002.

Darty SN et al: Cardiovascular magnetic resonance imaging, *Am J Nurs* 102(12):34-38, 2002.

Hendel RC: Interpreting noninvasive cardiac tests. In Alpert JS, editor: *Cardiology for the primary care physician*, ed 3, Philadelphia, 2001, Current Medicine, Inc, pp 25-36.

Ulstad VK: Cardiac testing. In Mladeovic J, editor: *Primary care secrets*, ed 2, Philadelphia, 1999, Hanley & Belfus, pp 115-120.

Invasive Cardiovascular Testing
(Angiography and Electrophysiology Studies)

Lisa A. Kiger and Kendra Hennings

1. What are the clinical indications for cardiac catheterization?

The indications for cardiac catheterization given by the American College of Cardiology (ACC) and the American Heart Association (AHA) are summarized as follows:
- Known or suspected coronary artery disease
- Positive exercise and/or pharmacological stress test
- Diagnostic evaluation of atypical chest pain and/or coronary spasm
- Stable and/or unstable angina
- Myocardial infarction
- Valvular heart disease
- Congenital heart disease
- Congestive heart failure
- Cardiomyopathy
- Sudden cardiac death
- Heart transplantation

2. What patients are considered "high risk" for cardiac catheterization?

Patients who are high risk (i.e., are more likely to have complications from the procedure) for cardiac catheterization include those with the following characteristics:
- Age of older than 60 years
- New York Heart Association Functional Class IV (symptoms of fatigue, palpitations, dyspnea, or angina at rest)
- Known left main disease
- Valvular heart disease
- Left ventricular dysfunction with ejection fraction (EF) of less than 30%
- Chronic comorbidity such as diabetes mellitus, renal insufficiency, peripheral vascular disease, or chronic lung disease

3. Describe the workup of a patient who is undergoing cardiac catheterization.

A cardiac catheterization may be performed, in most cases, after noninvasive tests such as echocardiography, exercise stress testing, or nuclear stress testing have been performed. Patients undergoing cardiac catheterization must have a recent electrocardiogram, chest radiograph, complete blood cell count, complete metabolic panel, and coagulation studies before the procedure. A serum pregnancy test is recommended for all females with child-bearing potential. A complete history and physical exam should be performed, as well as a review of previous lab data and the results of diagnostic studies and previous catheterizations. Heart sounds and carotid and peripheral pulses should be assessed before and after cardiac catheterization. Allergic reactions to dyes used in previous tests or procedures, iodine, shellfish (crab or shrimp), and strawberries should be noted. Antihistamines, corticosteroids, and histamine (H_1 and H_2) blockers may be administered prophylactically to decrease allergic and anaphylactic reactions to contrast agent. Informed consent is obtained after an explanation of the procedure and its purpose, potential benefits, and possible risks.

4. What preparation is needed for cardiac catheterization?

Patients should be NPO, except for medications, after midnight on the day before the scheduled procedure. Patients whose cardiac catheterizations are not scheduled until the afternoon may consume a light liquid breakfast. Certain medications may need to be discontinued or reduced. Insulin and food intake should be adjusted if the patient has diabetes. A patient usually receives half of his or her insulin dosage on the morning of the procedure. One class of oral hypoglycemic agents, Metformin, should be withheld the morning of the procedure and is typically not restarted for 48 hours after the procedure, if no dye-induced nephropathy occurs. Anticoagulants (e.g., warfarin) should be discontinued at least 48 hours before the cardiac catheterization. Before angiography is attempted, an acceptable target prothrombin time and international normalized ratio (INR) should be less than 15 seconds and 1.5 seconds, respectively. Antiplatelet medications need not be withheld before cardiac catheterization An intravenous line is required to administer fluids, medications, and conscious sedation. Catheter insertion sites (femoral, radial, or brachial vascular access) are shaved and prepared according to institution-specific protocols.

5. What occurs during the cardiac catheterization?

The patient is transported to the catheterization lab and transferred to an x-ray table. The patient is continuously monitored for signs of hypotension, arrhythmias, and angina. A mild sedative is usually administered intravenously. The patient is draped with sterile sheets. The area or areas where the sheaths and catheters will be inserted (groin, arm, or jugular) are cleaned thoroughly with an antiseptic solution. A local anesthetic is injected to numb the insertion site. A small incision is made in the skin, and a needle is used to puncture the vein or artery into which the sheath and catheters are inserted. The sheath protects the artery or vein and allows the insertion of multiple catheters. The catheters are then inserted through the sheath and positioned inside the heart. Dye is injected through the catheter and into the coronary arteries, and fluoroscopy is used to visualize blood flow through the coronary arteries. This allows the physician to determine vessel occlusion and the extent of coronary artery disease. A left ventriculogram (LV gram) is also performed to determine EF (see Question 12). Atropine and a transvenous pacer may be used if bradycardia occurs and persists as a reaction to contrast material.

6. What are the most common sites of vascular access for cardiac catheterization?

Catheters are introduced into the brachial, radial, or femoral artery and jugular or femoral vein. The percutaneous right femoral artery and vein are the sites most commonly used. The choice of access site depends on physician preference and extent of peripheral vascular disease of the patient.

7. What symptoms may the patient experience during the procedure?

- Slight burning or stinging from the medication used to numb the catheter insertion site
- Slight pressure at catheter insertion site on insertion of the catheter
- Nausea, headache, palpitations, and/or a warm flushed feeling as dye is injected into the coronary arteries
- Dizziness or lightheadedness
- Palpitations during insertion of diagnostic catheters into the heart
- Back and buttock soreness from lying flat during the procedure
- Dysrhythmias

8. What happens after a cardiac catheterization?

After the procedure is completed, the sheaths and catheters are removed. Timing for removal of sheaths or catheters may vary according to institution protocols. Firm pressure is applied to the arterial insertion site for 15-20 minutes and/or to the venous insertion site for 10 minutes, until hemostasis occurs. An adhesive bandage or clear dressing may be applied; the type of dressing depends on the type of closure mechanism that is used. Patients may be admitted to a short-stay unit or cardiac unit for close monitoring. The insertion site should be examined frequently for signs of bleeding. Vital signs and pulses in the extremity used for catheter insertion are monitored frequently. The usual protocol is every 15 minutes for 1 hour, every 30 minutes for 2 hours, and then every 1 hour for 4 hours. After 4 to 6 hours of bed rest, the patient may resume normal activity. Fluid volume may be replaced with oral hydration or intravenous replacement. After the cardiologist reviews the catheterization films, results and treatment options are discussed with the patient and family.

9. What closure techniques are used to achieve hemostasis after sheath removal?

Manual compression and mechanical devices, such as C-clamp and Femostop, are noninvasive techniques to achieve hemostasis at the insertion site. Percutaneous vascular devices such as AngioSeal, VasoSeal, Duett, Perclose, Clo-Sur P.A.D., and SyvekPatch are available options for wound closure. AngioSeal,

VasoSeal, and Duett are collagen-based devices that are inserted into the catheter site and seal the wound to prevent bleeding. Clo-Sur P.A.D. uses the cell-binding activity of Polyprolate as a hemostatic agent. Perclose uses a suture to close the tissue around the arteriotomy. SyvekPatch is an external device/dressing that is applied to the sheath access site. The use of sandbags, pressure dressings, and mechanical compression devices is not recommended with percutaneous vascular closure devices.

10. What are the minor and major complications of cardiac catheterization?

Minor Complications

- Vasovagal reactions
- Vascular complications at the access site, including bleeding and/or hematoma
- Cardiac arrhythmias (bradycardia, conduction disturbances, and heart block)
- Allergic reaction to contrast agent (dye)
- Renal insult from contrast agent (dye) (elevated blood urea nitrogen and creatinine)
- Hypovolemia and hypotension
- Perforation of blood vessel
- Perforation of the great vessels (aortic dissection)
- Air embolism or blood clot
- Infection

Major Complications

- Myocardial infarction (0.1%-0.3%)
- Stroke (0.1%-0.3%)
- Death (0.1%-0.2%)

11. What is the difference between a right-sided heart catheterization and a left-sided heart catheterization?

Right heart catheterization uses venous access and provides hemodynamic pressure measurements in the right atrium, right ventricle, and pulmonary artery and pulmonary capillary wedge pressure. Cardiac output and oxygen saturation may be calculated and measured. A right heart catheterization may be performed if a diagnosis of concomitant valvular heart disease, presumed pulmonary hypertension, or intracardiac shunts is suspected; otherwise, a right heart catheterization is not routinely performed. Left heart catheterization uses arterial access to visualize the left heart chambers and coronary arteries. It also measures systolic and end-diastolic pressures, stroke volume, and EF.

12. What does an LV gram measure?

The LV gram, which is commonly performed during a left heart catheterization, measures left ventricular wall motion. Wall motion can be defined as normal, hyperkinetic, hypokinetic, dyskinetic, or akinetic. The value of *normal* wall motion (i.e., EF) is 60%-75%. *Hyperkinesis* is defined as increased extent of contraction during systole. *Hypokinesis* is considered to be less-than-normal motion in systole. *Dyskinesis* is wall motion that bulges during systole. *Akinesis* is lack of wall motion. Mitral regurgitation, if present, can be assessed and graded as mild (1^+), moderate (2^+), moderately severe (3^+), or severe (4^+).

13. What does an aortogram measure?

The aortogram visualizes the aorta, aortic arch, great vessels, aortic valve, and saphenous vein grafts after coronary artery bypass graft (CABG) surgery. It can be used to determine or diagnose aortic valve insufficiency, aneurysms, dissections, coarctation of the aorta, and anomalous coronary and great vessels.

14. What is meant by a right or left dominant system?

Coronary dominance identifies the coronary artery that supplies the interventricular septum of the left ventricle. In approximately 85% of patients, the right coronary artery is dominant. In approximately 15% of patients, the left circumflex artery is dominant. However, a few patients will have co-dominance.

15. What information should a nurse obtain when receiving the report from the catheterization lab team?

Information about the procedure performed, type of wound closure, complications experienced (if any), amount of fluid and medications received, length of time to be on bed rest, most recent vital signs, and quality of pulses should be obtained from the nurse or technologist. Determine which ECG lead most predominantly displays ST-segment changes and monitor in that lead after the procedure.

16. What precautions should be observed after the procedure?

The duration of immobility depends on the type of closure device that is used. For example, a patient with a femoral insertion site should keep his or her leg straight and avoid bending at the hip for 2 to 6 hours. All patients should be instructed to hold the dressing firmly if they need to cough or sneeze. Patients should also be instructed to immediately report discomfort or sudden pain or swelling; a warm, moist, sticky feeling or bleeding at the insertion site; any discomfort in the chest, neck, jaw, arms, or upper back; shortness of breath; weakness; dizziness; or nausea.

17. In what circumstances should the nurse notify the physician, nurse practitioner (NP), or physician's assistant (PA)?

A physician, NP, or PA should be notified if the patient experiences oozing or bleeding at the insertion site, has a hematoma or pain/tenderness develop at the insertion site, has a decrease in peripheral pulses, has affected extremity pain or numbness, is hemodynamically unstable, or has chest pain (or chest pain equivalent).

18. What must a nurse do if a hematoma develops at the femoral insertion site?

For overt bleeding or hematoma, the nurse should apply continuous direct pressure $1/2$ to 1 inch above insertion site for a minimum of 15 minutes, without release. Once hemostasis is obtained, clean the site with alcohol, observe for bleeding, and apply an adhesive dressing. Monitor vital signs, insertion site, and extremity pulses, and maintain activity precautions. Mark the area of hematoma for later comparison.

19. What is the most important patient education for cardiac catheterization?

Patients should be informed of what will occur before, during and after the cardiac catheterization procedure. This would also include education about medication, diet, and activity. Modification of risk factors should be an integral component of education. Instructions should include control of high blood pressure, smoking cessation, a diet low in fat and cholesterol, weight reduction if overweight, regular exercise, stress reduction, and hyperglycemic control.

20. How long is the cardiac catheterization procedure?

A total of 1-1.5 hours may lapse from preprocedural preparation to post-procedural recovery, including transportation to and from the short-stay or cardiac unit. The process of obtaining the angiograms lasts approximately 20-30 minutes.

21. What treatments might follow a cardiac catheterization?

Depending on what is shown on angiography, the physician may recommend treatments such as medications, percutaneous transluminal coronary interventions (e.g., balloon angioplasty, intracoronary stents), or CABG surgery.

22. List common discharge instructions for a patient after cardiac catheterization.

- Make arrangements with a family member or friend to drive you home from the hospital.
- Avoid heavy lifting and perform only light activities for 2-3 days.
- Leave the dressing on until the day after the procedure.
- Keep the wound dry for at least 12 hours. Then you may shower. Do not bathe in a tub until the insertion site heals.
- A small bruise or lump under the skin at the insertion site is common and should go away within a few weeks.
- If bleeding or swelling occurs at the insertion site, place your fingers over the site and press firmly for 20 minutes. If bleeding continues, contact 911 or have someone drive you to the local emergency department, while maintaining pressure on the insertion site.

23. When should a patient contact the physician or NP/PA?

A patient should contact his or her physician or NP/PA if any of the following symptoms are noted:
- Bleeding, swelling, redness, or drainage at the insertion site
- Dizziness, shortness of breath, or chest pain or pressure
- Numbness, change in color, increase in temperature, or sensation in the arm or leg in which the catheter was inserted
- Fever

24. What is an electrophysiology study (EPS)?

An EPS is a diagnostic test that evaluates the electrical conduction system of the heart. It can determine the location and characteristic of an arrhythmia and help determine the type of therapy needed to correct the problem. The EPS can be used before implantation of a pacemaker or implantable cardioverter-defibrillator (ICD) or to identify the target tissue for a catheter ablation procedure. Information from the EPS can assist in programming the device and measuring device effectiveness. The EPS can also be used to evaluate the effectiveness of antiarrhythmic medications.

25. What are the clinical indications for an EPS?

The indications for an EPS provided by the ACC and the AHA are summarized as follows:
- Syncope
- Bradyarrhythmias (i.e., sinus bradycardia)
- Sinus node dysfunction (i.e., sinus pauses, sick sinus syndrome)
- Atrioventricular (AV) node dysfunction (i.e., heart block)
- Supraventricular tachycardias (i.e., AV node reentrant tachycardia [AVNRT], Wolff-Parkinson-White [WPW] syndrome, and atrial fibrillation/flutter)
- Ventricular tachycardia, ventricular fibrillation, and sudden cardiac death

26. Briefly describe the EPS procedure.

The EPS involves the insertion of special catheters into the heart that record electrical signals and pace the heart. Atrial and ventricular pacing thresholds are obtained and conduction intervals are measured. Various programmed electrical stimulation protocols are used to induce atrial and/or ventricular arrhythmias. The EPS helps identify the exact location or cause of the arrhythmia and determines the medications or treatments that are needed to correct the arrhythmia. The duration of the EPS can vary from 2 to 6 hours, sometimes longer. It can be done in a minimum amount of time if no arrhythmias are induced. The EPS may last for a number of hours if multiple medications are being evaluated.

27. What preparation is needed for an EPS?

Preparation of the patient for electrophysiology studies is the same as that for cardiac catheterization (see Question 5). In addition, antiarrhythmic medications are usually discontinued for at least five half-lives before the procedure. Discuss the discontinuation of antiarrhythmic medications before the procedure with the physician or NP/PA. The site where the catheters are inserted is shaved and prepared according to institution-specific protocols. In most cases, this area is the groin; in some cases, the neck, chest, or arm is used.

28. What happens during the EPS?

The EPS is performed in a specially equipped laboratory called an *EP lab*. The EP lab is equipped with a variety of monitoring devices, video monitors, and x-ray equipment. Transcutaneous pacing pads are placed in the event external cardioversion or defibrillation is required. Medication is usually administered to produce conscious sedation. Catheters may be introduced into the internal jugular, subclavian, brachial or femoral vein, and femoral artery. Catheters are commonly placed into the high right atrium (HRA), coronary sinus (CS), His bundle (HB), and right ventricular apex (RVA). Individual areas of the heart are then electrically stimulated in an attempt to induce an arrhythmia. Pacing catheters or defibrillation may be used to terminate arrhythmias. If an arrhythmia is induced, antiarrhythmic medications may be given through the intravenous line to test their effectiveness in stopping the heart rhythm.

29. What symptoms may the patient experience during the procedure?

Symptoms that patients may experience the same as those listed in Question 7, excluding a warm flushed feeling as dye is injected into the coronary arteries. This is not applicable to EPS. In addition, patients may experience palpitations during the insertion of catheters and during pacing.

30. Discuss the postprocedural care for EPS.

Postprocedural care is the same as that described in Question 8.

31. What precautions should be observed after the procedure?

Precautions are the same as outlined in Question 16.

32. What potential complications may occur during or after an EPS?

Complications are the same as those outlined in Question 10, excluding allergic reaction to contrast agent (dye) and renal insult from contrast agent. This is not applicable to EPS. In addition, the patient may experience oversedation and/or pericardial perforation.

33. What treatments might follow an EPS?

If an abnormal electrical pathway is causing an arrhythmia, radiofrequency catheter ablation (see Question 36) may be performed to remove the abnormal pathway and restore normal electrical conduction. Further treatment may include a prescription for antiarrhythmic medications or the implantation of a permanent pacemaker or ICD.

34. List common discharge instructions for patients after an EPS.

Discharge instructions are the same as those outlined in Question 22. However, heavy lifting and performance of light activities are permitted after 7-10 days.

35. When should a patient contact his or her physician or NP/PA?

A patient should contact his or her physician, NP, or PA if he or she notices any of the following symptoms:
- Bleeding or pain at the insertion site
- Dizziness, shortness of breath, or chest pain
- Numbness in the arm or leg in which the catheter was inserted
- Temperature of greater than 100° F
- Recurrence of the arrhythmia

36. What is radiofrequency catheter ablation?

Radiofrequency catheter ablation involves the application of radiofrequency energy to an anatomical abnormality that allows the arrhythmia to be palliated or cured. The radiofrequency energy causes a small lesion or burn that destroys the target tissue.

37. What are the clinical indications for radiofrequency catheter ablation?

Radiofrequency catheter ablation is used to treat tachyarrhythmias, such as supraventricular tachycardia, AVNRT, WPW syndrome, atrial fibrillation/flutter, and ventricular tachycardia.

38. Discuss the preprocedural care for radiofrequency catheter ablation.

The preprocedural care for radiofrequency catheter ablation is the same as that outlined in Questions 27.

39. Briefly describe the radiofrequency catheter ablation procedure.

The patient is brought to the EP lab and prepared in a similar manner as for an EPS. Sometimes an ablation is performed using general anesthesia. The location of the tachyarrhythmia is "mapped," or identified. Mapping is quite extensive and can take up to 6 hours or longer. The radiofrequency ablation catheter is positioned to the precise spot, and radiofrequency energy is delivered to the tissue for 10-120 seconds. After the ablation, the physician attempts to reinduce the tachyarrhythmia. If it can be induced, additional ablation burns can be administered to create more scar tissue. After a 30-minute monitoring period, the induction of the tachyarrhythmia is again attempted. Successful ablation occurs when the tachyarrhythmia cannot be induced.

40. What are the five common locations of catheters during the radiofrequency catheter ablation?

Catheters may be introduced into the internal jugular, subclavian, brachial, or femoral vein and femoral artery. Catheters are commonly placed into the HRA, CS, HB, and RVA. The fifth catheter is the ablation catheter, which is positioned in contact with the target tissue.

41. Discuss the postprocedural care for radiofrequency catheter ablation.

The postprocedural care for radiofrequency catheter ablation is the same as that given in Question 8. In addition, a chest radiograph is obtained to ensure there is no evidence of pneumothorax or cardiac tamponade. An echocardiogram may be performed before discharge to assess for any pericardial effusions or wall motion abnormalities.

42. Is radiofrequency catheter ablation safe?

Radiofrequency catheter ablation is a relatively low-risk procedure. In many cases, it permanently cures the arrhythmia. Depending on the location and type of abnormal pathway being ablated, there is a chance of damaging the electrical conduction system of the heart. A permanent pacemaker implant may be necessary. If the AV node is ablated, a permanent pacemaker implant is an expected part of the radiofrequency catheter ablation procedure.

43. What is the success rate of radiofrequency catheter ablation?

The following table identifies the common arrhythmias and associated success rates.

Common arrhythmias and associated success rates

Arrhythmia	Target	Cure or Palliation	Success Rate (%)
Atrioventricular node reentrant tachycardia	Atrial tissue	Cure	~95
Wolff-Parkinson-White syndrome	Accessory pathway	Cure	~95
Ectopic atrial tachycardia	Atrial tissue	Cure	~70
Atrial fibrillation	Atrioventricular node (permanent pacer implant)	Palliation	~99

Common arrhythmias and associated success rates *continued*			
Arrhythmia	**Target**	**Cure or Palliation**	**Success Rate (%)**
Atrial flutter	Atrial tissue	Cure	~90
Idiopathic ventricular tachycardia	Ventricular tissue	Cure	~90
Postinfarction ventricular tachycardia	Ventricular tissue	Cure	~50-70

Data from Parker DL, Kay GN: Radiofrequency catheter ablation. In Naccarelli GV et al, editors: *EPSAP II: electrophysiology self-assessment program,* Bethesda, Md, 2000, American College of Cardiology, pp 10.3-10.53.

44. Define common discharge instructions for a patient who underwent radiofrequency catheter ablation.

Discharge instructions for radiofrequency catheter ablation are the same as those outlined in Questions 22 and 34.

45. When should patients contact their physician, NP, or PA?

Palpitations lasting about two to four beats are normal and may be felt for 3-4 weeks after the procedure. Patients should contact the physician if they notice any of the following symptoms:
- Bleeding or pain at the insertion site
- Dizziness, shortness of breath, or chest pain
- Numbness in the arm or leg in which the catheter was inserted
- Fever (if temperature >101.5° F)
- Any symptom similar to that experienced before the ablation

 Key Points

- **Angiography is an invasive cardiovascular test that is indicated in patients with known or suspected coronary artery disease, stable or unstable angina, myocardial infarction, valvular heart disease, and other conditions.**

- It is imperative to understand the preprocedural, intraprocedural, and postprocedural care for patients undergoing angiography or for those undergoing electrophysiological procedures.

- Frequent assessment of the patient undergoing angiography is critical for safe patient care, because it involves recognizing and treating complications.

- Complications of angiography include vasovagal reactions, bleeding, hematoma, allergic reactions to contrast material, hypotension, and hypovolemia.

- An EPS is a diagnostic test that evaluates the electrical conduction system of the heart. It can determine the location and characteristic of an arrhythmia and determine the type of therapy needed to correct the problem.

- If an abnormal electrical pathway is causing an arrhythmia, radiofrequency catheter ablation may be performed to remove the abnormal pathway and restore normal electrical conduction.

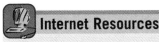

Internet Resources

American Heart Association:
www.americanheart.org

American College of Cardiology:
www.acc.org

NASPE Heart Rhythm Society:
www.naspe.org

Electrophysiology Lab: The EP Lab.com:
www.theeplab.com

FastHeartBeat.com: Dangerously Fast Heart Rhythms:
www.fastheartbeat.com

Bibliography

Attin M: Electrophysiology study: a comprehensive review, *Am J Crit Care* 10:260-273, 2001.

Blancher S, Main CC: Cardiac electrophysiology procedures. In Woods SL et al, editors: *Cardiac nursing,* ed 4, Philadelphia, 2000, JB Lippincott, pp 363-373.

Busch MM, Juel R, Newton KM: Cardiac catheterization. In Woods SL et al, editors: *Cardiac nursing,* ed 4, Philadelphia, 2000, JB Lippincott, pp 409-424.

Deelstra MH: Interventional cardiology techniques. In Woods SL et al, editors: *Cardiac nursing,* ed 4, Philadelphia, 2000, JB Lippincott, pp 541-559.

Norris TG: Principles of cardiac catheterization, *Radiol Technol* 72:109-144, 2000.

Parker DL, Kay GN: Radiofrequency catheter ablation. In Naccarelli GV et al, editors: *EPSAP II: electrophysiology self-assessment program,* Bethesda, Md, 2000, American College of Cardiology, pp 10.3-10.53.

Robertson RW, Miller WP: Cardiac catheterization and angiography. In Adair OV, editor: *Cardiology secrets,* ed 2, Philadelphia, 2001, Hanley & Belfus, pp 65-70.

Scanlon PJ, Faxon DP, Audet AM et al: ACC/AHA guidelines for coronary angiography: Executive summary and recommendations: a report of the American College of Cardiology/American Heart Association Task Force on Practice Guidelines (Committee on Coronary Angiography), *Circulation* 99:2345-2357, 1999.

Teplitz L: Treating tachyarrhythmias with radiofrequency catheter ablation, *Dimens Crit Care Nurs* 19:28-31, 2000.

Tracy CM, Akhtar M, DiMarco JP et al: Clinical competence statement on invasive electrophysiology studies, catheter ablation, and cardioversion, *J Am Coll Cardiol* 36:1725-1736, 2000.

Section III

Symptoms and Disease States

Chapter 8

Hypertension

Linda K. Daley

1. What is hypertension (HTN)?

The seventh report of the Joint National Committee on Prevention, Detection, Evaluation, and Treatment of High Blood Pressure (JNC VII) defines hypertension as a systolic blood pressure (SBP) of ≥140 mm Hg, a diastolic blood pressure (DBP) of ≥90 mm Hg. Anyone taking antihypertensive medication is also considered to have hypertension.

2. How is hypertension diagnosed?

Hypertension is diagnosed when the average of two or more systolic measurements made on two or more consecutive visits is >140 mm Hg or the average of two or more diastolic measurements made on two or more consecutive visits is >90 mm Hg.

3. How should the blood pressure be measured in order to ensure an accurate reading?

The patient needs to be seated with his or her back firm against a chair and have the arms resting on a surface supported at heart level. The patient should rest for 5 minutes before any reading is taken. The arms need to be bare for accuracy in hearing the Korotkoff sounds, and the cuff size must be appropriate. Two or more readings separated by a 2-minute wait period should be averaged.

4. How is appropriate cuff size determined?

A cuff that is too large or too small gives inaccurate readings. The bladder length within the cuff should encircle at least 80% of the arm circumference, or the bladder width of the cuff should approximate 40% of the arm circumference.

5. What if the blood pressure reading is different in each arm?

Differences of less than 10 mm Hg are considered normal. Differences greater than 10 mm Hg may not have significant meaning, however, they should be reported to a physician or to an advanced practice registered nurse (APRN) to determine the need for further evaluation. The difference might be indicative of a more serious problem (e.g., arteriovenous malformation or aortic aneurysm or dissection in a patient with Marfan syndrome).

6. What is considered "high blood pressure"?

According to JNC VII, blood pressure is classified into four different categories for individuals 18 years of age or older who are not taking blood pressure medication and are not experiencing an acute illness.

Category	Systolic Blood Pressure (mm Hg)	Diastolic Blood Pressure (mm Hg)
Normal	<120	<80
Pre-hypertension	120-139	80-89
Stage 1 hypertension	140-159	90-99
Stage 2 hypertension	≥160	≥100

7. Are there critical levels of hypertension?

Clinicians subdivide hypertension into two stages based on degrees of risk for associated morbidity and mortality.

Stage	Systolic Blood Pressure (mm Hg)	Diastolic Blood Pressure (mm Hg)
1	140-159	90-99
2	≥160	≥100

8. Are there differences among men and women, or ethnic groups with regard to individuals who are more prone to have hypertension?

Males tend to be affected more than women until about the age of 55, at which time females tend to catch up to their male counterparts. From age 75 on, more females than males have high blood pressure. Black Americans develop high blood pressure earlier in life than do non-blacks. Black males die from strokes at almost twice the rate of males in the total population. Blacks and whites in the Southeastern region of the United States have a greater prevalence of high blood pressure and a higher death rate from stroke than those in other regions of the United States.

9. What are the risk factors for hypertension?

The primary risk factors for hypertension include genetic predisposition, advanced age, obesity, diet high in sodium, increased consumption of alcohol, and lack of exercise. High blood pressure is two to three times more common in women taking oral contraceptives, particularly women who are obese or older.

10. How prevalent is hypertension?

Hypertension affects more than 50 million Americans age 6 or older; this represents roughly 1 in 5 Americans and 1 in 4 adults. About 60% of Americans age 60 or older have hypertension. Approximately 31% of individuals are unaware that they have hypertension.

11. What is primary hypertension?

Primary hypertension refers to elevated systolic and diastolic levels with no known cause. It is also known as essential or idiopathic hypertension. Researchers are examining three contributing factors: hyperactivity of the sympathetic nervous system, hyperactivity of the renin-angiotensin system, and endothelial dysfunction. More than 90% of individuals with high blood pressure have primary hypertension.

12. What is secondary hypertension?

Secondary hypertension results from alterations of other systems, such as the vascular system (e.g., arteriosclerosis), renal system (e.g., renal artery stenosis), endocrine system (e.g., hyperthyroidism) or neurological system (e.g., increased intracranial pressure). Pregnancy can also cause secondary hypertension

13. What is "white coat" hypertension?

White coat hypertension refers to the physiological response or elevation in blood pressure in individuals who become stressed in the presence of a health care provider but whose blood pressure is normal when taken at other times. There are wide variations in the literature in regards to the frequency of this phenomenon (5%-60%), with some studies suggesting that Black females and individuals with diabetes are more susceptible. Patients with suspected white coat hypertension might be asked to monitor their blood pressure at home or to wear an ambulatory blood pressure monitor in order to determine whether the findings are indeed benign.

14. What are the signs and symptoms of hypertension?

Unfortunately, during the early stages there are no signs or symptoms that would cause an individual to seek help. Some individuals experience un-explained headaches or nosebleeds, weakness or numbness in an extremity, or visual disturbances. Most clinical manifestations are the result of damage to other tissues and organs (referred to as end-organ damage) and are therefore system specific. For example, a funduscopic examination by an ophthalmologist might reveal changes in the retina. A cardiovascular examination might reveal a precordial heave, murmur, bruit, or extra heart sounds.

15. Do treatment goals differ for patients who already have established cardiovascular disease or diabetes?

Preventing stroke and heart disease and maintaining renal function are essential, but the overall goal for all individuals is to reduce morbidity and mortality through lifestyle modification, medication, or both. For individuals who have diabetes or other evidence of cardiovascular disease, stage 1 hypertension should be treated with medication in addition to lifestyle modification in order to reduce blood pressure to below 130/85 mm Hg.

16. What lifestyle changes can individuals make in order to lower their blood pressure?

Lifestyle Change	Purpose
Smoking cessation	Cardiovascular benefits of smoking cessation can be seen within a year. Cessation is essential for individuals to receive the full benefit of antihypertensive therapy.
Exercise	Exercise helps to achieve and maintain ideal body weight and is particularly beneficial to individuals who have been diagnosed with high normal blood pressure. Aerobic activity such as 30-45 minutes of brisk walking each day helps to improve stroke volume, which in turn lowers the heart rate and systolic pressure. Exercise has also been shown to be beneficial in reducing stress.
Follow recommended nutrition guidelines	Weight management and blood pressure control can be aided by limiting saturated fats, cholesterol, overall caloric intake, and caffeine, as well as limiting salt intake to no more than 2.4 grams of sodium per day.
Maintain ideal body weight	A body mass index of >27 is associated with increased blood pressure. A weight loss of 10 pounds has been found to be beneficial in reducing blood pressure.
Decrease and/or manage stress	Stress can be managed through relaxation techniques such as guided imagery, yoga, or biofeedback. These techniques help to reduce catecholamine levels, thereby reducing blood pressure.
Take prescription medication	When taken as prescribed, medications help to decrease cardiovascular morbidity and mortality. Health care providers need to be informed of all prescribed as well as over-the-counter (OTC) medications and herbal supplements.

17. Why are some patients prescribed more than one antihypertensive medication?

Pharmacological intervention often requires combined management strategies depending on age, race, or target organ problems; more than half of patients diagnosed with hypertension do not respond to single-drug therapy. Diuretics are often used to help reduce volume, but additional drugs are often needed to decrease peripheral vascular resistance. Furthermore, studies have shown that different populations require multidrug therapy. Black Americans tend to respond better to combination therapies due to a decreased sensitivity to angiotensin-converting enzyme (ACE) inhibitors. Pregnant women with hypertension require combination drugs as well as changes in pharmacological regime as the due date nears. Elderly persons often require lower dosages due to impaired drug clearance.

18. Are there any recommendations about alcohol that should be given to individuals with high blood pressure?

The JNC VII recommends the following: no more than two 12-ounce beers per day, two 4-ounce glasses of wine per day, or 2 ounces (maximum) of liquor per day (adjusted downward for women and those with lower body weight). Ethanol intake greater than 30 ml/day has been associated with a 3 mm Hg or more rise in blood pressure.

19. What is the DASH diet that is often recommended by the American Heart Association and JNC VII?

DASH stands for Dietary Approaches to Stop Hypertension. The DASH plan requires several servings of fish per week, increasing fiber to 30 grams per day, drinking plenty of water and eating a diet rich in fruits and vegetables. The diet also stresses low-fat dairy products and foods high in potassium, calcium, and magnesium. A helpful website for patients and health care providers can be found at **http://dash.bwh.harvard.edu.**

20. If a patient wants to measure his or her blood pressure at home, what type of device is recommended?

Devices that have proven to be accurate to standardized testing are recommended. Individuals should be made aware of the need for periodic calibration of these devices with a mercury sphygmomanometer. Patients should also be encouraged to periodically bring home monitoring devices with them to their physician or APRN in order to verify the accuracy of readings. Finger monitors have been found to be inaccurate. International guidelines for self–blood pressure monitoring are currently being revised.

21. How often should patients take their blood pressure at home?

This varies according to hypertension classification, etiology, and prescribed therapy. Two measurements in the morning and two in the evening for at least 3 working days have been suggested. For accuracy, individuals should wait 30 minutes following caffeine intake, smoking, or physical activity.

22. Are there any specific differences in accuracy between readings with an automatic blood pressure cuff and a manual cuff?

Automated monitoring devices provide accurate (± 10 mm Hg) readings in patients who are hemodynamically stable and are useful in clients who have difficulty with manual dexterity. However, in individuals with vascular disease or those with dysrhythmias, a manual device is preferred.

23. What strategies would enhance medication compliance for patients with hypertension?

A thorough assessment of lifestyle and socioeconomic needs is beneficial to understanding compliance issues. Quality of life, cost of medications, need for other medications, and adverse effects of the antihypertensive medication or the effects of combined medication therapy should be discussed with the individual. Having a clinician available for follow-up visits and counseling might be important to some patients. Having an actively involved, well-informed patient helps to reduce issues associated with compliance.

24. What is malignant hypertension?

Malignant hypertension is a rapidly progressing hypertension that can cause profound cerebral edema from a sustained intracranial pressure of 20 mm Hg or higher, with diastolic pressure rapidly rising to above 140 mm Hg. This hypertensive emergency requires fast action to prevent organ damage and death. The goal is to effectively lower blood pressure but not necessarily to within normal range as cerebral hypoperfusion can occur if blood pressure is lowered too rapidly. The nurse will need to be prepared for an arterial line (A-line) insertion (and transfer to an intensive care unit [ICU] if necessary) for continuous monitoring of blood pressure and administration of parenteral vasodilators such as sodium nitroprusside (Nipride, Nitropress) or diazoxide (Hyperstat). In individuals without end-organ damage, blood pressure may be lowered more slowly over a period of hours with oral agents. (*Alert!* Drugs often used to rapidly reduce blood pressure—such as IV labetalol and nonselective alpha- and beta-blockers—can cause hyperkalemia, especially in patients with renal failure. Nifedipine, sublingual, is no longer given because excessive hypotension, myocardial infarction, and sudden death have been reported). Common causes of death are cardiac failure, uremia, and strokes.

25. What are the causes of a hypertensive crisis?

The nurse must be aware that a hypertensive crisis may occur in individuals with no history of a problem or may be precipitated by individuals who are not compliant with diet or pharmacological management. Common causes in individuals with no known history include: acute renal failure, pregnancy-induced eclampsia, adrenal tumors, and use of cocaine or amphetamines.

26. What signs or symptoms should the nurse be alert for in order to prevent this crisis from occurring?

Neurological signs include mental confusion, stupor, seizures, and loss of consciousness or stroke. Cardiovascular system signs include chest pain, dysrhythmias, and severe back pain associated with aortic dissection. Decreasing urinary output and elevated serum creatinine and blood urea nitrogen might occur over several days.

27. What new research might provide some insight into why certain individuals are prone to problems with hypertension?

Recent studies are focusing on finding genetic clues to the cause of hypertension. Kallikrein, an enzyme produced by the kidneys, promotes actions that tend to lower blood pressure. Investigators in one study found that the B variant of this gene was more common in white than in black Americans. Finding the gene that controls kallikrein might be helpful in furthering our understanding of vulnerable populations. Another study involves the genes that control the production of transforming growth factor (TGF-beta$_1$). Investigators have determined that individuals with high blood pressure also have higher levels of TGF-beta$_1$ and that black Americans produce TGF-beta$_1$ at greater rates than whites. Other studies are looking at the relationship of sleep apnea to poor control of hypertension.

Key Points

- Proper assessment of blood pressure includes the following key points:
  - Make sure the cuff size is appropriate.
  - Ensure that the arm is resting at the heart level.
  - Make sure the patient has rested for several minutes before measuring BP.
- No patient should be medicated for hypertension based on inaccurate BP readings or readings from a single day.
- A period of silence or auscultatory gap is common in older and hypertensive patients.
- Korotkoff sounds often become inaudible during phase II or phase III.
- Maintaining a slow but steady release of the cuff until the reading reaches zero helps to correctly determine blood pressure measurements.

Internet Resources

The Seventh Report of the Joint National Committee on Prevention, Detection, Evaluation, and Treatment of High Blood Pressure (JNC VII)
www.nhlbi.nih.gov/guidelines/hypertension

National Heart, Lung, and Blood Institute: The DASH Eating Plan
www.nhlbi.nih.gov/health/public/heart/hbp/dash

Bibliography

American Heart Association: *High blood pressure,* available online: http://www.americanheart.org/statistics/02about.html.

Asmar R, Zanchetti A: Guidelines for the use of self-blood pressure monitoring: a summary report of the first international consensus conference, *J Hypertens* 18(5):493-508, 2000.

Fitzgerald WA: Observations on sleeping position and essential hypertension, *Med Hypotheses* 49(1):27-30, 1997.

Hamad A et al: Life-threatening hyperkalemia after intravenous labetalol injection for hypertensive emergency in a hemodialysis patient, *Am J Nephrol* 23(3):241-244, 2001.

Lilley LL, Aucker RS: *Pharmacology and the nursing process,* ed 3, St Louis, 2001, Mosby.

McCance K, Huether S: *Pathophysiology: the biologic basis for disease in adults and children,* ed 4, St Louis, 2002, Mosby, pp 1028-1036.

Multicultural Health Clearinghouse: Disease summary: hypertension, available online: http://mckinley.uiuc.edu.

National Heart, Lung, and Blood Institute: Federal government launches healthy people 2010, *Heart Memo* Spring 2000, available online: http://www.nhlbi.nih.gov/health/prof/heart/other/hm_sp00/index.htm.

National Marfan Foundation: Emergency diagnosis and treatment of aortic dissection, available online: http://www.marfan.org/pub/emergency.html.

Shepard R: *Aging, physical activity and health,* Champaign, Ill, 1997, Human Kinetics.

The Seventh Report of the Joint National Committee on Prevention, Detection, Evaluation, and Treatment of High Blood Pressure, *JAMA* 289(19):2560-2572, 2003.

Urden L, Stacy K, Lough M: *Thelan's critical care nursing,* ed 4, St Louis, 2002, Mosby, pp 433-435.

Acute Coronary Syndromes

Corinne M. Miller

1. What is an acute coronary syndrome (ACS)?

Acute coronary syndrome describes a group of clinical presentations that result from myocardial ischemia. Included in this group are unstable angina (UA) and acute myocardial infarction (AMI). AMI is subclassified into ST-segment elevation myocardial infarction (STEMI) and non–ST-segment elevation myocardial infarction (NSTEMI). Both STEMI and NSTEMI can be further classified as Q-wave (QMI) or non–Q-wave myocardial infarction (NQMI). The majority of patients with NSTEMI develop an NQMI (indicated by large arrows in the following figure); only a minority develop a QMI (indicated by small arrows in the following figure). The opposite is true for patients with an STEMI; the majority develop a QMI, and only a minority develop an NQMI.

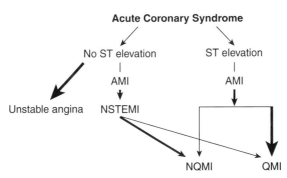

Nomenclature of acute coronary syndromes. *(Adapted from Braunwald EB, editor: Heart disease: a textbook of cardiovascular medicine, vol 2, Philadelphia, 2001, WB Saunders; Antman EM, Braunwald E: Acute myocardial infarction. In Braunwald EB, editor: Heart disease: a textbook of cardiovascular medicine, Philadelphia, 2001, WB Saunders.)*

2. What do typical ST-T wave changes on a 12-lead electrocardiogram (ECG) look like during an ACS?

Typical changes include ST-segment elevation or depression, or T-wave inversion (see the following figure). T-wave inversion is the most nonspecific ECG change and is less reliable in predicting whether an ACS is present.

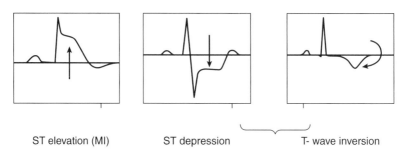

ST elevation (MI)   ST depression   T- wave inversion

Non–ST-elevation ACS

Examples of ST-T wave changes.

3. What are Q waves?

The Q *wave* on an ECG is defined as the first negative (downward) deflection of the QRS complex (see the following figure). Pathological Q waves represent transmural myocardial injury. This means the damage has affected the entire thickness of the heart muscle, from the endocardium through the myocardium to the epicardium. The absence of Q waves in a patient with positive cardiac markers (also called *cardiac enzymes*) indicates necrosis of the subendocardial layer of the endocardium and is called a *subendocardial infarction,* or NQMI.

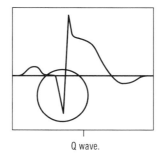

Q wave.

4. What causes an ACS?

ACSs are caused by myocardial ischemia, which is caused by a decrease in or interruption of blood flow to the myocardium. This results in the myocardium being deprived of oxygen and nutrients. The main cause of this imbalance of oxygen supply and demand is thrombus formation within the coronary artery. A thrombus usually forms on an existing atherosclerotic plaque that ruptures, causing damage to the endothelium and activation of the clotting cascade. As a result of this endothelial damage, platelets adhere to the vessel lining and become activated and secrete an array of substances, including fibrinogen. Fibrinogen then forms bridges between the platelets by binding to glycoprotein (GP) IIb/IIIa receptors located primarily on the platelet surface, causing platelet aggregation. These aggregated platelets accelerate the production of thrombin, which then converts fibrinogen to fibrin. The fibrin converts the loose platelet aggregation into a tightly woven thrombus. This thrombus can be occlusive (resulting in AMI) or nonocclusive (resulting in UA).

5. What are other causes of an ACS?

In an approach to management of the disease, Eugene Braunwald categorizes the following as etiologies of unstable angina (now commonly referred to as an ACS):

- **Dynamic obstruction:** Coronary vasospasm (Prinzmetal's angina) or coronary vasoconstriction
- **Progressive mechanical obstruction:** Progressive atherosclerosis or restenosis after a percutaneous coronary intervention (PCI)
- **Inflammation and/or infection:** Inflammation—possibly caused by or related to infection and mediated by macrophages and lymphocytes— triggers plaque instability, leading to thrombus formation.
- **Secondary unstable angina:** Patients with underlying coronary atherosclerotic narrowing can have ischemia precipitated by a condition outside of the coronary arteries. These conditions include those that cause a reduction in coronary blood flow, such as hypotension; a reduction in myocardial oxygen delivery, such as anemia or hypoxemia; or an increase in myocardial oxygen demand, such as fever or tachycardia.

6. What are the most common presenting symptoms in a patient with an ACS?

- Chest pain, pressure, tightness, or heaviness
  - May radiate to the neck, shoulders, back, jaw, and/or one or both arms
  - Usually central or substernal
- Associated symptoms
  - Indigestion or heartburn, nausea and/or vomiting
  - Persistent shortness of breath
  - Weakness, dizziness, lightheadedness, loss of consciousness
  - Diaphoresis
  - Palpitations

7. What other noncoronary presentations have symptoms similar to those of an ACS?

- Life-threatening presentations
  - Acute aortic dissection (sharp pain radiating through to the back, unequal pulses and/or blood pressure bilaterally, aortic regurgitation murmur)
  - Pulmonary embolism (sudden onset of dyspnea, tachypnea, tachycardia)
  - Pneumothorax (acute dyspnea, pleuritic chest pain, differential breath sounds)
  - Esophageal tear (sudden onset of vomiting followed by severe, sharp chest pain and possibly shortness of breath and upper gastrointestinal bleeding)
- Other common but non–life-threatening presentations
  - Musculoskeletal pain
  - Gastrointestinal disorders (gastroesophageal reflux, esophageal spasm, gastritis, peptic ulcer disease, cholecystitis)
  - Pulmonary disease (pneumonia, pleurisy)
  - Mitral valve prolapse
  - Acute pericarditis
  - Anxiety

8. **What questions must be answered quickly during an initial evaluation of a patient with a suspected ACS?**

   • Is the patient hemodynamically unstable?
   • Are the symptoms a result of an ACS?
   • Are there any other life-threatening complications present, such as lethal dysrhythmias or mechanical problems (severe valvular dysfunction, papillary muscle rupture, or ventricular septal defects)?

9. **What are the four components of the initial assessment used to answer Question 8?**

   The adage "Time is muscle" dictates that the following four steps of the assessment be done expeditiously. Treatment must not be delayed when evidence of an acute ischemic event is found or a life-threatening complication occurs.

   • **History** (especially prior history of coronary artery disease [CAD], MI, other vascular disease such as stroke or peripheral vascular disease, hypertension, or diabetes)
   • **Physical examination**
   • **ECG** (should be obtained within 10 minutes of the patient's presentation)
   • **Serial cardiac markers** (if the markers are negative within the first 6 hours of the onset of chest pain, another set should be obtained in the next 6-12 hours)

10. **How does the nurse evaluate a patient with anginal symptoms?**

   An easy way to remember the important points to cover when evaluating these symptoms is to use the "PQRST" mnemonic, as shown in the following table.

Chest pain assessment: PQRST

	Ask the Question	Examples
Provoke	What provokes or precipitates the pain?	Climbing the stairs, walking; may be unpredictable—comes on at rest
Quality	What is the quality of the pain?	Pressure, tightness, may have associated symptoms such as nausea, vomiting, diaphoresis
Radiation	Does the pain radiate to locations other than the chest?	Jaw, neck, scapular area, or left arm
Severity	What is the severity of the pain (on a scale of 1 to 10)?	On a scale of 1 to 10, with 10 being the worst, how bad is your pain?
Timing	What is the time of onset of this episode of pain that caused you to come to the hospital?	When did this episode of pain that brought you to the hospital start? Did this episode wax and wane, or was it constant? For how many days, months, or years have you had similar pain?

Modified from Chulay M, Guzzetta C, Dossey B: *AACN handbook of critical care nursing,* Stamford, Conn, 1997, Appleton & Lange; with permission from The McGraw-Hill Companies.

11. **List the key elements of a physical examination of a patient with a suspected ACS.**
    - **Vital signs,** including blood pressure taken in both arms (assess for hypotension or hypertension, tachycardia or bradycardia, pulsus paradoxus)
    - **Cardiac auscultation** (presence of a new or worsening mitral regurgitation murmur, S_3, pericardial friction rub)
    - **Breath sounds** (new or worsening rales, pulmonary edema)
    - **Skin** (diaphoresis, cool, clammy)
    - **Peripheral pulses** (diminished pulses, bruits, bilateral inequality)

12. **After the initial assessment, how does the nurse predict whether a patient has a low, intermediate, or high probability of having CAD as the etiology of the ACS symptoms? Why is this important?**

    It is very important to determine as soon as possible whether a patient's symptoms are from an ACS so that the correct site of care can be selected (coronary care unit, telemetry stepdown bed, or outpatient setting), appropriate therapy can be chosen, and the prognosis process can begin. Patients with an ACS are at higher risk for death or other adverse cardiac events. See the table on page 92.

13. **If a patient's symptoms indicate a low likelihood of an ACS, what is the treatment strategy?**

    The ECG and cardiac markers should be repeated in 4-8 hours. If the results remain negative and the patient does not have recurrent pain, he or she should undergo a stress test (either before discharge or as an outpatient). If the stress test is negative, it is unlikely that the pain is from cardiac ischemia. If the stress test is positive, the patient should be admitted to the hospital and managed via the Acute Ischemia Pathway (AIP) algorithm (see Questions 14 and 15).

14. **If a patient presents with recurrent or ongoing chest pain, ECG changes (ST-segment depression or T-wave inversion, not ST-segment elevation), and has positive cardiac markers, what initial steps should be taken?**

    The AIP algorithm should be initiated with the following steps:
    - Bed rest
    - Monitoring for signs of ischemia (symptoms and ECG)
    - Cardiac monitoring (telemetry) in the lead most likely to display ischemic changes
    - Intravenous access established
    - Oxygen if indicated (cyanosis, respiratory distress, hypoxemia)
    - Aspirin (ASA) (or clopidogrel if allergic to ASA)
    - Nitrates
    - Beta-blockers
    - Low-molecular-weight heparin (LMWH) or unfractionated heparin
    - GP IIb/IIIa inhibitor
    - Triage patient to either early invasive or early conservative management strategy

Likelihood that signs and symptoms represent an acute coronary syndrome secondary to coronary artery disease

Feature	High Likelihood: *Any of the Following*	Intermediate Likelihood: *Absence of High-Likelihood Features and Presence of Any of the Following*	Low Likelihood: *Absence of High- or Intermediate-Likelihood Features but May Have the Following*
History	Chest or left arm pain or discomfort as chief symptom reproducing prior documented angina Known history of coronary artery disease and/or myocardial infarction	Chest or left arm pain or discomfort as chief symptom Age >70 years Male sex Diabetes mellitus	Probable ischemic symptoms without any intermediate-likelihood characteristics Recent cocaine use
Exam	Transient mitral regurgitation, hypotension, diaphoresis, pulmonary edema	Extracardiac vascular disease (peripheral, carotid, and cerebral vascular disease)	Chest discomfort reproduced by palpation
Electro-cardiogram	New, transient ST-segment deviation or T-wave inversion with symptoms	Q waves Abnormal ST segments or T waves not documented to be new	T-wave flattening or inversion in leads with dominant R waves Normal electrocardiogram
Cardiac markers (creatine kinase [CK], CK-MB, troponin, and/or myoglobin)	Elevated	Normal	Normal

Adapted from Braunwald E, Mark DB, Jones RH et al: *Unstable angina: diagnosis and management,* Clinical Practice Guideline no 10 (amended), AHCPR pub no 94-0602, Rockville, Md, May 1994, Agency for Health Care Policy and Research and the National Heart, Lung, and Blood Institute, Public Health Service, U.S. Department of Health and Human Services.

15. **What is meant by an** *early invasive or early conservative* **management strategy? What determines the appropriate strategy for the patient?**

Pathways in the AIP algorithm for an early invasive strategy (proceeding directly to coronary angiography, also called a *cardiac catheterization*) or an early conservative strategy (noninvasive testing first) are depicted in the following figure. In general, patients who are thought to be at higher risk for having CAD are believed to benefit from an early invasive strategy. The availability of angiography at a hospital may also influence this decision.

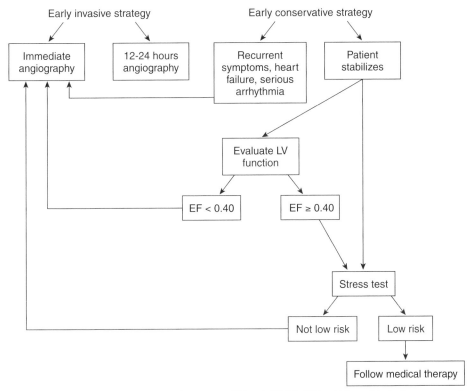

Acute ischemia pathway algorithm. *(Adapted from Braunwald E et al: ACC/AHA 2002 guideline update for the management of patients with unstable angina and non–ST-segment elevation myocardial infarction: a report of the American College of Cardiology/American Heart Association Task Force on Practice Guidelines (Committee on the Management of Patients With Unstable Angina), 2002; available online: http://www.acc.org/clinical/guidelines/unstable/ unstable.pdf, with permission from the American College of Cardiology Foundation.)*

16. What are the indicators that predict the patient is at high risk for death or a new or recurrent nonfatal MI?

- Age greater than 65 years
- Recurrent angina/ischemia despite aggressive antiischemia therapy
- Positive cardiac markers (creatine kinase [CK]-MB, troponin)
- New ST-segment depression on a 12-lead ECG
- Recurrent angina/ischemia associated with congestive heart failure (CHF) symptoms (S$_3$ heart sound, pulmonary edema, or new or worsening mitral regurgitation)
- Positive stress test
- Ejection fraction less than 40%
- Hemodynamic instability
- Sustained ventricular tachycardia (defined as ≥30 seconds in duration or causing the patient to be symptomatic)

- PCI within 6 months
- Prior coronary artery bypass graft (CABG) surgery

17. What medications are used to treat a patient with ACS?

The three goals of medical therapy for UA/NSTEMI are to (1) increase coronary perfusion, (2) decrease myocardial oxygen demand, and (3) decrease clot formation. The medications used to achieve these goals are as follows:

A. Antiplatelet drugs
- ASA
- Clopidogrel
- GP IIb/IIIa platelet inhibitors
  - Eptifibatide (Integrilin)
  - Tirofiban (Aggrastat)

B. Anticoagulants
- Unfractionated heparin (heparin)
- LMWH
  - Enoxaparin (Lovenox)
  - Dalteparin (Fragmin)

C. Antiischemia drugs
- Beta-blockers (e.g., metoprolol, atenolol)
- Nitrates (nitroglycerin [NTG])
- Calcium antagonists (used only as a second-line agent if the patient is unable to tolerate beta-blockers)
- Morphine

D. Other
- Angiotensin-converting enzyme inhibitors (e.g., captopril, enalapril)

18. What major complications may occur during an ACS?

- Arrhythmias (sustained ventricular tachycardia, ventricular fibrillation, atrial fibrillation/flutter, high-degree heart block such as second degree type II or complete heart block)
- Sustained hypotension
- Recurrent ischemia
- New mechanical defects (ventricular wall rupture, ventricular septal defect, ruptured papillary muscle)
- CHF

19. List the topics that need to be covered when discharging a patient after hospitalization for an ACS.

- Patient education topics for both patient and responsible caregiver
  - Use of NTG spray or sublingual tablets
  - Signs and symptoms of recurrent ACS (as indicated by symptoms that resemble those associated with prior documented angina), and instructions on what to do if they should occur

- Instructions for use of discharge medications, including purpose, dose, frequency, and important side effects (given in both verbal and written format)
- Resumption of regular exercise program and sexual activity (inclusion in a formal cardiac rehabilitation program recommended)
- Risk factor modification (see Chapters 35-39)
  - Smoking cessation
  - Weight loss if indicated
  - Control of hypertension if the blood pressure is higher than 130/85 mm Hg
  - Tight control of hyperglycemia in diabetic patients
  - Lipid management
- Follow-up appointment
  - Low-risk patients should be seen in 2-6 weeks.
  - Higher-risk patients should be seen in 1-2 weeks.

20. What are some controversies and unanswered questions associated with the diagnosis and treatment of an ACS?

1. What is the safest and most efficacious dose of ASA (81 versus 160 versus 325 mg) when treating UA/NSTEMI?
   - It is thought that a lower dose of ASA (81 mg) is effective as a platelet inhibitor and causes less bleeding, but a higher dose (325 mg) may be more effective in the initial treatment of an ACS. The actual dose of ASA that should be used to treat UA/NSTEMI has not been specifically studied.
   - The most important point to remember is that ASA should always be given unless contraindicated.
2. When a patient is treated according to an early invasive strategy (early cardiac catheterization), what is the most efficacious timing for coronary angiography: immediately or in 12-24 hours?
   - The advantages of immediate coronary angiography are that it offers immediate information regarding the extent of atherosclerotic obstruction and left ventricular function that can be used for prognosis and development of a treatment plan. Patients can proceed to earlier discharge, PCI, or CABG surgery, as indicated. This can lead to a shorter hospital stay and has the potential to decrease the risks of further ischemia.
   - The advantages of coronary angiography in 12-24 hours are that the waiting period allows for the use of antithrombotic and antiischemia therapies to medically stabilize the area of coronary occlusion and the patient's medical status. There have been some reports of fewer complications associated with angiography after this waiting period, but this issue has not been formally studied.

21. What are some of the new treatments under study?

- New antithrombotic medications that are being developed include direct thrombin inhibitors, factor Xa inhibitors, and new antiplatelet therapies.
- The role of inflammation in risk stratification of patients with ACS is being explored.

- The role of infection in atherosclerosis and plaque rupture is being studied.
- The potential role of therapies that target specific steps in the coronary inflammatory process, which has been proved to occur during an ACS, is under investigation.

Key Points

- The term *acute coronary syndrome* (ACS) is made up of a group of clinical presentations that include UA and acute STEMI and NSTEMI.

- ACSs are caused by myocardial ischemia, which is caused by a decrease in or interruption of blood flow to the myocardium.

- The main cause of myocardial ischemia or injury is thrombus formation within the coronary artery.

- Patients with an ACS are at higher risk for death or other adverse cardiac events and therefore must be diagnosed and treated quickly.

- Acute NSTEMIs are diagnosed using cardiac markers, not using ECG changes.

Internet Resources

The National Heart, Lung, and Blood Institute: Cardiovascular Information for Health Care Professionals:
http://www.nhlbi.nih.gov/health/prof/heart/index.htm

Heart Center Online for Patients: The Heart Attack Center:
http://www.heartcenteronline.com/The_Heart_Attack_Center.html?WT.srch=1

American College of Cardiology: ACC/AHA 2002 Guideline Update for the Management of Patients With Unstable Angina and Non–ST-Segment Elevation Myocardial Infarction:
http://www.acc.org/clinical/guidelines/unstable/update_index.htm

Family Practice Notebook.com: Ventricular Tachycardia Management in the Child:
http://www.fpnotebook.com/CV28.htm

American Heart Association website for professionals:
http://my.americanheart.org/portal/professional

Bibliography

Antman EM, Braunwald E: Acute myocardial infarction. In Braunwald EB, editor: *Heart disease: a textbook of cardiovascular medicine,* Philadelphia, 2001, WB Saunders.

Braunwald E: Unstable angina: an etiologic approach to management, *Circulation* 98:2219-2222, 1998.

Braunwald E et al: *ACC/AHA 2002 guideline update for the management of patients with unstable angina and non–ST-segment elevation myocardial infarction: a report of the American College of Cardiology/American Heart Association Task Force on Practice Guidelines (Committee on the Management of Patients With Unstable Angina),* 2002; available online: http://www.acc.org/clinical/guidelines/unstable/unstable.pdf.

Braunwald E, Mark DB, Jones RH et al: *Unstable angina: diagnosis and management,* Clinical Practice Guideline no. 10 (amended), AHCPR pub no. 94-0602, Rockville, Md, May 1994, Agency for Health Care Policy and Research and the National Heart, Lung, and Blood Institute, Public Health Service, U.S. Department of Health and Human Services.

Chulay M, Guzzetta C, Dossey B: *AACN handbook of critical care nursing,* Stamford, Conn, 1997, Appleton & Lange.

Gibbons RJ et al: ACC/AHA/ACP-ASIM guidelines for the management of patients with chronic stable angina: a report of the American College of Cardiology/American Heart Association Task Force on Practice Guidelines (Committee on the Management of Patients With Chronic Stable Angina), *J Am Coll Cardiol* 33:2092-2197, 1999.

Graham-Garcia J, Raines T: Acute coronary syndromes: current treatment strategies for acute coronary syndromes, *Adv Nurses* 2:20-21, 2000.

Granger B, Miller C: Acute coronary syndrome: putting the new guidelines to work, *Nurs 2001* 31:36-43, 2001.

Gylys K, Gold M: Acute coronary syndromes—new developments in pharmacologic treatment strategies, *Crit Care Nurse* (suppl):3-14, April 2000.

Koller C: The role of glycoprotein IIb/IIIa inhibition in the management of acute coronary syndromes, *Heart Lung* 30:321-329, 2001.

Kong D, Blazing M, O'Connor C: Advances in the approach to acute coronary syndromes, *Hosp Pract* April 15:61-82, 2000.

Siobhán O et al: Potential infectious etiologies of atherosclerosis: a multifactorial perspective, *Emerg Infect Dis* 7:780-788, 2001.

Chapter 10

Myocardial Infarction

Leslie Davis and Deborah D. Smith

1. What is a myocardial infarction (MI)?

A myocardial infarction (MI) is cardiac muscle death due to prolonged ischemia. The ischemia is caused by either diminished or absent blood flow to the cardiac muscle from the coronary arteries. Atherosclerotic plaques, which may exist for years, rupture suddenly. Most commonly a lipid-laden plaque with a thin fibrous cap ruptures, which causes a rough intimal surface. Next a monolayer of platelets covers the surface of the rupture (platelet adhesion). Additional platelets are recruited (platelet aggregation) and activated. Fibrinogen cross-links platelets, and the coagulation system is further activated by thrombin generation. This activation of the coagulation system causes a thrombus to partially or totally occlude the coronary artery, leading to cardiac ischemia and subsequent cardiac muscle death. Other theories for sudden rupture of plaque include shear stress, caused by catecholamine or sympathetic stimulation, or inflammatory components, which may predispose the plaque to rupture. A small percentage of MIs are caused by coronary artery spasm or hypoperfusion to the coronary arteries.

2. What are risk factors for developing an MI?

Major *non-modifiable* risk factors include the following:
- Family history of coronary artery disease (CAD) in a first-degree relative (male relatives younger than age 55, female relatives younger than age 65)
- Advancing patient age (males older than 45 years and females older than 55 years)
- Gender (males or postmenopausal women)

Modifiable risk factors include:
- Hyperlipidemia (high low-density lipoprotein [LDL], low high-density lipoprotein [HDL])
- Diabetes
- Hypertension
- Obesity and/or physical inactivity
- Cardiotoxic substance use (cocaine, tobacco, alcohol)
- Type A personality (specifically hostility and anger as associated with CAD)

Non-traditional risk factors include the following:
- Hyperhomocysteinemia
- High C-reactive protein (CRP) levels
- Hyperuricemia

Elements of previous medical history that contribute to risk include:
- Previous history of CAD
- Atherosclerotic disease of the aorta, arteries to limbs, or carotid arteries; or clinical signs of peripheral vascular disease
- Prior revascularization for CAD, such as percutaneous coronary intervention (PCI) or coronary artery bypass (CABG) surgery

3. Can cocaine use cause MI?

Yes. Cocaine causes alpha-adrenergic stimulation and therefore has a vaso-constrictive effect. Cocaine can cause an acute spasm that then blocks the coronary artery. Cocaine can also cause plaque rupture and therefore initiate the platelet aggregation/activation sequence (as described in Question 1). Accelerated arteriosclerosis may occur in young, otherwise healthy patients who use cocaine chronically. In addition, severe heart damage such as cardio-myopathy manifested by lowered ejection fractions may be present in chronic cocaine users. Therefore cocaine users who may be young and falsely assumed to be at low risk, are actually at high risk for MI.

4. How is MI diagnosed?

Parameters commonly used to diagnose an MI include the following:
- Patient history (current symptoms, risk factors, and health history)
- 12-lead electrocardiogram (ECG) findings
- Cardiac enzymes

5. What are the signs and symptoms of an acute myocardial infarction (AMI)?

Typical or "classic" signs and symptoms of AMI include crushing chest pain that may radiate to the arm or jaw and be associated with diaphoresis. Shortness of breath often is very common and may be a sign of cardiac ischemia. Atypical symptoms of AMI may include arm/back/jaw pain, dizziness, lightheadedness, syncope or near syncope, weakness, fatigue, tingling, nausea, and epigastric or stomach pain. Women, the elderly, and patients with diabetes often experience atypical symptoms.

6. Do some patients have "silent" MIs?

Yes, the initial presentation for many AMI patients may be asymptomatic. In fact between 20% and 30% of patients presenting with an AMI are completely asymptomatic at the onset of coronary occlusion. Diabetes and hypertension are frequently associated with silent infarction. For this reason a 12-lead ECG should always be done on those patients with suspected AMI. Continuous

ST-segment monitoring or Holter monitoring may be used in some facilities to detect ST segment changes. Otherwise serial ECGs should be done.

7. What is meant by *anginal equivalent*?

Anginal equivalent refers to the patient-specific symptom that is expressed during cardiac ischemia. In other words, whatever the patient's symptoms are, other than classic symptoms (i.e., chest pain) are that patient's "anginal equivalent." Since about one third of those presenting with MI have atypical MI symptoms, other symptoms may prevail. An example of anginal equivalent is shortness of breath. The nurse should also be aware that epigastric discomfort is a common anginal equivalent in some patients. One clue to assessing anginal equivalent in patients with a documented history of CAD is to inquire what symptoms were experienced with previous episodes of angina or MI. Then the nurse should ask if the current symptoms are similar to those previous "heart symptoms." It is important during future assessments to *use the words the patient uses* to describe the symptoms as a reference point for recurrent angina.

8. What are the hallmark ECG changes for AMI patients?

Classic AMI patients (that ultimately have ST segment elevation) start out in the *hyperacute phase* (typically pre-hospital) with giant positive T waves, which appear taller than normal R waves. These tall T waves are followed by the *acute phase* (typically seen in the hospital) in which ST segment is pronounced—at least 1 mm of ST segment elevation in two or more adjacent leads. As time passes (hours to days) the ST segment returns to normal, with T wave inversion. The R wave may be replaced with a pathologic Q wave (≥0.04 seconds) in the *chronic phase* (previously referred to as a "Q wave MI"). The Q wave may appear within hours of the infarct and may remain on the ECG permanently or eventually disappear. ST segment elevation may persist in some patients who develop left ventricular dyskinesis or akinesis (typically due to an aneurysm). ECG changes consistent with the classic findings above are represented in the portion of the 12-lead ECG that corresponds with the infarct-related artery. The ECG leads not representing the infarct-related artery (leads facing the area opposite the site of injury) typically show ST segment depression or T wave changes, often referred to as *reciprocal changes*.

9. Do all MI patients have ECG changes?

No, MI patients may have different types of ECG changes, or they may have none. The following are examples of ECG findings for MI patients:
- Normal ECGs
- New or persistent left bundle branch block (often represents a large anterior MI)
- Non–ST segment elevation ECG changes (such as T wave inversion, ST segment depression, or transient ST segment elevation)
- Classic ST segment elevation on the 12-lead ECG (see Question 8)

10. Why are MIs classified as either ST-segment elevation MI (STEMI) or non–ST-segment elevation MI (NSTEMI)?

For diagnostic and treatment purposes, an MI is classified as either an ST-segment elevation MI (STEMI) or a non–ST-segment elevation MI (NSTEMI). Patients with STEMIs, previously referred to as *Q wave* MIs, tend to have a more prolonged and complete coronary thrombus. Most commonly (but not always), a STEMI has more cardiac cell death (transmural cell necrosis), is larger in size, and tends to have higher in-hospital mortality as compared to a NSTEMI. Symptoms do not necessarily correlate with whether an MI is a STEMI or a NSTEMI.

THE REMAINDER OF THIS CHAPTER WILL FOCUS ON STEMIs.

Refer to Chapter 9, Acute Coronary Syndromes, for further information on NSTEMIs.

11. What cardiac enzyme markers are used to diagnose an AMI, and when would they become positive?

Acute myocardial infarction diagnosis using cardiac enzyme markers		
Cardiac enzyme marker	**Typical timing for rise and fall**	**Advantages/disadvantages**
Creatine kinase total (CK)	Starts to rise in 3-12 hours Peak: 24 hours Normalizes within 48-72 hours	Most facilities have the ability to measure this lab value Highly sensitive for MI diagnosis but not very specific (many false negatives) Should not be the sole lab value used to confirm diagnosis
Creatine kinase isoenzyme (CK-MB)	Starts to rise in 3-12 hours Peak: 24 hours Normalizes within 48-72 hours	Most facilities have the ability to measure this lab value Highly sensitive but not very specific since also found in skeletal muscle and small intestine More specific than CK total (if reaching 10% of CK) May be elevated by surgery, trauma, musculoskeletal diseases, hypothermia, diabetic ketoacidosis, seizures, IM injections, cerebrovascular accident, or strenuous exercise

Acute myocardial infarction diagnosis using cardiac enzyme markers *continued*

Cardiac enzyme marker	Typical timing for rise and fall	Advantages/disadvantages
Myoglobin	Starts to rise in 1-2 hours Normalizes within 6-12 hours due to rapid excretion in urine	Advantage in early rise with injury (rapidly released from necrotic tissue) Poor marker for those who delay seeking medical attention
	Doubling of the myoglobin level within 2 hours indicates MI Negative myoglobin 4-8 hours after symptom onset can rule out an MI	False positive in patients with skeletal muscle or renal disease
Cardiac troponins* Troponin I Troponin T	Both rise within 3-12 hrs after infarct Peak: 14-48 hours Normalize within 5-21 days (troponin I: 5-7 days; troponin T: up to 21 days)	Currently best cardiac sensitivity and specificity Available by bedside assay, so quick turnaround for results (20-30 minutes) is possible Troponin T affected by skeletal muscle injury and renal disease Troponin I very sensitive and specific; not influenced by skeletal muscle injury or renal disease

*Gold standard

12. Are bedside cardiac markers available?

Bedside markers for CK-MB, myoglobin, and troponin I are being successfully used to risk stratify patients, especially in the emergency department and for pre-hospital use. Early identification of high-risk patients is helping to decrease time to treatment and especially to prepare staff for hospital arrival. Although these markers are useful for initial risk stratification, specificity and sensitivity are lower than with standard laboratory assays. These bedside markers should therefore be rechecked using standard laboratory assays once the patient arrives at the hospital since false positives are common.

13. What are goals for treatment for STEMI patients?

All interventional strategies—from conservative medical treatment to aggressive reperfusion—target the following principles:
- Increasing oxygen supply to feed ischemic heart tissue
- Decreasing demand to decrease the workload of the heart
- Restoring blood flow to the heart to open the artery (reperfusion therapy)

- Maintaining perfusion to keep the artery open
- Preventing complications with early hospitalization and intensive monitoring
- Providing secondary prevention (preventing reinfarction and/or death)

14. What specific treatments are recommended for patients with a STEMI and why?

Treating a patient with a STEMI

Therapy	When to administer	Action/Effect
Oxygen 2-4 liters per minute by nasal cannula or face mask	Immediate and ongoing	Deliver more oxygen to ischemic cells
Aspirin 162-325 mg* Initially chewed (not enteric coated) followed by daily dose that may be enteric coated	Immediate and daily	Prevent platelet aggregation leading to coronary thrombosis
Nitroglycerin (nitrates): topical, sublingual, and intravenous	With ischemic symptoms, chest pain	Promotes peripheral vasodilation, decreasing preload and afterload of the heart; secondary effect of coronary artery vasodilation
Reperfusion therapy: either thrombolytics or primary percutaneous coronary intervention (PCI) depending on patient eligibility and facility capability	Goal for administration of thrombolytics is to begin within 30 minutes of hospital arrival or within 3 hours after symptom onset. May be given up to 12 hours after symptom onset. Goal for primary PCI (angioplasty with or without stent) is for catheter to be in within 60-90 minutes of hospital arrival or within 12 hours of symptom onset	Early reperfusion reduces infarct size and decreases morbidity and mortality. Thrombolytics break up fibrin in clots
Heparin	To be given with thrombolytics for ST-segment elevation myocardial infarction (STEMI). Should be given with fibrin-specific thrombolytics (alteplase or reteplase)	Forms a complex with antithrombin III, which inactivates thrombin. aPTT should be 1.5-2 times control for first 48 hours in STEMI patients

*Substitute clopidogrel if patient has allergy to aspirin.

Treating a patient with a STEMI   *continued*

Therapy	When to administer	Action/Effect
Heparin	Subcutaneous unfractionated heparin or low–molecular-weight heparin may be used if STEMI patient is not treated with thrombolytics	Low–molecular-weight heparins still being studied with STEMI patients who receive thrombolytic therapy
Beta-blockers	Administered intravenously within 12 hr of symptom onset, ideally followed by oral administration	Reduce myocardial oxygen consumption; Inhibit sympathetic nervous stimulation of the heart (reduces both heart rate and contractility) Decrease afterload Overall decrease acute and long-term morbidity and mortality Reduce infarct size and incidence of ventricular fibrillation and reinfarction
Angiotensin converting enzyme inhibitors	Indicated in patients with heart failure, large anterior myocardial infarction (MI), or an ejection fraction <40% Administer within first 24 hours post-MI	Reduce morbidity and mortality post-AMI Reduce remodeling from MI Decrease endothelial dysfunction
Glycoprotein IIb/IIIa inhibitors	Use with primary PCI, rescue angioplasty, and/or with thrombolysis is being studied	Prevents binding of fibrinogen to platelets and therefore blocks platelet aggregation Improves vessel patency rate and decreases early cardiac events related to thrombotic vessel closure

15. What are the most important initial actions for the nurse to take when caring for a patient with a STEMI?

Time is muscle; therefore every minute counts when the nurse is taking actions to assess and implement care for a patient with a STEMI. The nurse can "drive" the system. The following should be done when a patient with suspected MI presents to a facility:

- Rapid triage for suspected MI patients—*sound the alarm* for high-risk patients

- Rapid EKG—national guidelines call for ECG within 10 minutes of hospital arrival
- Facilitate rapid ECG interpretation by the physician or nurse practitioner for diagnosis
- Rapid initiation of reperfusion therapy (thrombolytic therapy or primary PCI)—thrombolytics to be started within 30 minutes of hospital arrival; primary PCI within 60-90 minutes of hospital arrival
- Facilitate cardiology consult as early as possible
- Alert the teams for reperfusion therapies (e.g., catheter laboratory [cath lab] team to be notified for possible primary PCI (especially in those patients with large anterior MI, those in cardiogenic shock, hypotension, or overt heart failure who are more likely to go for primary PCI)

16. What actions can nurses take when they are notified that a STEMI patient will arrive at their unit within the next 10 minutes?

Nurses should assume that the patient is unstable and be prepared for the following:

- Have oxygen and all resuscitation equipment available for use—cardiac monitor, code cart (including all cardiac drugs), defibrillator, and temporary pacemaker
- Mobilize staff—consider the need for at least two nurses in the patient's room to initiate reperfusion therapy if eligible (either providing thrombolytic therapy or preparing the patient for primary PCI)
- Anticipate the need for cardiologist or interventional cardiologist for potential coronary intervention in the cath lab
- Be prepared to obtain a stat 12-lead ECG and laboratory work
- Be prepared to initiate a minimum of two or three intravenous lines if not already in place
- Consider absolute and relative contraindications to thrombolytic therapy
- Anticipate need for and have available the following drugs: aspirin, nitroglycerin (intravenous and sublingual), thrombolytics, heparin, beta-blockers
- Upon patient arrival, place the patient on an ECG monitor and continuous ST segment monitoring if available

17. Does nursing care differ based on location of the patient's infarct-related artery?

The location of an MI, which depends on which coronary artery is occluded, is depicted on the 12-lead ECG by the various leads. Specific complications and symptoms based on type of MI are displayed in the following table. Anticipation by the nurse of potential patient complications based on location of ECG changes may lead to earlier recognition of problems and muscle-saving interventions.

Nursing care based on type of myocardial infarction

Type of myocardial infarction (MI)	Infarct Related Artery (IRA)	Lead changes on the 12-lead ECG	Damage location	Potential complications	Nursing considerations
Septal MI	Left anterior descending (LAD) or left circumflex (LCX)	Leads V_1-V_2	Septum, bundle of His, bundle branches	Infranodal and bundle branch blocks	Check ECG for widening QRS Repeat ECGs Watch for hemodynamic instability*
Anterior MI	LAD or LCX	Leads V_1-V_4	Anterior wall of left ventricle (LV)	LV dysfunction (acute pulmonary edema) Ventricular dysrhythmias Heart block Bundle branch block	Assess lungs frequently Careful IV fluid administration Continuous ECG monitoring to observe for dysrhythmias*
Lateral MI	LCX	Leads V_5-V_6 and/or I, aVL	Lateral wall of LV	LV dysfunction	Assess lungs frequently
Inferior MI	Right coronary artery (RCA)	Leads II, III, aVF	Inferior wall of the LV Posterior wall of the LV	Heart block Nausea	Monitor ECG continuously for heart block or bradycardia
Right ventricular infarct	RCA: proximal branches	II, III, aVF Also if using right sided chest leads: V4R	RV, inferior wall LV, posterior wall LV	Hypotension Jugular vein distention (JVD) with clear lungs Heart block Most commonly associated with either infero-posterior or true posterior MI	Subject to preload problems Fluids first-line treatment for hypotension Sensitive to nitroglycerin and morphine
Posterior MI	RCA	Normal ECG or ST segment depression and a large R wave in V_1-V_2	Posterior lateral wall of LV	Dysrhythmias	Monitor ECG continuously for dysrhythmias* ECG deceptively normal

*Standard for care of all types of MI.

18. What is different about caring for a patient with a right ventricular infarction?

A right ventricular (RV) infarction is usually associated with an inferior wall MI. Bradycardia, heart block, and atrial arrhythmias (such as atrial fibrillation) occur in a third of patients with RV infarction. Hypotension with the use of nitroglycerin, morphine, or diuretics should alert the nurse to suspect an RV infarction. Affected patients have a syndrome of low output failure characterized by hypotension and clear lung fields, and they typically require more volume by IV fluids as first-line therapy. However, this should be used cautiously since some patients will have LV dysfunction as well. For those patients with underlying LV dysfunction that experience cardiogenic shock, inotrope therapy or balloon pump support may be utilized.

19. What does it mean when a STEMI patient who has been stable and comfortable following reperfusion therapy (either PCI or thrombolytics) has recurrent chest pain or shortness of breath?

Recurrent symptoms (be they angina or dyspnea) are highly suspicious for a non-patent infarct related artery (IRA). Either the initial reperfusion strategy did not completely open the IRA, or the patient is experiencing reocclusion of the IRA. Coronary ischemia is a dynamic process. The coronary artery blood flow during treatment of an acute infarct may wax and wane depending on the size of the clot and stability of the plaque. Even in those patients who undergo primary PCI (with or without stent placement), reperfusion may be incomplete initially or may reocclude. Because prompt intervention is required for either an incomplete reperfusion or a reocclusion, the nurse is in a critical position to recognize early signs of ischemia. Alternatively recurrent chest pain and/or shortness of breath may indicate pericarditis; although this usually develops a few days after the MI.

20. What nursing actions should be taken when reocclusion is suspected?

Patients who have recurrent or prolonged signs of ischemia should be considered "time bombs" and reassessed frequently. Nurses should take the following actions:
- Notify the physician or advance practice registered nurse (APRN) stat
- Reassess vital signs, monitoring for evidence of hemodynamic instability
- Obtain a stat 12-lead ECG to assess for changes indicative of recurrent ischemia. ST segment elevation or ST depression, which may or may not occur on the same leads as on the previous ECGs, or new-onset bundle branch blocks are worrisome
- Assess symptoms in the patient's own words. Ask the patient if the present symptoms feel like they did before with a previous heart attack. Probing patient symptoms is imperative
- Administer nitroglycerin and/or morphine for recurrent symptoms, reassessing after each intervention
- Consider checking coagulation panels. If the patient is receiving IV heparin, check the activated partial thromboplastin time (aPTT) for a therapeutic range. If the patient is receiving low-molecular-weight heparin (LMWH),

did the patient miss a dose? Did the patient get the appropriate daily doses of ASA and clopidogrel?
- Prepare patient for possible cardiac catheterization to visualize the coronary artery for assessment of abrupt closure or reinfarction

21. What signs and symptoms may indicate a STEMI patient is having a complication?

The following signs and symptoms should alert the nurse that the patient may be experiencing a potential complication:
- Shortness of breath
- Decreased pulse oximeter oxygen levels
- Continued chest pain or other symptoms of ischemia
- Hemodynamic instability, that is, tachycardia, hypotension, change in skin color that may indicate poor skin perfusion, dysrhythmias (such as heart block or increased ventricular ectopy)
- Syncope
- Altered mental status
- An increased level of anxiety or the expressing a feeling of impending doom

22. What are the most common complications following a STEMI?

The most common complications of a STEMI are outlined in the following table.

Common STEMI complications

Complication	Signs and Symptoms	Nursing Actions
Recurrent ischemia	Recurrent angina or anginal equivalent symptoms with or without ECG changes	Obtain a stat 12-lead ECG Notify physician or advanced practice registered nurse (APRN) (See question 19)
Recurrent myocardial infarction (MI)	Signs of recurrent ischemia ST segment changes on the 12-lead ECG Reelevation of cardiac markers	Obtain a stat 12-lead ECG Notify physician or APRN Same as initial MI treatment (reperfusion therapy of either thrombolytics or primary percutaneous coronary intervention [PCI] if eligible)
Cardiogenic shock	Hypotension Tachycardia Pulmonary edema Decreased urinary output Altered mental status Dyspnea	Intraaortic balloon pump (IABP) Inotrope therapy Vasopressors Oxygen and/or mechanical ventilation for severe hypoxemia Diuretics for pulmonary edema Caution with IV fluids (See Chapter 19, Shock)

Common STEMI complications   *continued*

Complication	Signs and Symptoms	Nursing Actions
Mechanical complications such as cardiac rupture, ventricular septal defect, papillary muscle rupture	New murmur of mitral regurgitation Acute decompensation Cardiogenic shock Death May see on echo	Emergent surgery
Ventricular dysrhythmias	Ventricular tachycardia (V tach) or ventricular fibrillation (V fib) on the telemetry monitor Tachycardia Palpitations Dyspnea Angina Hypotension Syncope Cardiac arrest	Continuous ECG monitoring with defibrillator readily available Early defibrillation for unstable or pulseless V tach or V fib Amiodarone (especially in patients with LV dysfunction) Possible internal cardiac defibrillator placement if not periinfarct MI, V tach, or V fib (See Chapter 25, Implantable Cardioverter Defibrillators)
Other dysrhythmias: atrial and heart block	Irregular and/or slow pulse Change in cardiac rhythm on telemetry Hypotension	Continuous ECG monitoring Transcutaneous pacemaker available as a standby for advanced bradycardia or heart block Amiodarone for atrial dysrhythmias (especially in the setting of LV dysfunction) (See Chapter 34, Antiarrhythmic Agents)

23. What information should be included in discharge teaching for an STEMI patient?

Patient education should include teaching about the disease process, risk-factor modification, post-MI activity, and discharge medications. See Chapters 36 (Lipid-Lowering Strategies), 37 (Physical Activity), and 38 (Cardiac Rehabilitation). Patients should be warned *not to stop taking any cardiac medications abruptly* because this may result in major side effects or even death (stopping beta blockers abruptly). Additional patient education should include instructing patients to contact their physician or nurse practitioner or go to the closest emergency department if any of the following occur:

- Chest pain or their equivalent (see Question 7)
- Shortness of breath
- Irregular pulse rhythm
- Feeling weak, passing out
- Side effects from medication

If any of the above symptoms arise, patients should be encouraged to call 911 rather than driving because of the high risk of sudden cardiac death. Teaching the patient the importance of seeking medical attention early is critical. Despite extensive education, patients continue to delay seeking prompt attention when MI symptoms start. A family member should also be educated; this may make it easier for patients to seek medical care early.

24. Should patients older than 75 years of age receive the same reperfusion strategies as younger patients do?

Recent census data show a change in demographics that has increased the elderly (>75 year old) population by 10% since 1990. Nearly one third of all AMIs occur in patients older than 75 years of age, with a mortality rate of 30%. Of all MI deaths, 60% are in patients older than 75. Older patients are more likely to have strokes, renal failure, bleeding, and mechanical complications, yet limited data have shown greater benefit with successful reperfusion therapies in these patients. Tailored therapies for the elderly that consider the risk/benefit ratio need to be explored, and "gentle reperfusion" therapies that consider the high risk are being proposed. (See Question 25.)

25. What are the current controversies in the field of STEMI care?

- *Controversy #1:* Should STEMI patients be transferred to a site with primary PCI capability versus be given thrombolytics on site? Current thoughts are that if the STEMI patient can receive primary PCI within 90-120 minutes of arrival at the facility, primary PCI is preferred.
- *Controversy #2:* Should primary PCI be done without surgical backup? Some facilities are now considering offering primary PCI without surgical backup, but this is controversial because the risk for dissection or needing urgent surgical revascularization is much greater than for patients undergoing elective PCI.
- *Controversy #3:* Should thrombolytic therapy be given prehospital (in the field)? Newer rapid bolus type thrombolytic therapy will make this an option for some communities, especially those with long transport times to the hospital.
- *Controversy #4:* Should facilitated PCI (combining primary PCI with partial-dose thrombolytics) be first-line therapy for STEMI patients? Combination therapy is probably best for certain subgroups of STEMI patients, such as those younger than age 75 with a large anterior MI.
- *Controversy #5:* How can time to treatment be decreased? This question remains unanswered. Specifically, the time from symptom onset to hospital arrival is still an average of 2.5 hours in the United States, despite public educational. The REACT study showed that massive educational efforts to the public did not make a difference in symptom-to-door time.
- *Controversy #6:* The timing of prophylactic implantable cardioverter defibrillator (ICD) placement in STEMI patients with low ejection fraction (EF) is unclear. The MADIT II study demonstrated a mortality reduction in patients who underwent ICD placement >30 days post-MI in the setting of a low EF. Ongoing clinical studies are looking at placement of ICDs before the 30-day mark.

26. What is on the horizon for care of the STEMI patient?

- *Improving time to treatment:* Time to treatment for STEMI patients has not improved much since the 1990s despite emphasis in literature. Quality indicators and improvement measures now established by the Joint Commission on Accreditation of Healthcare Organizations (JCAHO) to reflect hospital performance will increase accountability. Hospitals will be held accountable for the standards of care as recommended by the American Heart Association/American College of Cardiology guidelines.
- *Myocardial protection mechanisms:* This is based on theory that damage occurs during reperfusion and can be prevented by adjunctive therapies such as antiinflammatory agents, endothelial targets, metabolic modulation, alteration of cellular sodium, hydrogen and calcium shifts, and physical cooling.
- *Use of adenosine:* Acute use provides antiinflammatory and metabolism-altering activities to reduce infarct size

 Key Points

- Women, diabetics, and the elderly often have atypical symptoms at presentation. Such symptoms are often referred to as *anginal equivalents* and may include shortness of breath, arm/back/jaw pain, dizziness, lightheadedness, syncope or near syncope, weakness, fatigue, tingling, nausea, and epigastric or stomach pain.
- When assessing the history in a patient with CAD, the nurse should inquire what symptoms were experienced with previous episodes of angina or MI and determine if the current symptoms are similar.
- Obtain a 12-lead ECG in all patients at risk for suspected MI. Up to 20% to 30% of patients presenting with an MI are completely asymptomatic at the onset of coronary occlusion.
- Diabetes and hypertension are frequently associated with silent infarction.
- Some patients do not have characteristic ECG changes of AMI like ST elevation or depression, T wave inversions or depressions.
- Once a 12-lead ECG is completed in patients with suspected AMI, the sooner the ECG is interpreted the better. Maintain a high level of suspicion for patients at high risk for coronary heart disease.
- Treatment goals for STEMI patients include the following:
  - Increasing oxygen supply to feed ischemic heart tissue
  - Decreasing demand to minimize workload of heart
  - Restoring blood flow to open the artery (reperfusion therapies)
  - Maintaining perfusion to keep the artery open
  - Preventing complications with early hospitalization and intensive monitoring
  - Providing secondary prevention (preventing reinfarction and/or death)

Key Points   *continued*

- Nurses are on the "front line" to rapidly facilitate efforts in the care of STEMI patients, which means ensuring that ECGs are performed and interpreted rapidly and that patients are either started on thrombolytic therapy promptly or prepped for the cardiac cath lab for primary PCI.
- Nurses should always be prepared for a STEMI patient to either be or become unstable; therefore they should anticipate complications. Standard STEMI treatments (oxygen, nitroglycerin, heparin, and beta-blockers) must be readily available. The patient care team should be mobilized and ready to begin treatment upon the patient's arrival at the facility.
- Patients with right ventricular infarction (RV infarct), usually associated with an inferior MI, may have a syndrome of low output failure characterized by hypotension and clear lung fields. Hypotension with nitroglycerin, morphine, and diuretics should alert the nurse to suspect RV infarct. Treatment for RV infarct includes increased fluid volume, although this must be provided with caution.
- The following may indicate a potential complication in a STEMI patient:
  - Shortness of breath
  - Decreased pulse oximeter oxygen levels
  - Continued chest pain or signs of ischemia
  - Hemodynamic changes: tachycardia, hypotension, change in skin color, dysrhythmias
  - Syncope
  - Altered mental status
  - Increased level of anxiety or expression of feeling of impending doom
- If the patient develops recurrent symptoms or has new symptoms of potential complications after stabilization, the nurse should take action quickly by obtaining an ECG and investigating the cause of symptom changes. Watchful waiting could mean loss of heart muscle!

Internet Resources

ACC/AHA Guidelines for the Management of Patients With Acute Myocardial Infarction:
http://www.americanheart.org/presenter.jhtml?identifier=2865

American College of Cardiology Professional Education:
http://www.meetingcast.com/acc02live/index.php3?l=faculty

Journal Article: A Comparison of Coronary Angioplasty With Fibrinolytic Therapy in Acute Myocardial Infarction:
http://content.nejm.org/cgi/content/short/349/8/733

American Heart Association:
www.americanheart.org

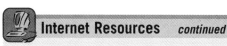

Internet Resources *continued*

American Heart Association Journals:
http://www.ahajournals.org

American Heart Association: Emergency Cardiovascular Care:
www.cpr-ecc.org

Genentech Patient Profiles:
www.gene.com/gene/products/profiles/tnkase.jsp

MEDLINE Plus: Health Information:
http://www.nlm.nih.gov/medlineplus

CardioSource: A collaboration of American College of Cardiology Foundation and Elsevier:
http://cardiosource.com

Bibliography

Becker R, Alpert J: *Cardiovascular medicine practice and management,* London, 2001, Arnold.

Braunwald E: *Essential atlas of heart diseases,* ed 2, New York, 2001, McGraw-Hill.

Braunwald E: *Atlas of heart diseases, acute myocardial infarction and other ischemic syndromes,* vol VII, Philadelphia, 1996, Mosby.

Brown D: *Cardiac intensive care,* Philadelphia, 1998, WB Saunders.

Burnett L, Adler J: *Cocaine toxicity,* 2000, available online: http://www.emedicine.com/emerg/topic.

Cohn P: *Silent myocardial ischemia and infarction,* ed 4, New York, 2000, Marcel Dekker.

Granger CB: Reperfusion therapy for acute myocardial infarction. In Topol EJ, editor: *Textbook of cardiovascular medicine UPDATES,* vol 5, no 2, New York, 2002, Lippincott Williams & Wilkins Healthcare.

Hudson M, Granger C et al: Clinical investigation and reports early reinfarction after fibrinolysis, *Circulation* 104:1229, 2001.

Keeley E, Boura J, Grines C: Primary angioplasty versus intravenous thrombolytic therapy for acute myocardial infarction: a quantitative review of 23 randomized trials, *Lancet* 361:13-20, 2003.

Kroll C, Ohman M: Should reperfusion strategies in myocardial infarction be modified in the elderly? *Am Heart J* 143:373-376 (editorial), 2002.

Nagle B, Nee C: Recognizing and responding to acute myocardial infarction, *Nursing* 2002 32: 50-54, 2002.

Roettig M, Tanabe P: Emergency management of acute coronary syndromes, *J Emerg Nurs* 26(6 suppl): S1-S42, Dec 2000.

Ryan TJ, Antman EM, Brooks NH et al: 1999 update: ACC/AHA guidelines for the management of patients with acute myocardial infarction: executive summary and recommendations: a report of the American College of Cardiology/American Heart Association Task Force on Practice Guidelines (Committee on Management of Acute Myocardial Infarction), *Circulation* 100:1016-1030, 1999.

Smith D: Care of the acute MI patient: what's on the horizon? *Am J Nurs* 5(suppl):4-11, 1998.

Topol E: *Acute coronary syndromes,* ed 2, New York, 2001, Marcel Dekker.

Topol E: *The textbook of cardiovascular medicine,* ed 2, Philadelphia, 2002, Lippincott Williams & Wilkins.

Van De Werf F: Reperfusion for ST-segment elevation myocardial infarction: an overview of current treatment options, *Circulation* 105:2813, 2002.

Chapter 11

Heart Failure

Margaret T. Bowers

1. What is heart failure?

Heart failure is a complex clinical syndrome. It is the only cardiac disorder that continues to increase in prevalence and incidence in the United States. Survival rates from acute myocardial infarction (MI) have improved over the years, resulting in an increased number of older adults with damaged myocardium and the potential for development of heart failure. Heart failure can result from cardiac or chronic metabolic disorders. The heart is unable to pump effectively to meet the metabolic needs of the body or may require elevated filling pressures to meet this demand. Therefore based on the cause, congestion may or may not be present. Systolic dysfunction is most common and occurs when the ejection fraction (EF) is less than 50%.

2. What is an ejection fraction?

An EF is an estimate of the amount of blood pumped from the left ventricle to the rest of the body with each heartbeat. It is used as a determinant of left ventricular function and reflects systolic performance of the heart. An EF can be obtained from an echocardiogram (echo), a multigated acquisition scan (MUGA), or a left heart cardiac catheterization. A normal EF ranges between 50% and 75%.

3. What is systolic dysfunction?

Systolic dysfunction is the inability of the left ventricle to effectively pump blood to the rest of the body. The stroke volume decreases, and the body compensates with retaining water and sodium, which ultimately leads to an increase in stroke volume and results in pulmonary congestion. The EF in systolic dysfunction is less than 50%, which is not considered normal.

4. What is preserved systolic dysfunction?

In preserved systolic dysfunction, more commonly referred to as diastolic dysfunction, the EF is normal or greater than 50% to 55%. The left ventricle is unable to fill because of the inability to completely relax. This condition is most often seen with hypertension. Differentiation between systolic and diastolic dysfunction guides the pharmacological treatment and prognosis for patients with heart failure.

5. What are the precipitating causes of heart failure?

See the following box.

Most Common	Least Common
Coronary artery disease	Viral
Hypertension	Anemia
Valvular dysfunction	Dysrhythmias (atrial fibrillation)
Idiopathic	Peripartum
	Endocrine (thyroid and diabetes)
	Restrictive (amyloid, sarcoid, and hemochromatosis)
	Cardiotoxic substances (alcohol, chemotherapy, cocaine)

6. How do neurohormones affect heart function?

Research has brought to attention the role of neurohormonal activation in the development and progression of heart failure. Prolonged exposure to catecholamines (epinephrine and norepinephrine) with resulting vasoconstriction can worsen volume overload and myocardial ischemia in patients with heart failure. In addition, these catecholamines stimulate cellular pathways, which can lead to apoptosis (programmed cell death). This adrenergic nervous system stimulation triggers the renin-angiotensin-aldosterone system. This stimulation causes vasoconstriction, which is initially beneficial but ultimately results in excessive left ventricular wall stress that diminishes systolic function.

7. What is cardiac remodeling?

- Remodeling is structural changes that occur in the cardiac myocytes (heart muscle cells). These changes may occur locally or globally as a result of MI or cardiomyopathy. Activation of the renin-angiotensin-aldosterone system and stimulation of the sympathetic nervous system contribute to the process of remodeling.
- Remodeling results in physical changes in the ventricle, impacting its ability to pump effectively.

8. Is remodeling beneficial?

Cardiac remodeling is detrimental because it creates physical changes in the heart with resulting changes in EF. The goal of therapy in the management of heart failure is minimization and possible reversal of the areas of remodeling for preservation of ventricular function. Reversal of the remodeling process can occur with the use of medications, which modulate the renin-angiotensin-aldosterone and sympathetic system. These medications include angiotensin-converting enzyme (ACE) inhibitors, angiotensin receptor blockers, and beta-blockers.

9. What signs and symptoms are likely to be present in heart failure?

Signs	Symptoms
Jugular venous distention	Orthopnea
Rales or crackles	Paroxysmal nocturnal dyspnea
Tachypnea	Fatigue
Unexplained weight gain	Dyspnea on exertion
Ascites	Depression
Edema	Cough
Nocturia	Decreased exercise tolerance
Pallor	Anxiety
Diminished peripheral pulses	Palpitations
Hepatomegaly	Nausea/vomiting
Hepatojugular reflux	Abdominal fullness
Extra heart sounds (S3 or S4)	Chest pain
Orthostasis	Early satiety
Right upper quadrant tenderness	Anorexia or loss of appetite

Most of the signs and symptoms are familiar with respect to heart failure. However, fatigue and early satiety are also signs of cardiac decompensation. As heart failure progresses, symptoms of fatigue and early satiety result from the shunting of blood to vital organs. Poor perfusion of the gut may result in symptoms of abdominal fullness, constipation, nausea, and even vomiting.

10. How is heart failure classified?

New York Heart Association Functional Class	American Heart Association/ American College of Cardiology Guidelines	Recommendations
	Stage A: People at high risk for heart failure (HF) but without structural heart disease or symptoms of HF	Treat lipid disorders, hypertension, and diabetes. Encourage smoking cessation and regular exercise. Discourage use of illicit drugs and alcohol. Use of angiotensin-converting enzyme (ACE) inhibitor if indicated.

continued

New York Heart Association Functional Class	American Heart Association/ American College of Cardiology Guidelines	Recommendations
Class I: Patients with cardiac disease without limitations of physical activity. Ordinary physical activity does not cause undue fatigue, dyspnea, palpitations, or anginal pain.	**Stage B:** People with structural heart disease but no symptoms of HF.	All stage A therapies. ACE inhibitor unless contraindicated. Beta-blocker unless contraindicated.
Class II: Patients with cardiac disease who have slight limitations of physical activity and are comfortable at rest. Ordinary physical activity results in fatigue, palpitations, anginal pain, or dyspnea.	**Stage C:** People who have structural heart disease with current or prior symptoms of HF.	All stage A and B therapies. Sodium-restricted diet. Diuretics. Digoxin. Avoidance of or withdrawal from antiarrhythmic agents, most calcium channel blockers, and nonsteroidal anti-inflammatory drugs. Consideration of aldosterone antagonists and angiotensin receptor blockers.
Class III: Patients with cardiac disease who have marked limitation of physical activity and are comfortable at rest. Less than ordinary physical activity causes fatigue, dyspnea, palpitations, or anginal pain.		Addition of hydralazine and nitrates.
Class IV: Patients with cardiac disease who cannot carry out any physical activity without discomfort. Symptoms of cardiac insufficiency or of the anginal syndrome may be present even at rest. Any physical activity increases discomfort.	**Stage D:** People with refractory heart failure that necessitates specialized interventions.	All therapies for stages A, B, and C. Mechanical assist device such as biventricular pacemaker or left ventricular assist device. Continuous inotrope therapy. Hospice care.

Adapted with permission from Caboral M, Mitchell J: New guidelines for heart failure focus on prevention, Nurse Pract J 28(1):13-23, 2003.

11. Why does edema occur?

Increased central venous pressure results in a rise in capillary pressure that causes transudation of fluid from the intravascular space to the interstitial space. Tissue edema occurs and often is seen in both the periphery and the sacral regions as a result of gravitational forces. In patients with heart failure, reduced cardiac output causes a decreased arterial blood pressure (BP) that then activates the renin-angiotensin-aldosterone system, resulting in the retention of sodium and water and predisposing the patient to edema.

12. How is edema assessed?

Assessment of edema is a subjective evaluation. Quantification of pitting edema is described in the following table.

1+	Mild edema	2-mm induration	Rapidly resolves
2+	Moderate edema	4-mm induration	Resolves within 10-15 s
3+	Moderately severe edema	6-mm induration	Lasts up to 1 min
4+	Severe pitting edema	8-mm induration	Resolves within 2-5 min

13. What should be anticipated with auscultating the lungs?

Often "crackles" or rales may be heard from secretions that clear with coughing. Rales that persist may be a sign of heart failure. Pulmonary congestion may or may not be present as evidenced by the fact that 80% of patients with chronic heart failure who are hospitalized do not have rales.

14. What does it mean when an S3 or S4 is auscultated?

- An S3 results from decreased myocardial contractility, heart failure, or ventricular volume overload. It is heard immediately after S2 at the apex with the bell of the stethoscope. Placing the patient in the left lateral recumbent position may enhance the ability to auscultate an S3.
- An S4 is most often the result of an increase in resistance to ventricular filling immediately after atrial contraction and is often present in patients with hypertension. It is indicative of decreased compliance in the left ventricle and is heard immediately before S1. An S4 is best heard with the bell of the stethoscope with the patient in the left lateral recumbent position.

15. What are the primary treatment goals in heart failure?

The primary goal of treatment is helping the patient to "Feel better, live longer, and stay out of the hospital." This is done with both pharmacological and nonpharmacological therapies. First-tier therapy includes pharmacological and nonpharmacological interventions. Pharmacological treatment usually includes the following classes of medications: ACE inhibitors, beta-blockers, diuretics, angiotensin II receptor blockers (ARBs), and digoxin. Nonpharmacological treatments include a variety of lifestyle changes including dietary restrictions, weight monitoring, and monitoring of fluid intake.

Second-tier treatment includes the addition of aldosterone inhibitors such as spironolactone. Third-tier therapy is usually related to advancing symptoms and includes patients in New York Heart Association (NYHA) Functional class III and IV. Inotropic therapy, left ventricular assist device (LVAD), and cardiac transplantation are treatment options. Results from the Multicenter Automatic Defibrillator Implantation Trial II (MADIT II) trial in November 2001 revealed a 30% mortality rate reduction in patients with a history of MI and EF of 30% after an implantable cardioverter defibrillator (ICD) was implanted.

16. How do ACE inhibitors work in patients with heart failure?

Angiotensin-converting enzyme inhibitors prevent the conversion of angiotensin I to angiotensin II, which is a potent vasoconstrictor and stimulator of sodium and water retention. These drugs result in decreased peripheral vascular resistance, increased diuresis, vasodilation, and lower BP, without any change in heart rate. Clinical benefits include improved NHYA functional class, exercise tolerance, and symptoms.

Angiotensin-converting enzyme inhibitors should be used in all patients with heart failure within the following parameters:
- Blood pressure more than 90 mm Hg systolic.
- No evidence of hyperkalemia or bilateral renal artery stenosis.
- Stable renal function (blood urea nitrogen [BUN], creatinine, potassium).

Development of a nonproductive cough may be a sign of intolerance to an ACE inhibitor. Using another medication in the same class or of an ARB is recommended. Mortality benefits of both ACE inhibitors and ARBs have been well researched. With intolerance to both an ACE inhibitor and ARB, a combination of hydralazine and isosorbide dinitrate should be used. Patient response to treatment with an ACE inhibitor may be influenced by genetic factors from polymorphisms. (Refer to Chapter 46, Genetics.)

17. Why are beta-blockers used in patients with heart failure?

For years beta-blocker use in heart failure was contraindicated. Several clinical trials support the use of beta-blockers in patients with low EF to reduce mortality rates by up to 35%. As previously stated, excess circulating catecholamines are beneficial in the initial phase of heart failure. Chronic exposure to this stimulation results in decreased systemic perfusion as a result of an increased afterload. It manifests in the patient as worsening fatigue or exercise intolerance. Initiation of beta-blocker use reduces these effects. Beta-blocker use should not be initiated if the patient has volume overload or if NYHA class IV symptoms are present. "Start low and go slow" is the motto to follow with beta-blocker initiation. Patients with diabetes should be cautioned that beta-blockers may mask signs of hypoglycemia (i.e., tachycardia).

18. How are diuretics used in patients with heart failure?

Diuretics promote water and sodium excretion at various sites of the nephron in the kidney. They reduce both intravascular (blood) and extravascular (edema) fluid. Worsening renal function reduces the effectiveness of a diuretic. When ascites (abdominal edema) is present, torsemide may be more effective as a diuretic. Intravenous diuretics, such as furosemide, should be considered in a patient in whom ascites may preclude absorption of oral diuretics. Monitoring for electrolyte abnormalities—potassium, sodium, magnesium, calcium, and glucose—is necessary, as is monitoring for orthostatic hypotension and oto-toxicity. Potassium sparing diuretics are used more often in heart failure, so diligence in monitoring potassium levels is critical. For details regarding diuretic therapy, refer to Chapter 30, Diuretics and Nitrates.

19. How is digoxin used in patients with heart failure?

Digoxin is indicated for patients with systolic dysfunction (low EF) who continue to have symptoms despite treatment with diuretics and ACE inhibitors. Digoxin has been shown to reduce hospitalization rates but has no mortality benefit. Digoxin increases myocardial contractility, reduces systemic vascular resistance (SVR), and improves cardiac output. Because digoxin has a narrow therapeutic range, caution must be taken to monitor renal function. Dose reduction is recommended for the elderly and those with worsening renal function and concomitant amiodarone use. Adverse effects include: bradycardia, dysrhythmias, nausea, anorexia, vomiting, and visual disturbances. Refer to Chapter 33, Digoxin and Other Positive Inotropic Agents, for further details.

20. What type of nonpharmacologic interventions should be used?

- Diet: sodium restriction to less than 2 g/d allows diuretics to work more effectively.
- Fluids: restrictions of less than 2 L/d are primarily recommended when hyponatremia is present. When advanced stages of heart failure develop, fluid restrictions may need to be reduced to 1000 to 1500 mL/d.
- Weight monitoring: daily weight monitoring is critical for early identification of fluid retention. A weight gain of 2 to 4 lbs within a 1- to 2-day period is clinically significant and should be reported to the healthcare team.
- Smoking cessation.
- Avoidance of alcohol and other cardiotoxic substances.
- Weight reduction with obesity.

21. What type of patient education should be provided?

- Pathophysiology of heart failure on the basis of the etiology for the individual patient.
- Symptom identification: orthopnea, paroxysmal nocturnal dyspnea (PND), dyspnea, cough, edema, chest discomfort.

- Daily weight monitoring with instructions to weigh at the same time in the morning in the same amount of clothing and to report significant weight gain to members of the healthcare team.
- Dietary modifications, including details for a sodium-restricted diet.
- Medication instructions should include indications, dosing, frequency, side effects, and financial assistance for medications.
- Activity modifications to reduce cardiac workload. When the patient is sitting, the legs should be elevated to promote venous return.
- Low-level aerobic activity to the level of perceived exertion is the current recommendation until further research can evaluate the role of exercise in heart failure.
- Self care of other chronic illnesses, such as diabetes, asthma, and hypertension.
- Avoidance of over-the-counter (OTC) products and herbal supplements.
- Who and when to contact if symptoms develop.

22. What precipitates an episode of heart failure?

The precipitants of heart failure exacerbations include:
- Excess salt intake.
- Cardiac arrhythmias. Atrial fibrillation is most common.
- Medication noncompliance.
- Uncontrolled hypertension.
- Myocardial infarction or new ischemia.
- Inadequate therapy: too much or too little.
- Drugs that may cause fluid retention: steroids, nonsteroidal antiinflammatory drugs (NSAIDs), hormones.
- Financial limitations.
- Psychological issues.

23. What is the prognosis for heart failure?

Heart failure is a chronic illness, and the trajectory is often unpredictable. The mortality rate for all patients with heart failure is approximately 50% in 5 years. Therefore discussion of the possibility of sudden death and completion of advanced directives are important topics to address. The diagnosis of heart failure often elicits fear, anxiety, and depressive symptoms in patients and their family members. Evaluation of the patient's social support, quality of life, and psychological state is a valuable piece of the care and management of the patent with heart failure.

24. What physiologic markers indicate a poor prognosis in a patient with heart failure?

- Advancing age.
- Hyponatremia (sodium level less than 133 mEq/L).
- Tachycardia.
- Worsening hepatomegaly.
- Ischemic etiology.

- Refractory to optimal medical management.
- Increasing frequency of hospitalization.
- Declining NYHA status.

25. What are current controversies in the medical management of heart failure?

- Only two beta-blockers are approved by the US Food and Drug Administration (FDA) for use in patients with heart failure and are supported by randomized clinical trials in the heart failure population. The concept of "class effect" regarding beta-blocker use has not been determined. The two approved beta-blockers are carvedilol and metoprolol.
- If a patient has decompensation, the recommendation is that the beta-blocker dose be reduced during the exacerbation period. Whether or not patients should remain on beta-blocker therapy if they need inotropic support for the management of heart failure is controversial.
- Treatment with inotropic medications, such as milrinone or dobutamine, remains controversial because of their proarrhythmic effect and associated high mortality rate in patients with heart failure. Previous attempts with oral inotropes such as enoximone were not successful, and evaluation continues. (Refer to Chapter 33, Digoxin and Other Positive Inotropic Agents.)
- Whether to guide the medical team's treatment decisions in patients in acute heart failure (class IIIb to IV) with insertion of a pulmonary artery catheter or with use of clinical signs and symptoms (without a pulmonary artery catheter) is currently the focus of a research trial, Evaluation Study of Congestive Heart Failure and Pulmonary Artery Catheterization Effectiveness (ESCAPE). Debate exists on whether such an invasive procedure is beneficial or detrimental to patients with heart failure.

26. What does the future hold for heart failure management?

- Biventricular pacing is being studied as a method of resynchronization in patients with an intraventricular conduction delay (QRS >150 ms). The aim of this therapy is to provide synchronous biventricular contraction and relaxation, resulting in an improved hemodynamic response.
- Nesiritide is an intravenous form of brain natriuretic peptide (BNP), which is a naturally occurring hormone found in the ventricles. It increases cardiac output and stroke volume without affecting the heart rate. Nesiritide promotes natriuresis, diuresis, and vasodilation. BNP is secreted from the atria and ventricles as a result of cardiac dilation. The level rises in proportion to the severity of heart failure. Monitoring of BNP levels as a point of care test is currently used in emergency departments as a tool in differentiating cardiac from pulmonary etiologies. A level greater than 100 pg/mL supports the diagnosis of symptomatic heart failure or left ventricular dysfunction.
- Enoximone is a phosphodiesterase inhibitor that is under investigation as an oral form of an inotrope for use in advanced heart failure.
- Vasopressin receptor antagonists and endothelin receptor antagonists are also being studied for their effect at the neurohormonal level for the treatment of heart failure.

- The role of exercise in patients with heart failure is the focus of an up-and-coming research study known as HF-ACTION (**H**eart **F**ailure and **A** **C**ontrolled **T**rial **I**nvestigating **O**utcomes of Exercise Trai**N**ing).

 Key Points

- Fatigue and early satiety are often early signs of cardiac decompensation associated with heart failure. As heart failure progresses symptoms of fatigue and early satiety result from shunting of blood to vital organs. Poor perfusion of the gut may result in symptoms of abdominal fullness, constipation, nausea and even vomiting.
- The primary goals of treatment for heart failure focus on helping the patient to "feel better, live longer and stay out of the hospital." This is done through both pharmacologic and nonpharmacologic therapies.
- Pharmacologic treatment for heart failure usually includes the following classes of medications: ACE inhibitors, beta-blockers, diuretics, Angiotensin II receptor blockers and Digoxin.
- Nonpharmacologic treatments include a variety of lifestyle changes including dietary restrictions, weight monitoring and monitoring fluid intake.
- Beta-blockers should not be initiated if the patient is volume overloaded or if NYHA Class IV symptoms.
- Heart failure is a chronic illness and the trajectory is often unpredictable. Mortality for heart failure patients is approximately 50% in 5 years. Therefore, discussion of the possibility of sudden death and completion of advanced directives are important topics to address.
- The diagnosis of heart failure often elicits fear, anxiety and depressive symptoms in patients and their family members. Evaluating the patient's social support, quality of life and psychological state are a valuable piece of your care and management of the patient with heart failure.

 Internet Resources

Journal Article: ACC/AHA Guidelines for the Evaluation and Management of Chronic Heart Failure in the Adult:
http://circ.ahajournals.org/cgi/content/full/104/24/2996

Heart Failure Society of America: Heart Failure Practice Guidelines:
http://hfsa.org/hf_guidelines.asp

Doctor's Guide:
http://www.docguide.com

Heart Failure Online:
http://heartfailure.org

Heartmates: Resources for the Spouse, Family, and Loved Ones of a Heart Patient:
http://heartmates.com

Bibliography

Adams K et al: Heart Failure Society of America (HFSA) practice guidelines, *J Card Fail* 5:357-382, 1999.

Baig M et al: The pathophysiology of advanced heart failure, *Heart Lung* 28(2):87-101, 1999.

Bates B et al: *A guide to physical examination and history taking,* Philadelphia, 1999, JB Lippincott.

Caboral M, Mithcell J: New guidelines for heart failure focus on prevention, *Nurs Pract J* 28(1):13-23, 2003.

Carelock J, Clark A: Heart failure: pathophysiologic mechanisms, *Am J Nurs* 101(12):26-33, 2001.

Cazeau S et al: Effects of multisite biventricular pacing in patients with heart failure and intraventricular conduction delay, *N Engl J Med* 344(12):873-880, 2001.

Cianficci LJ: Cardiac assessment. In Schell H, Puntillo K: *Critical care nursing secrets,* Philadelphia, 2001, Hanley & Belfus.

Colucci WS et al: Intravenous nesiritide, a natriuretic peptide, in the treatment of decompensated heart failure: nesiritide study group, *N Engl J Med* 343:246-253, 2000.

Greenberg G: Heart failure awareness 2002—and beyond, *J Card Fail* 8(1):6-7, 2002.

Nohria A, Lewis E, Stevenson LW: Medical management of advanced heart failure, *JAMA* 287(5):628-640, 2002.

Remme WJ, Swedberg K: Task Force for the Diagnosis and Treatment of Chronic Heart Failure, European Society of Cardiology Guidelines for the diagnosis and treatment of chronic heart failure, *Eur Heart J* 22(17):1527-1560, 2001.

Taylor G: *Primary care management of heart disease,* St Louis, 2000, Mosby.

Tsuyuki R et al: Acute precipitants of congestive heart failure exacerbations, *Arch Intern Med* 161(19):2337-2342, 2001.

Uretsky B et al: Beyond drug therapy: nonpharmacologic care of the patient with advanced heart failure, *Am Heart J* 135(6):264-284, 1998.

Yusuf S, Negassa A: Choice of clinical outcomes in randomized trials of heart failure therapies: disease-specific or overall outcomes? *Am Heart J* 143(1):22-28, 2002.

Chapter 12

Presyncope and Syncope

Rachel Tunstall

1. Define presyncope.

Presyncope is the sensation of lightheadedness or dizziness accompanied by at least one of the following symptoms: nausea, vomiting, pallor, weakness, diaphoresis, diminished vision, delayed response time to verbal stimuli, headache, dyspnea, chest pain, palpitations, or abdominal pain. The condition usually occurs without warning and may or may not lead to actual syncope.

2. What is the definition of syncope?

Syncope is the sudden and transient loss of consciousness and loss of postural tone with spontaneous recovery. Syncope usually lasts from seconds to minutes. Other terms used synonymously with syncope include fainting, blackout, and loss of consciousness. Syncope is a common disorder that accounts for between 3% and 5% of emergency department visits and between 1% and 6% of hospital admissions. It occurs in all age-groups, from pediatric to elderly. Estimates are that 30% of the population will have at least one episode of syncope in their lifetime.

3. List some common causes of syncope.

Cardiovascular	Hypotensive	Metabolic	Neurological	Psychiatric	Other
Coronary disease	Vasovagal	Hypoglycemia	Seizures	Anxiety	**Medications**
Congenital and	carotid sinus	Hyperglycemia	Migraines	Conversion	Diuretics
valvular heart	Hypersensitivity	Hyponatremia	Subarachnoid	disorders	Nitroglycerin
disease	Volume depletion	Hypokalemia	hemorrhage	Depression	Beta-blockers
Cardiomyopathy	or dehydration	Hypocalcemia	Transient	Panic	Angiotensin-
Arrhythmias (heart	Autonomic	Hypoxia	ischemia	disorders	converting
block, brady-	insufficiency			Somatization	enzyme (ACE)
arrhythmias,				disorders	inhibitors
and tachy-					Vasodilative or
arrhythmias)					sympatholytic
Conduction system					anti-
disorders					hypertensives

Cardiovascular	Hypotensive	Metabolic	Neurological	Psychiatric	Other
Aortic stenosis					Antidepressants
Pulmonary					
embolism					**Neuroleptics**
					Amiodarone
					Sotalol
					hydrochloride
					Procainamide
					Recreational
					drugs
					Cocaine
					Alcohol
					Trauma

4. How is syncope evaluated?

Syncope is a symptom that signals an underlying pathology. Therefore the goal for patients with syncope is determination of the cause of the syncope. The history and physical exam are essential to this process because studies have shown that their results yield a cause about 45% of the time. If the history and physical exam do not elicit a cause, they do guide risk stratification and choice of diagnostic tests. However, the etiologies of 50% of syncopal events are unknown.

5. What are some common diagnostic tests used in determining the cause of syncope?

Although no single diagnostic test is considered the gold standard for syncope, the following tests are commonly used in patient work-ups.

Electrocardiography (ECG). A 12-lead ECG is recommended for all patients because of its low risk and fairly low cost and because it can provide useful information to direct further evaluation and diagnostic testing. Examples of ECG findings or diagnoses made with ECG include previously undiagnosed bundle branch block, previous myocardial infarction, left ventricular hypertrophy, ventricular tachycardia, and bradyarrhythmia.

Holter monitor. This test is used to rule out arrhythmia as the cause of syncope. 24-hour Holter monitoring is recommended for patients with frequent episodes of syncope and a healthy heart. The monitor is also recommended for patients with abnormal ECG results, heart disease, or symptoms indicative of arrhythmias.

Loop recorder. Patients with frequent episodes of syncope or presyncopal symptoms and structurally healthy hearts are candidates for this test. However, this test requires patient compliance; the test includes turning on the recorder in the mornings and pushing a button after an episode for reliable results. In addition, implantable loop devices are available for use. It is important to note that patients who have organic heart disease and are at risk for fatal ventricular arrhythmia are deferred to electrophysiologic testing (see Chapter 7, Invasive Cardiovascular Testing).

Echocardiogram (echo). Echocardiograms are useful in the determination of whether a structural problem exists with the heart. Therefore an Echo is performed if heart disease, such as a valve abnormality, is suspected. This test is also useful for patients with abnormal ECG results, known or suspected heart disease, suspected arrhythmia, and a family history of sudden death. However, routine use of this test is not recommended.

Intracardiac electrophysiological studies. Current guidelines have outlined two situations in which electrophysiological testing is beneficial with syncope. The first is in patients with unexplained syncope and documented structural heart disease. The second is in patients with syncope, no structural heart disease, and negative head-tilt table testing. Therefore the underlying guideline is that if cardiac syncope is suspected but all other noninvasive test results show no abnormalities, then proceed with this study.

Head-tilt table testing. This test is useful in diagnosis of neurocardiogenic syncope. This type of syncope is common in patients with suspected cardiovascular syncope but without structural or ischemic heart disease. Typically a patient is placed at a 60-degree angle for at least 45 minutes. The following parameters are monitored during a tilt table test: ECG, pulse oximeter, and blood pressure. Patients may also be connected to a defibrillator and/or pacemaker during the procedure. Signs and symptoms to expect during the test include symptoms they had before the test (e.g., nausea, dizziness), or fainting, although patients may experience no symptoms at all. In addition, if patients are given Isuprel during the test they may feel nervous or feel that their heartbeat is faster or stronger than normal.

Exercise stress testing. This test is important in the work-up of exertional, exercise-induced, or postexertional syncope to determine whether ischemia or tachyarrhythmia is the culprit. However, an echo should be performed in patients with exertional syncope before exercise stress testing to rule out hypertrophic cardiomyopathy.

Neurological testing. Computed tomography, magnetic resonance imaging, carotid or transcranial Doppler ultrasonographic studies, and electroencephalography are examples of neurological tests for syncope. These tests are done depending on the patient history (e.g., seizures, diplopia, headaches) and physical exam (e.g., focal neurologic signs) warranting further investigation.

Basic laboratory tests: complete blood cell count, electrolytes, toxicology screen, thyroid tests. These tests should be ordered depending on the patient history, review of symptoms, and physical exam. Otherwise laboratory tests are not routinely performed or recommended.

Pregnancy test. This test should be considered in women of childbearing age, particularly if head-tilt table or electrophysiological tests are being pursued in the work-up.

6. What areas should nurses focus on with assessments?

Topic	Tips
Vital signs	• Orthostatic vital signs assessment: search for a systolic blood pressure drop of 10 to 20 mm Hg or more from a lying to standing position or an increase in heart rate of at least 20 bpm. • Monitor vital signs routinely for any variations in pulse and blood pressure throughout the day, any association between medications given and these variations, and any difference in blood pressure measurements between arms.
History	• Assess the patient history surrounding the event (such as exertion, time of day, any seizure activity, and associated signs and symptoms).
Medical history	• Assess for any contributory medical history, such as any structural cardiac abnormalities, coronary artery disease, congestive heart failure, arrhythmias, pacemaker or implantable cardiac defibrillator, seizures, diabetes mellitus, family history of cardiac disease or sudden death, and psychiatric disorders like anxiety, depression, or panic disorders.
Cardiovascular assessment	• Know the baseline value and note any changes throughout the shift or between clinic visits and report to the physician or advanced practice registered nurse (APRN) in charge. • Particular areas to focus on are heart sounds, pulse rate, and blood pressure measurements. • Monitor the patient for any presyncope or syncope symptoms. Remind patients to report signs of any other cardiac symptoms, such as chest pain. • Monitor telemetry and assess rhythm strips throughout the shift for any changes. These abnormalities can include tachycardia, bradycardia, or heart block. Monitor patients for the presence of symptoms associated with these changes.
Neurological assessment	• Do a quick assessment at baseline and note any changes throughout the shift or between clinic visits and report to the physician or APRN.
Medications	• Note the patient's medications and their potential side effects. Also note any new patient medications. Particularly be aware that certain classes of drugs are culprits for syncope, such as diuretics, antihypertensives, antidepressives, and herbal preparations, as is polypharmacy in elders.
Fluid and electrolytes	• Monitor patient intake and output and any recent lab values.
Risk of falls assessment	• Assess the patient for the potential for falls while hospitalized or at home.

7. **What are some patient education tips for patients with presyncope or syncope?**

- Provide counseling on recognition of presyncope symptoms. Review with the patient what the symptoms are and what other potential symptoms occur in the presyncope stage.
- Advise the patient if presyncope symptoms occur to sit down and put the head between the knees or to lay down flat with legs elevated and to ask for help.
- Remind the patient to report any symptoms to the nurse (while hospitalized) or to contact his or her health care provider or call 911 (if at home).
- Counsel patients, family members, friends, and significant others about appropriate actions to take after a syncopal event, such as elevating the patient's feet and legs.
- If orthostatic hypotension is the suspected cause, educate the patient about some prevention measures. For example, patients should change positions slowly. When moving from a supine position to a sitting position, patients should dangle or exercise their legs for few minutes before standing. Maintaining hydration by avoiding alcohol, avoiding hot environments, drinking plenty of water, and eating small frequent meals is also important.
- If vasovagal syncope is the cause and a situational stimulus is identified (e.g., stressful situation, site of blood), then counsel on stress management or avoidance of stimulus if possible.
- Provide patient education on any diagnostic tests as appropriate, such as Holter monitoring or use of the loop recorder.
- Counsel the patient on prevention of falls at home and in the hospital.

8. **Describe special population issues in regard to syncope.**

- Syncope occurs more frequently in the elderly, who account for 80% of the hospital admissions for syncope. Because of physiological changes that are age related, along with chronic illness and polypharmacy, the elderly are more prone to syncope. Therefore syncope in the elderly is usually multifactorial. The work-up for this group of patients focuses on history, physical exam (with close attention to cardiac, neurological, and psychiatric symptoms), and any situational stresses. Diagnostic tests focus first on whether or not any associated heart disease exists, which includes the use of echo and ECG and potentially an exercise stress test if myocardial infarction is ruled out.
- Athletes with syncope need a complete cardiovascular work-up to determine whether or not a risk for sudden death exists (e.g., supraventricular tachycardia (SVT), Wolff-Parkinson-White (WPW) syndrome, or coronary disease).
- Syncope is rare in the pediatric population, but when it occurs, a thorough evaluation is needed to determine risk for sudden death or underlying cardiac cause. Common etiologies in the pediatric population include: vasovagal, orthostatic hypotension, WPW syndrome, SVT, other tachyarrhythmias, and cardiomyopathy.

Key Points

- Syncope is a symptom that signals an underlying pathology. Therefore the goal for patients with syncope is determination of the etiology that produces syncope.

- The history and physical exam results yield a cause for syncope 45% of the time. If the history and physical exam do not yield a cause, they do guide risk stratification and choice of diagnostic tests.

- No single diagnostic test is considered the gold standard for syncope.

- Nursing assessments should focus on the following areas: vital signs, history, medical history, cardiovascular assessment, neurological assessment, medications, fluid and electrolytes, and risk of falls assessment.

- One key patient education topic to review with patients and their families is presyncope symptoms and what to do when they occur.

Internet Resources

NASPE Heart Rhythm Society:
www.naspe.org

American College of Cardiology:
www.acc.org

National Institute of Neurological Disorders and Stroke Syncope Page:
http://www.ninds.nih.gov/health_and_medical/disorders/syncope_doc.htm

Neurocardiogenic Syncope:
www.syncope.co.uk

Bibliography

Farewell D, Sulke N: How do we diagnose syncope? *J Cardiovasc Electrophysiol* 13(1 suppl):S9-S13, 2002.

Fenton AM, Hammill SC, Rea RF et al: Vasovagal syncope, *Ann Intern Med* 133:714-725, 2000.

Graham MV, Uphold CR: *Clinical guidelines in child health,* ed 2, Gainesville, Fla, 1999, Barmarrae Books.

Grubb BP, Kosinski DJ: Cardiovascular evaluation of patients with syncope of uncertain etiology, *Cardiac Electrophysiol Rev* 1(2):159-167, 1997.

Hackney T: Syncope. In Godsby MJ, editor: *Nurse practitioner secrets: questions and answers reveal the secrets to successful NP practice,* Philadelphia, 2000, Hanley & Belfus, pp 85-88.

Linzer M, Yang EH, Estes NA III et al: Diagnosing syncope. Part 1: value of history, physical examination, and electrocardiography. Clinical Efficacy Assessment Project of the American College of Physicians, *Ann Intern Med* 126:989-996, 1997.

Linzer M, Yang EH, Estes NA III et al: Diagnosing syncope. Part 2: unexplained syncope. Clinical Efficacy Assessment Project of the American College of Physicians, *Ann Intern Med* 127:76-86, 1997.

Massie BM, Amidon TM: Heart. In Tierney LM, McPhee SJ, Papadakis MA editors: *Current medical diagnosis & treatment 2000,* ed 39, New York, 2000, Lange Medical Books/McGraw Hill, pp 351-443.

Mathias CJ, Deguchi K, Schatz I: Observations on recurrent syncope and presyncope in 641 patients, *Lancet* 357(9253):348-353, 2001.

Nehgme R: Evaluation and treatment of other arrhythmic causes of syncope in children and adolescents with an apparently normal heart: Wolff-Parkinson-White syndrome and right ventricular cardiomyopathy, *Prog Pediatr Cardiol* 13(2):111-125, 2001.

Rose MS, Doshman ML, Spreng S et al: The relationship between health-related quality of life and frequency of spells in patients with syncope, *J Clin Epidemiol* 53(12):1209-1216, 2000.

Sim V, Pascual J, Woo J: Evaluating elderly patients with syncope, *Arch Gerontol Geriatr* 35(2):121-135, 2002.

Sisson SD, Kramer PD: Dizziness, vertigo, motion sickness, syncope and near syncope, and disequilibrium. In Barker LR, Burton JR, Zieve PD editors: *Principles of ambulatory medicine,* ed 5, Baltimore, 1999, Williams & Wilkins, pp 1252-1273.

Steinberg LA, Knilans TK: Costs and utility of tests in evaluation of the pediatric patients with syncope, *Prog Pediatr Cardiol* 13(2):139-149, 2001.

Arrhythmias

Kimberly Vitale-Sheldon, Pauline A. Gearing,
and Leslie Davis

1. What is the normal conduction pathway for a heartbeat?

Cardiac depolarization normally begins at the sinoatrial (SA) node and travels to the atrioventricular (AV) node through a variety of intraatrial pathways. At the AV node, the impulse pauses momentarily for the ventricles to fill. Next the electrical impulse travels from the AV node to the ventricles by way of the bundle of His and down through the Purkinje fibers. See the following figure.

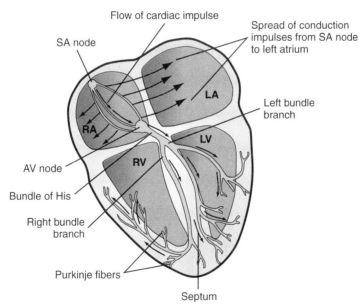

Conduction system of the heart. *AV*, Atrioventricular; *LA*, left atrium; *LV*, left ventricle; *RA*, right atrium; *RV*, right ventricle; *SA*, sinoatrial.

2. What is the normal intrinsic heart rate for each of these parts of the conduction pathway?

The intrinsic rate for the SA node is 60 to 100 bpm. The AV node fires at a rate of 40 to 60 bpm, and the His bundle and the Purkinje fibers at 20 to 40 bpm.

The AV node or the ventricles usually initiate a heartbeat only if the SA node does not fire or if the impulse is blocked from reaching that area.

3. What constitutes a normal cardiac cycle?

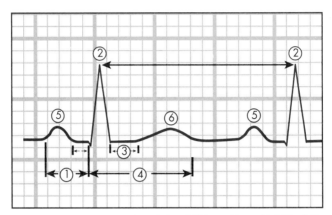

The electrocardiogram complex as seen in a normal sinus rhythm. *1*, PR interval (normal is 0.12 to 0.20 sec); *2*, QRS complex (normal is 0.04 to 0.12 sec); *3*, ST segment; *4*, QT interval (normal is 0.35 to 0.43 sec); *5*, P wave; *6*, T wave.

The cardiac cycle refers to the period from the end of one heart contraction to the end of the next contraction. See the figure in Question 3. This repetitive electrical stimulation causes a mechanical contraction of the heart muscle that pumps blood through the heart. This electrical activity is seen on the electrocardiogram (ECG) as a P wave, a QRS complex, and a T wave. The cardiac cycle is divided into two parts: a period of relaxation called diastole and a period of contraction called systole. In a normal cardiac cycle, the atria are electrically stimulated (depolarized), which causes the muscle to contract and thus eject blood to the relaxed ventricles. The P wave reflects the impulse through the atria. The atria prepare to be restimulated (repolarized) and relax while the ventricles, now filled with blood, contract and pump blood to the systemic and pulmonary circulation (QRS) complex. After the ventricular contraction, the ventricles repolarize and relax, recorded as the T wave. The cycle then begins again at the end of ventricular repolarization.

4. What does each wave represent?

- Each beat manifests as five major waves: P, Q, R, S, and T. The P wave represents depolarization of both atria and has a normal measurement at the P-R interval of less than or equal to 0.20 seconds. The P-R interval should not exceed a large box.
- The QRS wave represents depolarization of the ventricular myocardium, and the normal measurement is less than or equal to 0.12 seconds. The QRS complex should not be greater than half a large box.

- The measurement from the S wave to the end of the T wave is ventricular repolarization, a complete resting state.

5. How do you calculate the heart rate from an ECG strip?

The methods used to measure the cardiac rate are as follows:
- Because each large block on the ECG paper represents 0.20 seconds, five large blocks equal 1 second. The number of complexes in a 6-second rhythm strip are counted and multiplied by 10.
- Because each large block on the ECG paper represents 0.20 seconds, 300 large blocks equal 1 minute (0.20 × 300 = 60 seconds). If the rhythm is regular, one should divide 300 by the number of large blocks between two R waves (QRS complexes). For example, if two large boxes are between R waves, division of 300 by two large blocks gives a rate of 150 bpm. (If three blocks were found, the rate would be 100; four blocks, 75).
- A prepared rate ruler may also be used.

6. What cardiac rhythms originate above the ventricles?

- From the sinus node: sinus rhythm, sinus bradycardia, sinus tachycardia, sinus arrhythmia.
- From the atrium: atrial fibrillation, atrial flutter, premature atrial contractions (PACs), and atrial tachycardia.
- From the AV junction: junctional escape rhythm, junctional rhythm, junctional tachycardia, and premature junctional contractions (PJCs; sometimes called nodal beats).
- Wandering pacemaker: the pacemaker activity "wanders" away from the SA node to a nearby focus somewhere in the atria. Because the focus originates from somewhere other than the SA node, the P-R interval will differ and the P wave configuration may appear different.

7. Differentiate unique qualities about rhythms that originate from the sinus node.

Rhythm	Heart Rate (bpm)	Unique Quality
Sinus rhythm	60-100	None
Sinus bradycardia	<60	Heart rate
Sinus tachycardia	>100	Heart rate
Sinus arrhythmia	60-100 (average around 70-80)	Slightly irregular in pattern; usually associated with sleeping

8. Differentiate unique qualities about rhythms that originate from the atrium.

Rhythm	Heart Rate (bpm)	Unique Quality
Atrial fibrillation	Atrial: 350-600	No distinct P waves
	Ventricular: no set rate	Irregular rhythm

Rhythm	Heart Rate (bpm)	Unique Quality
		Atrioventricular node usually controls electrical stimulation to ventricles, preventing ventricular tachycardia and ventricular fibrillation
Atrial flutter	Atrial: 250-350	No distinct P waves
	Ventricular: no set rate	Flutter waves
		Typically regular rhythm, but not always
Paroxysmal atrial tachycardia	Ventricular: 150-250	Unable to distinguish P waves
		Narrow complex QRS waves
		Sudden onset
Premature atrial contractions	No set rate; typically sinus rhythm as underlying rhythm with ectopic beats from atrium	QRS comes earlier than expected
		P wave precedes early QRS
		P wave may look different than other P waves

9. What is the difference between atrial fibrillation and atrial flutter?

When atrial fibrillation occurs, the atria initiate the electrical beat in a rapid or disorganized manner, between 350 and 600 times per minute. Several atria foci originate from the electrical conduction, which may come from either atria. This causes the ventricles to beat irregularly in response to the multiple foci in the atrium, in an attempt to "keep up with" the atria. Normal P waves are replaced by irregular rapid waves, and the appearance of the atrial activity is that of a chaotic "fib"-type waveform or almost straight line. See the following figure.

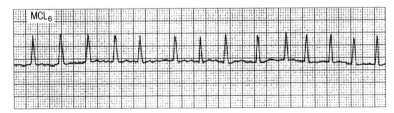

Atrial fibrillation with rapid ventricular response.

Atrial flutter, although similar to atrial fibrillation, begins the electrical conduction from one specific foci in the atrium. These atrial contractions are less rapid and more organized, causing the atrium to initiate an electrical current between 250 to 300 times per minute. The atrial contractions appear as "saw-tooth" P waves, best seen in leads II, II, and AVF on the 12-lead ECG. However, the ventricular response rate is still a concern because it may become accelerated in an attempt to "keep up with" the atrial conductions as well. See the following figure.

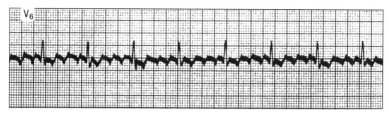

Atrial flutter with a constant 4:1 conduction ratio.

10. What are the differences between paroxysmal, persistent, and chronic atrial fibrillation?

Atrial fibrillation can occur intermittently, known as paroxysmal atrial fibrillation (a paroxysm is usually a self-terminating episode and has sudden onset), or it can be persistent (does not stop on its own). When atrial fibrillation has been present for more than 6 months, it is known as permanent or "chronic atrial fibrillation."

11. What causes atrial fibrillation and atrial flutter?

Causes of atrial fibrillation and atrial flutter include dysfunction of the sinus node (the natural pacemaker of the heart) and a number of cardiac disorders such as: coronary artery disease (CAD), including myocardial infarction (MI); rheumatic heart disease; valvular disorders; congestive heart failure; pericarditis; and hypertension. Other causes include pulmonary disorders (such as chronic obstructive pulmonary disease [COPD] or cor pulmonale), hyperthyroidism, hypokalemia, and alcohol abuse, or the conditions may occur after cardiac or pulmonary surgery.

12. What are complications from atrial fibrillation or flutter?

- Decreased cardiac output. If the atria fibrillate rather than contract fully, they are not able to completely eject the blood volume they are holding. This leads to less blood being emptied into the ventricles, which in turn means less overall cardiac output from the ventricles.
- Thromboembolic disorders. About 15% of strokes occur with atrial fibrillation. This is a result of venostasis. The complete volume of blood is not fully ejected from the atria because of inadequate atrial contraction; the blood pools in the atria, and small clots form. These small clots may dislodge and travel to parts of the brain and pulmonary system as an embolus.
- Rapid ventricular response rate. The danger of atrial fibrillation or flutter is a rapid ventricular response rate. This condition may occur because many rapid discharges from numerous foci in the atria occur with atrial fibrillation. These multiple foci then travel to the AV node. The AV node in response may allow an increased number of stimuli to pass through to the ventricles, thereby increasing the overall heart rate.

13. What are the treatment goals for atrial fibrillation/flutter?

Although treatment varies, depending on the cause of the arrhythmia, the three overall treatment goals are:
- Control of the ventricular heart rate or slowing of conduction of the impulses to the ventricles (AV conduction) with beta-blockers, calcium channel blockers, digitalis, or other medications (see Chapter 34, Antiarrhythmic Agents). Ensuring adequate electrolyte balance is important.
- Prevention of thromboembolic events with anticoagulants such as heparin or warfarin.
- Restoring normal sinus rhythm if possible via electrical cardioversion or chemical cardioversion (antiarrhythmic medications; see Chapter 34, Antiarrhythmic Agents). Also radiofrequency catheter ablation may be a treatment option for patients without severe underlying heart disease or patients with persistent or chronic atrial fibrillation.

14. When it is appropriate to use cardioversion to treat atrial fibrillation or flutter?

If the patient at any time has atrial fibrillation/flutter and an unstable condition (shortness of breath, hypotension, decreased level of consciousness, diaphoresis, or paleness), he or she should be prepared for immediate cardioversion. For stable episodes of atrial fibrillation/flutter, the patient should first undergo anticoagulation therapy (unless contraindicated because of a serious risk of bleeding) with heparin, followed by warfarin for at least 3 weeks, before cardioversion or until a transesophageal echocardiogram (TEE) shows no signs of atrial clots. Whether atrial fibrillation/flutter continues or frequent episodes of intermittent atrial fibrillation/flutter after cardioversion are seen determines how long anticoagulant therapy (such as warfarin) is maintained.

15. Differentiate unique qualities about rhythms that originate from the AV junction.

Rhythm	Heart Rate (bpm)	Unique Quality
Junctional escape beats	Usually within normal range but depends on underlying rhythm	Rhythm is regular with late beats. P wave is inverted (negative) preceding or following QRS or absent.
Junctional escape rhythm	Between 40 and 60	Rhythm may be irregular as result of escape beats. P wave is inverted (negative) before, during, or after QRS or absent. QRS is normal. P-R interval <0.12 sec if present.
Premature junctional contractions (PJCs)	Usually within normal range but depends on underlying rhythm	PJCs occur early in cycle of baseline rhythm. Full compensatory pause may occur. If PJCs are occasional, they are insignificant. If PJCs are frequent, junctional tachycardia may result.

continued		
Rhythm	**Heart Rate (bpm)**	**Unique Quality**
Junctional tachycardia	When junctional rate increases to >100	Rhythm is regular. QRS normal or widened with aberrant ventricular conduction. P waves are inverted, as are in junctional rhythm. P-R interval is shorter than normal (<0.12 sec if present).

16. What are causes of junctional rhythms?

When the SA node does not function as the originating pacemaker in the conduction system, the AV node has potential pacemakers that will "kick in" and take over in the absence of regular pacing stimuli starting from the atria. The most common cause of this rhythm in healthy individuals is sinus bradycardia. It may also be seen in the presence of a high-degree or complete AV block. If the ventricular rate is slow, hemodynamic compromise may occur.

17. In which situations would a junctional rhythm require treatment, if any?

Because the inherent rate of the AV node is 40 to 60 bpm, for some patients this rate may be too slow and could produce symptoms such as weakness, lethargy, syncope, or hypotension. The treatment administration therefore would be to increase the heart rate chemically or with an external pacemaker.

18. What is heart block?

Heart block is a disorder of the electrical conduction system of the heart. It occurs when the atria electrical conduction system fails to coordinate (or conduct) to the ventricles. This interrupts the passage of impulses from the atria to the ventricles. The three degrees of AV block are first, second, and third. This classification is based on the ECG characteristics. See the following table and figure.

Degree of Heart Block	Description	Symptoms	Diagnosis
First-degree block	Delay in conduction from sinoatrial node to ventricles. PR interval is >0.20 sec on electrocardiogram.	Typically no symptoms exist.	Normally benign but may progress to second-degree block, usually Mobitz type I. PR interval should be carefully monitored.

continued

Degree of Heart Block	Description	Symptoms	Diagnosis
Second-degree block: Mobitz type I (Wenckebach)	Progressive prolongation of PR interval is seen until beat is blocked. P wave fails to conduct to ventricle (QRS is missed), and then cycle repeats. Rhythm (R-R interval) is irregular, and more P waves than QRS complexes are seen.	Symptoms of second degree heart block may include complete absence of symptoms or symptoms in manifested any slow irregular rhythm.	Occurs commonly after inferior myocardial infarction and tends to be self-limiting. Does not normally require treatment, although hemodynamic instability may develop with 2:1 block.
Second degree block: Mobitz type II (occasional blocked beats)	Most beats are conducted normally, but occasionally atrial contraction without subsequent ventricular contraction is seen. Characterized by unexpected blocked P waves (P wave not followed by QRS) without prolongation of PR interval.	One consequence of Mobitz type II can be slow ventricular rate resulting in low cardiac output. This diminished output can produce myocardial or cerebral ischemia. Early indications of cerebral insufficiency include restlessness, mental confusion, or agitation.	Often progresses to complete heart block and if recognized needs expert assessment. Second degree block of any type requires pacemaker if symptomatic bradycardia exists.
Third degree block: complete heart block	Complete absence of atrioventricular conduction; no atrial impulses (P waves) conduct or reach ventricle, and flow of oxygenated blood to brain and rest of body is insufficient.	Rarely a person can tolerate slow heart rate associated with third degree block; inherent ventricular rate is 20-40 bpm, and syncope may result.	Temporary transvenous pacing may be required. Permanent pacemaker is required if block is chronic.

First-degree AV block

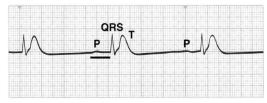

A

Heart block. **A,** First-degree AV heart block.

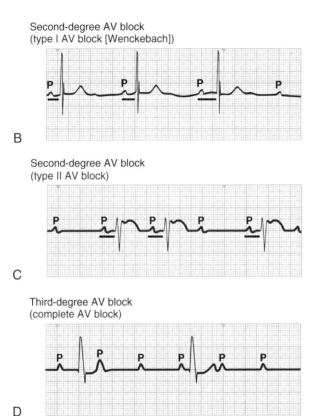

Heart block. **B,** Second-degree AV heart block, type I (Wenckebach). **C,** Second-degree AV heart block, type II. **D,** Third-degree AV block (complete AV block).

19. What are causes of the various types of heart block, and how are they treated?

Heart block may be caused by CAD, inflammation of the heart muscle, rheumatic fever, hyperkalemia, or acute MI. Reversible causes may occur because of use of medications (i.e., digoxin, beta-blockers, calcium channel blockers, and amiodarone). When necessary, the offending medications should be discontinued. However, this is not always plausible if the medication is necessary to control the tachyarrhythmia.

20. What cardiac rhythms originate at the ventricles?

- Premature ventricular contraction (PVC)
- Ventricular escape rhythm
- Ventricular tachycardia (V Tach)
- Ventricular fibrillation (V Fib)

21. Differentiate unique qualities about rhythms that originate from the ventricles.

Rhythm	Heart Rate (bpm)	Unique Quality
Premature ventricular contraction	May be many per min	Causes irregular rhythm Premature QRS complexes that are wide (>0.12 sec)
Ventricular escape rhythm	20-40	Occurs only if patient's inherent pacemaker is not stimulated from above ventricles
Ventricular tachycardia	100-250	Ventricular complexes continuously Typically regular rhythm Usually heart rate >150/min QRS complexes are wide (>0.12 sec) Can not identify P waves
Ventricular fibrillation	350-450	Ventricles do not provide mechanical pumping; if not treated immediately death will ensue Chaotic rhythm Can not identify P waves or QRS complexes

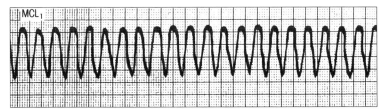

Ventricular tachycardia.

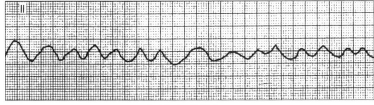

Ventricular fibrillation.

22. What are the causes of ventricular arrhythmias?

Most ventricular arrhythmias are associated with serious heart disease such as coronary artery blockage, cardiomyopathy, or valvular heart disease. V tach is often triggered by an extra beat that originates in either the right or the left ventricle. It also occurs frequently in connection with a MI. V tach commonly occurs within the first 24 hours of MI. It must be treated quickly to prevent V fib. After 48 to 72 hours of the MI, the risk of V tach is diminished. However, people who have had severe damage to the larger anterior wall of the heart have a second danger period because V tach often occurs during convalescence from this type of heart attack.

23. What are the treatment options for V tach and V fib?

- Any episode of V tach that causes symptoms needs to be treated. An episode that lasts more than 30 seconds, even without symptoms, also needs to be treated. Drug therapy can be given intravenously to suppress episodes of V tach. See the following table.

| Amiodarone (first choice) | 300 mg intravenous (IV) push. May repeat once at 150 mg in 3-5 min (maximal cumulative dose: 2.2 g IV/24 hr). |
| Lidocaine | 1.0-1.5 mg/kg IV. May repeat in 3-5 min (maximal loading dose: 3 mg/kg). |

- If drug therapy is ineffective and the patient becomes unconscious and pulseless, cardiopulmonary resuscitation (CPR) and defibrillation (shock) should be instituted immediately. Pulseless V tach and V fib are treated the same way. Shock should be administered immediately to stop the abnormal electrical signals and rapidly restore a normal rhythm.
- Other treatments for a ventricular tachyarrhythmia include the following:
  - Medications to reduce the heart rate (see Chapter 34, Antiarrhythmic Agents).
  - Implantable cardioverter defibrillator (ICD). Such devices are capable of defibrillating the heart back into normal rhythm if the arrhythmia reoccurs (see Chapter 25, Implantable Cardioverter Defibrillators).
  - Additional options include electrophysiologic testing and ablation of the arrhythmia focus (area of the heart causing the arrhythmia; see Chapter 7, Invasive Cardiovascular Testing).

24. In which situations (if any) do PVCs need to be treated?

Treatment of PVCs depends on many factors: cause, patient symptoms, and presenting clinical situation. Most patients with PVCs do not need treatment with antiarrhythmic medications. Currently, no clinical evidence suggests that the suppression of PVCs reduces mortality in patients with no known structural heart disease. However, in the immediate postinfarction period, the presence of PVCs that occur frequently or in pairs or groups of three (V tach) is associated with an increase in the risk of symptomatic or fatal dysrhythmias (V fib).

25. What is torsades de pointes?

Torsades de pointes is a life-threatening arrhythmia, marked by polymorphic V tach. It is characterized by onset with an early complex that follows a long pause and changes in the shape of the QRS complexes. The QRS complexes during this rhythm tend to show a series of complexes points up followed by complexes points down. Torsades occurs during a prolonged QT interval (greater than one half of the R-R interval), which can occur from drug therapy, slow rate arrhythmias, electrolyte imbalance, and ischemic conditions. Torsades de pointes is often self-limiting but may progress to V fib. Alertness for a prolonged QT interval is the most important aspect of prevention. The QT interval should not exceed one half of the R-R interval. The treatment is prompt cardioversion if the rhythm is sustained, followed by intravenous magnesium, avoidance of agents that prolong the QT interval, and correction of myocardial ischemia, hypoxia, and electrolyte abnormalities.

26. How do you measure the QT interval?

Measure the QT interval from the beginning of the Q wave (or the onset of the R wave if no Q wave is seen) until the end of the T wave. If the QT is less than one half the R-R interval, the QT is normal. If the QT is clearly more than one half the R-R interval, the QT is prolonged. If the QT is about half the R-R interval, the QT is borderline.

27. What is the difference between supraventricular tachycardia (SVT) and V tach?

Supraventricular tachycardia is a type of tachycardia (ventricular heart rate of more than 100 bpm) that originates from cardiac tissues above the ventricles of the heart ("supra" meaning "above"). The term SVT is a generic one that refers to many different kinds of arrhythmias, which may include sinus tachycardia or atrial tachycardia such as atrial fibrillation or atrial flutter. Often the SVT is so rapid that it is difficult to distinguish between sinus tachycardia or a type of atrial tachycardia. SVT may have a wide QRS complex if the patient has a bundle branch block (BBB) or has a rate induced wide QRS.

Ventricular tachycardia on the other hand originates in the ventricles. V tach may be defined as a series of multiple (three or more) consecutive PVCs occurring at a rate usually between 150 and 200 bpm. V tach is a life-threatening situation. Sustained V tach, which lasts more than 30 seconds, can easily convert to V fib if left untreated, which is the most common cause of sudden cardiac death.

28. How is V tach differentiated from SVT with aberrancy?

Differentiating V tach from SVT with aberrancy can be done with careful assessment of a 12-lead ECG or rhythm strip. However, an electrophysiology study is the only way to differentiate these two arrhythmias with complete accuracy. Some general criteria can help differentiate V tach from SVT with aberrancy:
- QRS complex greater than 0.14 seconds suggests V tach.
- A regular wide complex rhythm suggests V tach. An irregular wide complex

rhythm that manifests as either a right or a left bundle branch pattern suggests SVT with aberrancy.
- If AV dissociation is seen (P waves marching through at a constant rate with variable relationship to the QRS complex), the rhythm is V tach.

29. What is meant by an ectopic focus?

The term ectopic indicates that depolarization originated in an abnormal place (i.e., not the SA node), hence the abnormal shape of the P wave. An ectopic focus is an area of myocardial tissue that takes over pacemaker functions because it spontaneously discharges more rapidly than the SA node, usually because of injury. If such a focus depolarizes early, the beat produced is called an extrasystole or premature contraction and may be followed by a compensatory pause. If the underlying SA node rate is slow, sometimes a focus in the atria takes over and the rhythm is described as an atrial escape because it occurs after a small delay. Extrasystoles and escape beats have the same QRS appearance on the ECG, but extrasystoles occur early whereas escape beats occur late.

30. What are the most serious cardiac arrhythmias?

The most serious cardiac rhythm disturbance is V fib, in which the ventricles fibrillate or "quiver." There is no distinct ventricular contraction; therefore collapse of the cardiovascular system with subsequent sudden cardiac death follows unless medical help is provided immediately. In some cases, sustained V tach may result in inadequate ventricular filling and loss of adequate contraction, resulting in a markedly decreased cardiac output. This results in loss of blood pressure/pulse and leads to a loss of consciousness. Sustained V tach is the most common cause of sudden cardiac death.

31. What is Wolff-Parkinson-White (WPW) syndrome?

Wolff-Parkinson-White syndrome is an AV reentrant tachycardia from an accessory connection between the atria and ventricles. This accessory connection allows for a reentrant circuit, resulting in a reentrant tachycardia. Usually WPW is considered insignificant if tachycardia does not exist or if the patient has no associated cardiac disease. If tachycardia does occur in WPW syndrome, decreased cardiac output may develop. The three characteristic findings in WPW are: *1*, QRS widening (duration greater than 0.10 seconds); the QRS width varies depending on how much of the impulse travels down the AV node versus the accessory pathway; *2*, A delta wave is the hallmark of WPW syndrome; the beginning of the QRS complex may be positive (upright), negative (pseudo Q wave), or isoelectric (not apparent) and *3*, PR interval varies; when the P wave is present, the PR interval may be normal or shortened.

32. What are the essential components nurses should include in assessment of arrhythmias?

A careful assessment and risk stratification are the essential components in determining the interventions needed. Clinical manifestations of a fast heartbeat (tachycardia) usually are a combination of palpitations, faintness, or shortness of breath. In some cases, the person will notice only "pounding" of the heart. In other cases, the person may pass out with little warning. The symptoms of a slow heartbeat (bradycardia) are similar except that people usually do not notice palpitations or "pounding." It is essential that a complete and detailed history and physical examination be taken, and it is often necessary to perform blood work, a chest radiograph, a 12-lead ECG, or an echocardiogram as a part of the initial evaluation. Careful clinical judgment must be exercised. Causes of symptoms other than arrhythmias must be considered, and appropriate additional studies obtained. In some circumstances, particularly in patients with exertional symptoms, an exercise test might give a higher yield for correlation between symptoms and cardiac rhythm. Electrophysiological studies and tilt-table testing also may be considered in certain circumstances. If symptoms are severe, monitoring may need to be performed in-hospital continuously on telemetry. If arrhythmias are thought to be a causative factor in patients with transient symptoms, the crucial information needed is the recording of an ECG during the exact time the symptom is occurring. With such a recording, one can determine whether the symptom is related to an arrhythmia.

 Key Points

- Normal ECG parameters include:
  Heart rate: 60 to 100 bpm.
  Heart rhythm: regular.
  P waves: upright.
  PR interval: 0.12 to 0.20 seconds.
  QRS duration: 0.06 to 0.12 seconds.
  QT interval: <0.40 seconds.

- Waveforms and what they represent:
  The P wave represents atrial depolarization.
  The QRS wave represents ventricular depolarization.
  The T wave represents ventricular repolarization.

- Tips for interpreting AV block
  AV blocks delay or prevent the atrial impulse from reaching the ventricles.
  First degree AV blocks are characterized by a prolonged PR interval of more than 0.20
    seconds (one large square).
  Second degree AV blocks are characterized by some P waves with a dropped QRS.
  Second degree type I blocks have PR intervals that are progressively longer until a QRS is
    dropped.
  Second degree type II blocks have PR intervals that are constant but occasionally drop a QRS.
  Third degree blocks are "complete" AV blocks; P waves are completely dissociated from the
    QRS waves; the typical ventricular heart rate is 30 to 40 bpm.

Key Points   *continued*

- Characteristics of atrial fibrillation:
  Atrial rate is greater than 350 to 450 bpm.
  Atrial and ventricular rhythms are usually irregular.
  Instead of P waves to represent atrial activity, a chaotic pattern of "fib waves" is seen.

- Characteristics of atrial flutter:
  Atrial rate is between 250 to 350 bpm.
  Atrial rhythm is regular.
  Instead of a P wave, a continuous "saw-tooth" baseline between the QRS waves is seen.

- Characteristics of V tach
  QRS complexes are wide and typically regular.
  Ventricular rate is rapid (greater than 250 to 350 bpm).
  Looks "more organized" than V fib.
  Patients may or may not have a pulse with the rhythm.

- Characteristics of V fib
  Lethal, chaotic, disorganized ECG activity is seen.
  No clearly identifiable QRS complexes or P waves are found.
  V fib requires immediate defibrillation or CPR if defibrillator is not readily available. The nurse should "call a code."

Internet Resources

New York Emergency Nurse RN: Arrhythmias, Dysrhythmias, EKG, Echocardiograms:
http://www.nyerrn.com/h/a.htm#rhythm

The Alan E. Lindsay ECG Learning Center in CyberSpace: ACC/AHA Clinical Competence in ECG Diagnosis:
http://www-medlib.med.utah.edu/kw/ecg/ACC_AHA.html

Essential Information for Physicians: Physicians:
http://www.themdsite.com/physicians.cfm

Bibliography

Braunwald E, Fauci AS, Hauser SL, et al: Harrison's principles of internal medicine, ed 15, 2002, New York, McGraw Hill.

Falk RH: Atrial fibrillation, *N Engl J Med* 344:1067-1078, 2001.

Fenton JM: The clinician's approach to evaluating patients with dysrhythmias. In Morton PG, Manno D, Apple S: Cardiovascular nursing, *AACN Clin Issues Adv Pract Acute Crit Care Cardiovasc Nurs* 12(1):72-86, 2001.

Go AS, Hylek EM, Phillips KA et al: Prevalence of diagnosed atrial fibrillation in adults: national implications for rhythm management and stroke prevention: the AnTicoagulation and Risk Factors in Atrial Fibrillation (ATRIA) study, *JAMA* 285:2370-2375, 2001.

Gregoratos G et al: ACC/AHA guidelines for implantation of cardiac pacemakers and antiarrhythmia devices, executive summary, *Circulation* 97:1325-1335, 1998.

Hayes DL: Indications for pacemakers and ICDs. In Hayes DL, Lloyd MA, Friedman PA: *Cardiac pacing and defibrillation: a clinical approach,* Armonk, NY, 2000, Futura, pp 87-124.

Josephson ME, Zimetbaum P, Marchlinski FE et al: The bradyarrhythmias: disorders of sinus node function and AV conduction disturbances. In Braunwald E, Fauci AS, Isselbacher KI et al: *Harrison's principles of internal medicine,* 2001, New York, McGraw-Hill, pp 1253-1278.

Jung F, DiMarco J: Treatment strategies for atrial fibrillation, *Am J Med* 104(3):272-286, 1998.

Kosinski D, Grubb BP, Wolfe DA, Mayhew H: Catheter ablation for atrial flutter and fibrillation, *Postgrad Med* 103(1):103-106, 1998.

Levy S, Breithardt G, Campbell RWF et al: Atrial fibrillation: current knowledge and recommendations for management, *Eur Heart J* 19:1294-1320, 1998.

Chapter 14

Valvular Heart Disease

John Stover

1. What is the purpose of the mitral, aortic, tricuspid, and pulmonic valves?

The purpose of each of the four cardiac valves is to provide a one-way valve or doorway to maintain a forward flow of blood through the heart and to prevent mixing of unoxygenated blood with oxygenated blood and to prevent stasis.

Valve	Purpose: to provide one-way valve or doorway between:	Normally open during:
Mitral valve	Left atrium and left ventricle	Ventricular diastole
Aortic valve	Left ventricle and aorta and systemic circulation	Ventricular systole
Tricuspid valve	Right atrium and right ventricle	Ventricular diastole
Pulmonic valve	Right ventricle and pulmonary artery	Ventricular systole

2. What are common terms to describe a diseased valve?

Because the valve supplies a doorway for blood to flow through, several problems can occur in any of the four valves. Valvular regurgitation or insufficiency is referred to as a "leaky valve" because blood is allowed to flow back through the valve during the time it should be closed, therefore allowing blood to backup when higher pressures are achieved. Valvular stenosis is referred to as a "tight valve" because the valve remains partially blocked when it should be fully opened, therefore restricting blood flow. Another term used to describe valvular disease is sclerosis. Sclerosis refers to the thickening of the valve *without* obstruction of blood flow, causing a murmur but no symptoms.

3. What are the most common valvular disorders in adults?

Mitral valve prolapse is the most common valvular heart disease in adults, affecting 2% to 6% of the population. However, more mitral valve disease than is reported is possible because of the lack of symptoms of mitral valve disease and the characteristics of a "flow murmur," which may decrease the likelihood of a diagnostic study for these patients.

4. What are causes of valvular heart disease?

The incidence rate of congenital valvular heart disease has remained nearly constant in recent decades at about 0.6% of births, but acquired valvular heart disease has increased despite improved prevention of rheumatic heart disease. Part of the increase in acquired heart disease is the increase in the elderly population and better diagnostic techniques for identification of valvular heart disease. The following table lists some of the common causes of valvular heart disease.

Causes of valvular heart disease

Pulmonary Valve Disease	Aortic Valve Disease	Mitral Valve Disease	Tricuspid Valve Disease
Congenital heart disease			
Bicuspid valve Quadracuspid valve Valve prolapse from ventricular septal defect Tetralogy of Fallot Absent pulmonary valve Atrial septal defects Hypoplastic right ventricle	Bicuspid valve Tricuspid valve Storage diseases, such as Hurler's syndrome or xanthomatoses Ehlers-Danlos syndrome	Cleft leaflet Transposed valve Storage diseases, such as Hurler's syndrome or xanthomatoses	Ebstein's anomaly Congenital atresia Ehlers-Danlos syndrome
Inflammatory/Infective			
Rheumatic heart disease (rare) Syphilis (extremely rare) Endocarditis (extremely rare)	Rheumatic heart disease Bacterial endocarditis Ankylosing spondylitis Syphilis Rheumatoid arthritis (rare)	Rheumatic heart disease Systemic lupus erythematosus Anticardiolipin syndrome Endocarditis Rheumatoid arthritis (rare)	Infective endocarditis Rheumatic heart disease
Myocardial/Vascular disease			
Pulmonary hypertension Idiopathic dilation of pulmonary artery Carcinoid syndrome	Aortic dissection Idiopathic dilation (annuloaortic ectasia)	Myocardial infarction/ ischemia Chordae rupture Cardiomyopathy	Pulmonary hypertension Right ventricular failure Mitral valve disease Carcinoid syndrome

Causes of valvular heart disease *continued*			
Pulmonary Valve Disease	**Aortic Valve Disease**	**Mitral Valve Disease**	**Tricuspid Valve Disease**
Degenerative			
	Calcification of valve Marfan syndrome Myxomatous degeneration Arteriosclerosis	Myxomatous degeneration Mitral valve prolapse Traumatic mitral regurgitation	Myxomatous degeneration (tricuspid valve prolapse)
Other			
	Diet drugs	Diet drugs	Diet drugs

5. How is valvular heart disease most commonly diagnosed?

Valvular heart disease is most commonly diagnosed with cardiac auscultation by an experienced health care provider. A murmur heard with auscultation may help to identify valvular heart disease (see Chapter 2, Physical Examination of the Cardiovascular Patient). However, physical exam is not enough to diagnose the lesion with certainty or to determine the degree of involvement. During the past two decades, the diagnosis of valvular heart disease has improved dramatically. Several different techniques are currently used in the diagnosis of valvular heart disease:

- Transthoracic echocardiogram (TTE)
  - Noninvasive
  - Painless
  - Limited by body habitus
- Transesophageal echocardiogram (TEE)
  - Invasive
  - Requires sedation
  - Potential complications
- Cardiac catheterization
  - Should not be the first line test
  - Invasive with potential complications
  - Radiotracers and fluoroscopy
  - Visualization of the coronary arteries at the same time
  - More accurate than TTE
- Radionuclide ventriculogram
  - Uses radiotracer and nuclear medicine
  - Measures flow through valves; no actual visualization of valves
  - Mildly invasive

6. What is mitral regurgitation (MR)?

Mitral regurgitation occurs when blood from the left ventricle moves back across the closed but misaligned mitral valve into the left atrium during ventricular systole (a leaky valve). MR can occur when the leaflet of the mitral valve becomes misaligned from multiple causes (see the table in Question 4). These causes can be grouped into primary and secondary causes and congenital or acquired causes. The primary causes of MR occur when any of the four components of the mitral valve apparatus (the mitral annulus, the chordae tendineae, the papillary muscles, or the mitral leaflets) are abnormal. Common causes of primary regurgitation include rheumatic heart disease, mitral valve prolapse (frequently hereditary), endocarditis, spontaneous rupture, or infarct of the chordae tendineae. Secondary causes of MR occur when the shape of the left ventricle dilates and causes misalignment of the papillary muscles. Secondary causes of mitral valve disease include left ventricular hypertrophy from hypertension, idiopathic cardiomyopathy, and congestive heart failure. Acquired heart disease occurs at any time after birth when the mitral valve was previously healthy without abnormalities. The most common cause of acquired mitral valve prolapse is rheumatic heart disease. Congenital heart disease occurs in fetal development and causes misalignment of the valves before birth.

7. Why is the left ventricular ejection fraction (LVEF) falsely elevated in MR?

In MR, the LVEF may be falsely elevated because part of the volume of the ventricle is forced back into the left atrium instead of progressing to the aorta. This condition decreases the efficiency of the left ventricle while initially increasing preload, which is wasted or ineffective cardiac output that causes a backup of volume into the left atrium, the pulmonary system, and subsequently the right ventricle.

8. What are the consequences of MR if untreated?

In acute causes of MR, the left atrium and ventricle do not have time to compensate by becoming larger (dilated) or thicker (hypertrophic), which usually causes acute right ventricular failure and eventually increases afterload. In chronic MR, the atrial and ventricular hypertrophy is a compensatory mechanism of the heart causing remodeling in an attempt to compensate for the higher atrial volumes presented to the left ventricle as preload. However, the forward stroke volumes from the left ventricle actually decrease. During compensation, MR may be asymptomatic and left ventricular function may be normal. However, the compensation may cause a worsening of the secondary causes of regurgitation as the ventricle enlarges causing worsening alignment of the valve from papillary displacement; therefore the condition is likely to become symptomatic. Also, if the ventricle becomes hypertrophic (thicker) without dilating, worsening diastolic dysfunction may develop. The stretching and remodeling of the atrium predisposes the patient to atrial arrhythmias such as atrial fibrillation or flutter.

9. What is mitral valve stenosis (MS)?

Mitral valve stenosis causes narrowing of the opening created by the mitral valve (a tight valve) during ventricular filling in early ventricular diastole. The normal cross-sectional area of the mitral valve is 4 cm^2. Most patients are not symptomatic until the mitral valve area is decreased by 75% to less than 1.0 cm^2. Blood flow builds up in the left atrium and backs up into the pulmonary system and subsequently to the right ventricle. With MS, a pressure gradient develops as the pressure in the left atrium becomes higher than that of the left ventricle during ventricular diastole. The smaller the opening in the mitral valve, the higher the pressure gradient. Unlike MR, MS does not initially cause an increased demand on the left ventricle, so left ventricular hypertrophy does not develop until much later.

10. What are the consequences of MS if untreated?

Some pulmonary hypertension and right ventricular hypertrophy are likely. The LVEF remains high, but the stroke volume decreases as the stenosis worsens because the volume presented or available to the left ventricle (preload) is significantly reduced. The left atrium is also likely to become enlarged (hypertrophy). Fortunately, sudden cardiac death from *asymptomatic* MS or regurgitation has not been reported.

11. What are symptoms of MR and MS?

The symptoms of MR and MS are related to the congestion of the pulmonary system and the remodeling of the heart. Although MS is more likely to cause pulmonary hypertension, the symptoms are virtually identical. The symptoms are not necessarily related to the severity of the disease. Some people may have symptoms with moderate disease, and others may not have symptoms with severe disease. Many people with MR/MS do not have symptoms until many years after valvular disease develops.

12. What is the treatment for MR and MS?

Treatment for mitral valve dysfunction depends on the severity of the symptoms. Treatments are most likely to focus on the diminishment of the symptoms and the prevention of deterioration of the valve from secondary causes, such as endocarditis. MS or MR may lead to systemic emboli that cause myocardial infarction, cerebrovascular accidents, or ischemia wherever the emboli lodge. Emboli are more common for MS than for MR, unless atrial fibrillation exists with the MR. However, both MR and MS have higher rates of systemic emboli than any other *native* valve diseases. Therefore systemic anticoagulation therapy may be needed for patients with MS or MR (see Chapter 29, Chronic Anticoagulation). Patients with MR and MS also need to take prophylactic antibiotics to prevent subacute bacterial endocarditis (SBE) before nonsterile procedures (see Question 29). Rate control is needed if atrial fibrillation develops. Beta-blockers, digoxin, or calcium channel blockers may be used for rate control.

Diuretics are used to decrease dyspnea caused by congestion of the pulmonary system. Some other medical therapies being studied include afterload reduction with angiotensin-converting enzyme inhibitors, angiotensin II blockers, or hydralazine. These agents may help reduce the left ventricular pressure by reducing systemic vascular resistance to decrease the amount of regurgitation into the left atrium for MR but would not be as helpful in MS alone. Also, surgery for valve replacement or repair in either MS or MR or balloon valvuloplasty for MS is recommended for the patients who are symptomatic patients and need medical treatment. Valvuloplasty is less invasive than surgery but is not effective for MR.

13. What is mitral valve prolapse?

Mitral valve prolapse is caused by an anatomic abnormality of the mitral valve leaflets, supporting chordae, or both, causing the leaflets to buckle back into the left atrium during ventricular systole. This causes a mid to late systolic click to be heard as the chordae are stretched tight and may allow for MR. The exact cause is unknown, but evidence exists for a hereditary cause, which is more common in females.

14. What is mitral valve prolapse syndrome?

Some patients with mitral valve prolapse have chest pain without ischemia. The exact mechanism is not fully known, but beta-blockers are the drug of choice to decrease symptoms. Other symptoms of mitral valve prolapse syndrome include fatigue, shortness of breath, dizziness, and anxiety.

15. What is aortic stenosis (AS)?

Aortic stenosis may be caused by valvular AS (70%), subvalvular (14%), supravalvular (8%), or mixed stenosis (8%). AS causes restriction of the blood flow from the left ventricle, which increases the workload of the ventricle during systole and increases end diastolic pressures and stress.

16. What are the consequences of aortic stenosis (AS)?

Aortic stenosis leads to compensatory and noncompensatory remodeling of the left ventricle. Compensatory remodeling increases the muscle of the left ventricle to help create the increased pressure needed to overcome the level of stenosis. Unfortunately, as the ventricular muscles continue to become larger (hypertrophy), the capacity for volume of the left ventricle also decreases, creating diastolic dysfunction. The ventricle may also attempt to increase its volume, creating dilated cardiomyopathy that can lead to systolic dysfunction. Frequently the heart rate also increases in an attempt to increase cardiac output with smaller forward stroke volumes. Patients may also have a wide pulse pressure from the high systolic pressure necessary to pass blood through the valve followed by a sharp decline in the diastolic pressure from closure of the valve.

17. Why can AS lead to myocardial ischemia and chest pain?

The aortic sinuses supply the coronary arteries (giving oxygen to the heart itself) and are located just distal to the aortic valve. These arteries fill during diastole and are closed during the higher pressure systole. In AS, the pressure in the aorta around the aortic sinuses during diastole (when the coronary arteries are filling) is lower than normal, which means that a risk of less blood flow to the coronary arteries exists. When this condition is combined with tachycardia (decreased filling time), coronary artery disease, or acute changes in the cardiac demand, one can see why AS is the most dangerous valvular disease. This is the mechanism that may lead to angina with AS. Sudden death has been associated with symptomatic AS. No reported studies show sudden death in asymptomatic AS. However, anecdotal reports of athletes dying of asymptomatic subaortic stenosis are found.

18. What is the treatment for AS?

The medical treatment for AS is limited to antibiotic prophylaxis for SBE in patients who are asymptomatic. For patients with symptoms, surgery is the treatment of choice. From the onset of symptoms until surgery, nitrates may be used to relieve angina; vasodilators may be used to decrease systemic vascular resistance, and oxygen may be necessary. After the onset of symptoms of AS, the average survival is less than 3 years without surgery; therefore prompt surgical intervention is recommended for patients with symptomatic AS. Balloon valvuloplasty is used in the pediatric population but has only a limited role in adult AS.

19. What is aortic valve insufficiency (AI) or regurgitation (AR)?

Aortic insufficiency or AR refers to the leaking of blood back through a closed but incompetent aortic valve (leaky valve). AI or AR causes a portion of the cardiac output to flow back into the left ventricle, thereby increasing the diastolic volumes and stress on the ventricle.

20. What are the consequences of untreated AI?

The retrograde flow leads to compensatory and noncompensatory left ventricular remodeling as with AS. This condition also leads to signs of diastolic and systolic congestive heart failure.

21. What is the treatment for AI?

The medical treatment for AI is vasodilators in patients who are symptomatic with dilated left ventricles for reduction of systolic blood pressure to normal, which theoretically improves the forward flow of blood by reducing systemic vascular resistance. So far, nifedipine and hydralazine have been used, but angiotensin-converting enzyme inhibitors may also be of benefit, especially in congestive heart failure. No evidence supports treatment of patients who are asymptomatic. Patients who are symptomatic with AR are also recommended to undergo surgical replacement of the aortic valve when possible.

22. What are some causes of tricuspid dysfunction?

Tricuspid disease is much less common than either aortic or mitral valve disease. Tricuspid disease frequently is caused by mitral valve disease or occurs concurrently with mitral valve disease. The common causes of tricuspid valve disease include pulmonary hypertension, right ventricular dysfunction, MS, and rheumatic heart disease (see the table in Question 4). The clinical presentation of tricuspid disease is similar to that of mitral and aortic valve disease. With tricuspid disease, the right atrium is likely to enlarge from congestion of the blood flow. Right atrial pressures may also rise.

23. Why is mitral valve disease frequently associated with tricuspid stenosis (TS)?

Tricuspid stenosis is almost always related to rheumatic heart disease, which is why the mitral valve is usually also affected.

24. What is the treatment for tricuspid regurgitation (TR) or TS?

Treatment of the underlying cause of TR may be enough to resolve the regurgitation. For example, treatments to improve MS or MR may decrease the pulmonary congestion and therefore decrease the pulmonary vascular resistance, allowing for more forward progression of the blood flow. Frequently, the tricuspid valve is repaired when the mitral valve is repaired or replaced if needed. For TS, the choices of treatment are balloon valvuloplasty or surgery (annuloplasty or replacement). Balloon valvuloplasty, however, may cause severe TR. In cases in which the tricuspid valve is not amenable to annuloplasty, a tricuspid replacement may be performed. Use of a bioprosthetic valve is recommended because of higher rate of thromboembolic events reported with mechanical valves in the tricuspid position.

25. What are common problems associated with the pulmonic valve?

Disease of the pulmonic valve is most commonly congenital and stenotic and only rarely occurs from acquired causes. As with AS, the outflow tract (in this case, the pulmonary artery) may be the cause of subvalvular, supravalvular, or branch pulmonary artery stenosis. This condition occurs with congenital disease and mimics valvular stenosis. Pulmonary insufficiency can also occur, but it is more rare and frequently occurs as a result of balloon valvuloplasty of the pulmonic valve.

26. What are symptoms of pulmonary stenosis and insufficiency?

Patients with pulmonary stenosis may remain asymptomatic even when disease is moderate to severe. Some patients may have symptoms of right heart failure with peripheral edema because of severe right ventricular dysfunction, syncope, lightheadedness, or chest pain. If an intraatrial or intraventricular shunt exists, the patient may have cyanosis from a right to left shunt of unoxygenated blood. Patients with pulmonary insufficiency may also be asymptomatic or have mild dyspnea with exertion.

27. What is the management for pulmonary stenosis and insufficiency?

Management for pulmonary stenosis depends on the symptoms. Diuretics and digoxin may be useful to decrease venous congestion until surgery or balloon valvuloplasty can be performed. Congenital pulmonary stenosis may be treated with surgery or balloon valvuloplasty. Diuretics or digoxin or surgical replacement if needed can be used to treat pulmonary insufficiency.

28. What are some key nursing assessments for patients with valvular heart disease?

The assessment of the patient with valvular heart disease is the same for each type of valvular disease, although the findings differ according to the valve involved. The subjective history is useful in determination of the severity of the disease on the patient's ability to accomplish daily activities and gives a sense of quality of life. The subjective history should include information about exercise tolerance, symptoms, duration of the disease, characteristics of the disease, and factors that affect symptoms. When symptoms are discussed, whether the patient is able to lie down flat at night or whether the patient needs to elevate the bed or sleep on two or more pillows to prop up the chest (orthopnea) should be determined. Orthopnea is more common with mitral or aortic valve disease but can be seen with any valvular disease. Whether the patient has symptoms of paroxysmal nocturnal dyspnea, which is more common in tricuspid or pulmonic disease but can also occur with mitral or aortic disease, is also important. Other symptoms for inquiry include swelling in the ankles or feet (or along the back if the patient is on bed rest), fatigue, syncope, palpitations or fluttering in the chest, chest pain, dizziness, a feeling of abdominal bloating (which may represent liver or spleen congestion or ascites), or a history of atrial fibrillation or flutter. A history of the disease itself should also be obtained. Does the patient know the results of the last echocardiogram or cardiac study? What is the current treatment for valvular heart disease? Is there a history of emboli or endocarditis?

29. When are prophylactic antibiotics prescribed in valvular heart disease?

For most patients with acquired or congenital heart disease, prophylactic antibiotics are recommended before an invasive procedure that may produce bacteremia. Prophylactic antibiotics are ordered to prevent fatal, although rare, endocardial infections. These infections may occur when the endothelial lining of the valves are damaged, especially when a high-velocity jet is present (which is created by severe stenosis of the high pressure valves). When the endothelial lining is damaged, platelets and fibrin deposit on the area of damage and present an area where bacteria can adhere and multiply, causing endocarditis. SBE does not present an immediate problem, but if left untreated, it does progress to fatal cardiomyopathy. Acute endocarditis is a medical emergency and requires prompt intravenous treatment to prevent infectious emboli and permanent heart damage. Patients with trivial regurgitation or stenosis and some patients with mitral valve prolapse without regurgitation are not given prophylactic antibiotics because the risk of side effects outweighs the risk of development of endocarditis. In general, prophylactic antibiotics are needed only for nonsterile procedures in which the respiratory, genitourinary, or gastrointestinal tracts are interrupted and for dental procedures in which bleeding is likely to occur.

30. What are the current guidelines for SBE prophylaxis?

The American Heart Association (AHA) has published guidelines for the prevention of endocarditis. Treatment is needed for procedures that are likely to introduce bacteria into the bloodstream (bacteremia). For this reason, some of the less invasive procedures (dental extractions, cystoscopy, rigid bronchoscopy) *do* require prophylactic antibiotics although more invasive procedures (abdominal aortic aneurysm repair, coronary artery bypass grafting, craniotomy) *do not* require prophylactic antibiotics for the prevention of SBE.

The bacterial flora of the upper gastrointestinal tract and oropharynx and respiratory tract are similar and respond to the same antibiotics (generally amoxicillin or ampicillin). Procedures involving the genitourinary tract or lower gastrointestinal tract may require additional antibiotics for high-risk valvular disease (generally ampicillin and gentamicin). See the AHA guidelines to prevention of SBE for full details.

See the following boxes for a brief summary of the current antibiotic guidelines of the AHA for SBE prophylaxis. See the Internet Resource Box for a link to the AHA website.

Dental procedures for which endocarditis prophylaxis is recommended (for patients with moderate and high-risk cardiac conditions)

- Dental extraction
- Periodontal procedures, including surgery, scaling and root planing, probing, and recall maintenance
- Endodontic (root canal) instrumentation or surgery only beyond the apex
- Subgingival placement of antibiotic fibers or strips
- Initial placement of orthodontic bands but not brackets
- Intraligamentary local anesthetic injections
- Prophylactic cleaning of teeth or implants in which bleeding is anticipated

Other procedures for which endocarditis prophylaxis is recommended

Respiratory tract
- Tonsillectomy or adenoidectomy
- Surgical operations that involve respiratory mucosa
- Bronchoscopy with a rigid bronchoscope

Gastrointestinal tract (prophylaxis is recommended for patients at high risk; it is optional for patients at moderate risk)
- Sclerotherapy for esophageal varices
- Esophageal stricture dilation
- Endoscopic retrograde cholangiography with biliary obstruction
- Biliary tract surgery
- Surgical operations that involve intestinal mucosa

Genitourinary tract
- Prostatic surgery
- Cystoscopy
- Urethral dilation

Cardiac conditions associated with endocarditis

High-risk category
- Prosthetic cardiac valves, including bioprosthetic and homograft valves
- Previous bacterial endocarditis
- Complex cyanotic congenital heart disease (e.g., single ventricle states, transposition of the great arteries, tetralogy of Fallot)
- Surgically constructed systemic pulmonary shunts or conduits

Moderate-risk category
- Most other congenital cardiac malformations (other than previously mentioned)
- Acquired valvar dysfunction (e.g., rheumatic heart disease)
- Hypertrophic cardiomyopathy
- Mitral valve prolapse with valvar regurgitation or thickened leaflets

Antibiotic guidelines for patients at risk who undergo dental, oral, respiratory tract, or esophageal procedures

Standard general prophylaxis*
- Amoxicillin: adults, 2.0 g (children, 50 mg/kg) orally 1 hour before procedure

Antibiotic guidelines for patients at risk who undergo dental, oral, respiratory tract, or esophageal procedures *continued*

For patients unable to take oral medications
- Ampicillin: adults, 2.0 g (children, 50 mg/kg) intramuscularly (IM) or intravenously (IV) within 30 minutes before procedure

For patients allergic to amoxicillin/ampicillin/penicillin
- Clindamycin: adults, 600 mg (children, 20 mg/kg) orally 1 hour before procedure
-OR-
- Cephalexin* or cefadroxil*: adults, 2.0 g (children, 50 mg/kg) orally 1 hour before procedure
-OR-
- Azithromycin or clarithromycin: adults, 500 mg (children, 15 mg/kg) orally 1 hour before procedure

For patients allergic to amoxicillin/ampicillin/penicillin and unable to take oral medications
- Clindamycin: adults, 600 mg (children, 20 mg/kg) IV within 30 minutes before procedure
-OR-
- Cefazolin†: adults, 1.0 g (children, 25 mg/kg) IM or IV within 30 minutes before procedure

*Children's dose should not exceed adult doses; follow-up doses are no longer recommended for this category.
†Cephalosporins should not be used in patients with immediate-type hypersensitivity reactions to penicillins.

For patients at risk who are undergoing genitourinary/gastrointestinal procedures

Patients at high risk:
- Ampicillin plus gentamicin: Ampicillin: adults, 2.0 g (children, 50 mg/kg) plus gentamicin 1.5 mg/kg (for both adults and children, not to exceed 120 mg) IM or IV within 30 minutes before procedure; follow-up dose: 6 hours later, ampicillin (adults 1.0 g; children, 25 mg/kg) IM or IV or amoxicillin (adults, 1.0 g; children, 25 mg/kg) orally

Patients at high risk and allergic to ampicillin/amoxicillin:
- Vancomycin hydrochloride plus gentamicin: Vancomycin (adults, 1.0 g; children, 20 mg/kg) IV for 1 to 2 hours plus gentamicin 1.5 mg/kg (for both adults and children, not to exceed 120 mg) IM or IV; complete injection/infusion within 30 minutes before start of procedure

Patients at moderate risk:
- Amoxicillin: adults, 2.0 g (children, 50 mg/kg) orally 1 hour before procedure
-OR-
- Ampicillin: adults, 2.0 g (children, 50 mg/kg) IM or IV within 30 minutes before procedure

Patients at moderate risk and allergic to ampicillin/amoxicillin:
- Vancomycin: adults, 1.0 g (children, 20 mg/kg) IV for 1 to 2 hours; complete infusion within 30 minutes of start of the procedure

Note: for patients already taking an antibiotic or for other special situations, refer to the full statement included in the reference of this chapter "Prevention of Bacterial Endocarditis: Recommendations by the American Heart Association."

31. **When is anticoagulation therapy necessary for patients with valvular heart disease?**

Not all valvular disease necessitates anticoagulation therapy. Damage to the mitral valve from rheumatic heart disease is more likely to cause a thrombus and produce emboli than any other damage to the native valves. This may be partially because the left atrium has a lower pressure that allows blood to pool for longer periods of time than in the ventricles. Some evidence exists that platelet survival times may also be affected by rheumatic MS or regurgitation, which may also lead to clotting. Atrial fibrillation in mitral valve disease increases the risk for systemic emboli by 700%. AS or AR without associated mitral valve disease does not usually require long term anticoagulation. Evidence does support use of long-term anticoagulation therapy for mechanical prosthetic valves in any position but especially with tricuspid or mitral positions. A wide degree of variation is found in the methods of anticoagulation therapy used to prevent emboli (see Chapter 29, Chronic Anticoagulation). For bioprosthetic valves, an aspirin may be sufficient to prevent thromboembolic events. As the bioprosthetic valve becomes older, it may become rougher and degenerated and may require additional anticoagulation therapy for prophylaxis. Again, if the patient has atrial fibrillation, the risk of emboli even with bioprosthesis increases. Anticoagulation therapy is a delicate balance of management of the risks of bleeding against the risks of emboli.

32. **What signs should not be missed for patients with newly diagnosed valvular heart disease?**
    • Conditions that may cause increased workload to the heart, which may mimic or exacerbate valvular disease, should be checked. These conditions include hyperthyroidism, arrhythmias, pregnancy, exercise, and anemia. Patients can have loud cardiac murmurs with any of these hyperdynamic states, with or without valvular disease.
    • Patients with subaortic stenosis may have sudden death, so they need to undergo annual or biannual evaluation for assessment of risks and for appropriate treatment and management.
    • Patient weight should be monitored. One of the first signs of deterioration in a patient's condition may be an abrupt increase in weight.
    • Signs of bleeding in patients undergoing anticoagulation therapy should always be monitored. Also, signs of thromboemboli, especially in patients who have been removed from anticoagulation therapy for prior bleeding or for an upcoming procedure or surgery, should be monitored.
    • The physical assessment findings of murmurs should always be documented for comparison of the findings with future findings for determination of whether a change in condition has occurred.
    • One should practice, practice, practice listening to heart sounds to become familiar with both normal and abnormal heart sounds and timing of the heart sounds.

33. **What is important patient or family teaching for valvular heart disease?**
    • Activity/exercise
      • Patients need to know in what exercises they can participate.

- Patients should pace activities to decrease fatigue.
- Patients with aortic valve disease should limit exercise and activities to prevent sudden death or cardiac ischemia. However, they should continue to be active with walking and activities that do not produce symptoms.
- Fluid balance
  - The head of the bed should be elevated on stable supports as needed.
  - The patients should be instructed on how to weigh themselves each morning at the same time with an empty bladder wearing the same clothes or naked for early signs of deterioration.
  - The legs should be elevated several times during the day to prevent peripheral edema of the legs and to decrease the likelihood of paroxysmal nocturnal dyspnea by allowing the heart more time to deal with fluid levels.
  - The patients need to understand the importance of following fluid restrictions, sodium restrictions, and medications if ordered to improve symptoms.
  - Smaller, more frequent meals are necessary when symptoms of bloating or gastric fullness appear from venous congestion.
- Prevention of SBE
  - The appropriate use of prophylactic antibiotics to prevent SBE is essential. (Preprinted wallet-sized cards are available for this purpose.)
  - The importance of dental hygiene and regular dental restoration and prophylactic cleanings by a dentist to help prevent complications should be discussed.
- Signs that should be reported immediately
  - Patients should be instructed to immediately call 911 if symptoms of a stroke or cerebrovascular accident develop.
  - Patients should be instructed to promptly report any symptoms of atrial fibrillation to their health care provider.

34. What are new advances on the horizon?

Transvascular echocardiography is an invasive form of ultrasound currently being developed and tested in the United States. This new procedure promises to give much clearer images than TEE or TTE with placement of the transducer directly into the vessels of the heart, thereby reducing the distance that the sound waves must travel. Transvascular echocardiography may also allow for less or no sedation of the patient when compared with the TEE. It also limits the interference in placement caused by obesity. The potential complications of this new device are similar to the risks of angiography (injury to the myocardium or vasculature, infection, and bleeding) but do not involve radiation or radiographic contrast, which some patients may be allergic to or may not tolerate.

Key Points

- The four valves of the heart act as one-way doors to maintain the forward flow of blood through the heart.
- Damage or dysfunction of the valves may lead to thrombosis or emboli, infection, or congestive heart failure symptoms.
- Of all valvular disease, AS is the most likely to cause myocardial ischemia or infarction from anatomic factors related to filling the coronary arteries.
- People with valvular heart disease likely need some form of anticoagulation therapy and prophylaxis against SBE.

Internet Resources

AHA Subacute bacterial endocarditis prophylaxis wallet card:
http://www.americanheart.org/downloadable/heart/1023826501754walletcard.pdf

Valvular Heart Disease Overview:
http://www.heartcenteronline.com/myheartdr/common/articles.cfm?ARTID=187

ACC/AHA Guidelines for the Management of Patients With Valvular Heart Disease
http://www.acc.org/clinical/guidelines/valvular/dirIndex.htm

Bibliography

Alpert JS, Dalen JE, Rahimtoola SH, editors: *Valvular heart disease*, ed 3, Philadelphia, 2000, Lippincott Williams & Wilkins.

Arnold R, Kitchiner D: Left ventricular outflow tract obstruction, *Arch Dis Child* 72(2):180-183, 1995.

Bonow RO, Carabello B, de Leon AC Jr et al: ACC/AHA guidelines for the management of patients with valvular heart disease: a report of the American College of Cardiology/American Heart Association Task Force on Practice Guidelines (Committee on Management of Patients with Valvular Heart Disease), *J Am Coll Cardiol* 32(5):1486-1588, 1998.

Carabello BA: Aortic stenosis, *N Engl J Med* 246(9):667-682, 2002.

Carabello BA: Indications for valve surgery in asymptomatic patients with aortic and mitral stenosis, *Chest* 108(6):1678-1682, 1995.

Dajani A et al: Prevention of bacterial endocarditis: recommendations by the American Heart Association, *JAMA* 277(22):1794-1801, 1997.

Gould KL: Angina pectoris in aortic stenosis? *Circulation* 95(4):790-792, 1997.

Lester SJ, Heilbron B, Gin K et al: The natural history and rate of progression of aortic stenosis, *Chest* 113(4):1109-1114, 1998.

Otto CM: Evaluation and management of chronic mitral regurgitation, *N Engl J Med* 345(10):740-746, 2001.

Rose AG: Etiology of valvular heart disease, *Curr Opin Cardiol* 11(2):98-113, 1996.

Salem D, Daudelin DH, Levine HJ et al: Antithrombotic therapy in valvular heart disease, *Chest* 119(suppl 1):207S-219S, 2001.

Scordo K: Factors associated with participation in a mitral valve support group, *Heart Lung* 30(2):128-137, 2001.

Deep Vein Thrombosis and Pulmonary Embolism

Penelope Ann Crisp

1. Define deep vein thrombosis (DVT).

Deep vein thrombosis is a blood clot that has formed in a vein. Venous thrombi commonly form at sites of slow or disturbed blood flow. Thrombosis begins as a small deposit of platelets, fibrin, and red cells in valve cusp pockets of a vein, intramuscular sinuses of the leg veins, or venous segments that have been exposed to direct trauma (the femoral vein after hip replacement surgery). When the thrombus enlarges, it occludes the lumen of the vein, blocking blood flow.

2. What are the signs and symptoms of DVT?

The signs and symptoms of DVT are determined by several factors: the location of the venous obstruction, the size of the thrombus, whether the vein lumen is partially or totally obstructed, and the adequacy of the collateral circulation. If the vein lumen is partially obstructed or if collateral flow exists around the obstruction, physical symptoms may be absent. This situation accounts for the 50% of DVTs that are silent and difficult to detect. Patients often have unilateral edema, resulting from congestion of venous, lymphatic, and capillary beds distal to the thrombotic occlusion. Patients have a sudden onset of pain in the calf or foot described as a dull throbbing sensation or a feeling of tightness. If a patient is seen with these symptoms, a DVT should be suspected and ruled out. A positive Homans' sign (calf pain on dorsiflexion of the foot) is not a sensitive or specific test for DVT; the results are positive in 50% of patients with DVT and in 40% without DVT.

3. What are the risk factors for DVT?

- Age >40 years
- Recent surgery
- Obesity
- Malignant disease
- Recent long travel (airplane, car)
- Prolonged bed rest
- Paraplegia
- Birth control pills/estrogen
- Previous history of deep vein thrombosis/pulmonary embolism
- Hypercoagulable states

- Low cardiac output
- Trauma/fracture

4. Which surgical patients are more prone to development of a DVT?

Orthopedic patients are especially prone to thrombosis, particularly those patients with hip fractures or those undergoing hip replacement surgery or knee reconstruction. However, the highest risk group is patients greater than 40 years old, undergoing major surgery of any type, with a history of thromboembolism, malignant disease, or hypercoagulable state.

5. What tests are used in the diagnosis of DVT?

Duplex ultrasonography (the determination of venous flow with a combination of Doppler analysis and B-mode ultrasound) has largely replaced venography for clinical purposes. More than 80% of symptomatic venous thrombi involve the easily interrogated proximal veins. Uniformly high sensitivities of 93% to 97% and specificities of 94% to 99% have been reported for the ultrasound diagnosis of proximal DVT. The Doppler probe can be used at the bedside. Doppler tracks sound waves created by blood moving through the vessel. It can detect the lack of flow, the effect of compression on venous flow, and changes in flow velocity. Magnetic resonance imaging (MRI) is excellent for detection of pelvic and lower extremity thrombi; however, MRI is much more costly than duplex ultrasound.

6. What are the treatment goals for DVT?

The foremost treatment goal is prevention of propagation of the thrombus with anticoagulation or thrombolytic therapy. Patients typically remain on anti-coagulation therapy for 6 months to a year after uncomplicated DVT. Resolution of existing thrombi is accomplished with limiting leg edema with leg elevation at rest. Early ambulation increases venous flow and reduces venous stasis. Graduated compression stockings are useful in prevention of a recurrent DVT; these stockings have the highest amount of compression at the ankle with a gradual decrease in pressure up the leg to the knee level. The stockings are fitted individually to each patient and the level of compression prescribed by a health care provider.

7. What are the complications of DVT?

Two serious complications from DVT include pulmonary embolism (PE) and venous gangrene of the extremity. PE occurs in 35% of patients with untreated DVT. Venous gangrene, specifically called phlegmasia cerulea dolens or "blue leg," represents near total obstruction of venous outflow; this occurs when the leg becomes blocked by the thrombotic process, causing massive swelling and a purple discoloration. Cardiovascular failure is caused by the entrapment of fluids in the extremity; gangrene develops unless venous outflow is established.

8. Define PE.

A PE is a free-floating particle (thrombus) that lodges in a pulmonary artery or arteriole. PEs in most cases (90%) originate from thrombi in the deep venous system of the legs. The clinical significance of PE depends on the size of the embolus and the cardiorespiratory reserve of the patient.

Venous thromboembolism is a single disorder. Therefore the diagnostic approach may be directed toward the legs or the lungs, starting with the least invasive testing and proceeding to more invasive tests. The treatments of venous thrombosis and PE are essentially the same. The risk factors are the same for DVT.

9. What are the complications of PE?

The outcome of a PE is dependent on the size of the embolus. The PE causes severe pulmonary obstruction, which leads to acute hemodynamic complications, right-sided heart failure, and hypoxemia. The obstruction causes a modest increase in pulmonary pressure but a large increase in right atrial and ventricular pressure, which causes right ventricular dilatation and failure. A massive PE is often fatal. Without treatment, approximately 33% of patients who survive an initial PE die of a future embolic episode. This is true regardless of the size of the embolism. Massive PE is one of the most common causes of unexpected death and is second only to coronary artery disease as a cause of sudden unexpected natural death at any age. The diagnosis is unsuspected until autopsy in approximately 80% of cases.

10. What are the signs and symptoms of PE?

PEs are often silent and difficult to detect. The clinical diagnosis of PE is highly unreliable. The classic triad of signs and symptoms of PE (hemoptysis, dyspnea, and chest pain) are neither sensitive nor specific. They occur in fewer than 20% of patients with diagnosis of PE. Of the patients who die of a massive PE, only 60% have dyspnea, 17% have chest pain, and 3% have hemoptysis. However, if these symptoms cannot be proven to have another cause, a diagnosis of PE should be investigated with an objective diagnostic evaluation. Massive PEs that lodge in a major pulmonary artery cause acute hemodynamic collapse, with jugular venous distention (JVD), shortness of breath, tachycardia, hypotension, and chest pain.

11. What tests are used in the diagnosis of PE?

Pulmonary angiography remains the gold standard for the diagnosis of PE. Positive pulmonary angiogram results provide 100% certainty that an obstruction to pulmonary arterial blood flow does exist. Negative pulmonary angiogram results provide greater than 90% certainty in the exclusion of PE. The sensitivity and specificity of MRI are comparable with those of spiral computed tomography (CT; 73% and 97%, respectively). The limitations of MRI include poor sensitivity in subsegmental branches. The major advantage of MRI is its ability in scanning the lungs, inferior vena cava, and lower extremities at the same time.

A chest radiograph, electrocardiogram (ECG), arterial blood gas, and echo-cardiogram (Echo) should be obtained in patients who are hemodynamically stable because all these tests are useful in ruling out other causes of the clinical symptoms or in further supporting the diagnosis of PE. However, these are not diagnostic in and of themselves.

12. What are the treatment goals of PE?

Goals of treatment for PE include: hemodynamic stability, oxygenation, and prevention of recurrent PE by:
- Anticoagulation.
- Thrombolytic therapy.
- Surgical or catheter embolectomy.
- Oxygen, intubation, and mechanical ventilation if needed.

13. How do the goals of anticoagulation and thrombolytic therapy differ?

A DVT is much more likely to produce a PE and should be treated with thrombo-lytics. Thrombolytic therapy is used for treatment of an existing thrombus, in particular an ileofemoral DVT. Anticoagulation, on the other hand, is used as preventative treatment.

14. What is an inferior vena cava (IVC) filter?

An IVC filter creates a vena cava interruption. The most popular technique of vena cava interruption is the endovascular approach with the Greenfield, Nitinol, or Bird's Nest IVC filters. These filters are mesh-like and shaped like a basket cone of wires. This procedure is done in the operating room or in the interventional radiology suite. Local anesthetic is used. A filter is placed percu-taneously through the femoral vein and placed in the vena cava inferior to the renal veins to avoid obstruction of blood from the kidneys. The jugular approach is a second choice of insertion but is used infrequently because of the risk of air embolus, pneumothorax, and carotid artery puncture. Complications after filter placement include air embolism, recurrent PE, or migration of the device.

15. What are the indications for an IVC?

Documented iliofemoral vein thrombosis and:
- Contraindication to anticoagulation therapy (active hemorrhage, brain injury).
- Documented PE during full anticoagulation.
- Free-floating iliofemoral thrombus.
- High-risk condition for fatal PE (severe lung disease).

16. Why is a higher dose of heparin needed in some patients?

In the presence of a large thrombus, more heparin may be needed to achieve effective anticoagulation (partial thromboplastin time, 1.5 × normal) because of the large amount of thrombin in the clot. Body weight, hereditary resistance to anticoagulants, and the amount of heparin binding to the plasma and endothelial cell proteins also affect heparin dosing.

17. What are the nursing interventions for patients with DVT or PE?

- Prevention of DVT/PE by having the patient engage in regular physical activity, avoid extended periods of sitting or standing, and elevate legs to the level of the heart with prolonged sitting.
- If the patients are hospitalized, they should ambulate early and perform active range-of-motion (ROM) leg exercises every hour while awake or perform passive ROM exercises if immobile.
- Identification of risk factors present in the patient that predispose the patient to DVT/PE (trauma, surgery, older age, malignant disease).
- Assessment of all extremities for pain, unilateral edema, erythema, and warmth.
- Monitoring for low-grade fever for detection of thrombophlebitis.
- Patient education about early recognition of DVT/PE.

18. What is the role of sequential compression devices (SCDs) in DVT prevention?

Sequential compression devices are mechanical devices used to prevent DVT. SCDs improve venous pressure and flow, reducing venous stasis in the lower extremities. External compression is applied intermittently with the application of two inflatable sleeves that are connected via air tubes to a pump to the patient's lower leg. This action mimics the pumping action of the musculo-venous pump. Venous pooling and stasis are reduced with the compression device's increase in the velocity of venous flow. SCDs are indicated for patients who cannot use anticoagulant therapy because of bleeding risk. SCDs are often initiated at the time of surgery and continued until the patient is ambulatory and are often combined with anticoagulant therapy in patients at high risk.

 Key Points

- Classic symptoms of DVT include sudden onset of pain in the calf or foot described as a dull throbbing sensation or a feeling of tightness. If a patient is seen with these symptoms, a DVT should be suspected and ruled out.

- A positive Homans' sign (calf pain on dorsiflexion of the foot) is not a sensitive or specific test for DVT. Its results are only positive in 50% of patients with DVT and in 40% without DVT.

- Pulmonary emboli in most cases (90%) originate from thrombi in the deep venous system of the legs. Therefore a patient with DVT has a high index of suspicion for PE.

Internet Resources

Arteriosclerosis, Thrombosis, and Vascular Biology (American Heart Association Journal):
http://atvb.ahajournals.org/

Guide to Anticoagulant Therapy:
http://www.americanheart.org/presenter.jhtml?identifier=1263

DVT Information for Patients:
http://www.svmb.org/patients/dvt.html

Vascular Disease Foundation:
http://www.vdf.org

Bibliography

Aquila A: Deep vein thrombosis, *J Cardiovasc Nurs* 15(4):25-44, 2001.

Byrne B: Deep vein thrombosis prophylaxis: the effectiveness and implications of using below knee or thigh-length graduated compression stockings, *Heart Lung* 30(4):277-284, 2001.

Clagett G: What's new in vascular surgery, *J Am Coll Surg* 194:165-193, 2002.

Feied C, Handler J: Pulmonary embolism, *E Med J* 3(1):1-30, 2002.

Greenfield L: Pulmonary embolism. In Cronenwett J, Rutherford R, editors: *Decision making in vascular surgery,* Philadelphia, 2001, WB Saunders.

Hull R, Pineo G: Venous thromboembolism and chronic venous disorders. In Loscalzo J, Creager M, Dzau V, editors: *Vascular medicine: a textbook of vascular biology and diseases,* Boston, 1996, Little, Brown, pp 1051-1069.

Kahn S: The clinical diagnosis of deep venous thrombosis: integrating incidence, risk factors and symptoms and signs, *Arch Intern Med* 158:2315-2323, 1998.

Kelly K, Rudd A, Hunt B et al: Anticoagulation in acute pulmonary embolism, *Arch Intern Med* 162(10):2148-2153, 2002.

Chapter 16

Congenital Heart Disease

Kari L. Crawford

1. What is congenital heart disease (CHD), and how common is it?

Congenital heart disease (also called congenital heart defect) is a group of diseases in which heart defects may affect heart chambers, valves, and the great vessels and veins arising from the heart. One aspect of the heart may be affected, or combinations of multiple abnormalities/anomalies may be seen.

CHD is the leading cause of birth defect–related deaths in children and affects eight of every 1000 newborns. The cause of these defects is unknown in about 90% of the cases.

2. What are some of the important events in the history of CHD that have helped these patients to survive?

In late 1930s, Dr. R. Gross successfully ligated a patent ductus arteriosus (PDA) and opened the era of congenital heart surgery. Another important event was the creation of the Blalock-Taussig shunt in 1945. This aorta-pulmonary shunt augmented pulmonary blood flow and allowed children with cyanotic heart disease to survive once the PDA closed. And in the 1970s, the use of alprostadil (prostaglandin E_1 [PGE_1]) rose to the forefront of pediatric cardiology and changed the field dramatically. Alprostadil is an intravenous medication that vasodilates vascular and ductus arterious smooth muscle, which allows the PDA to stay open and provide pulmonary or systemic blood flow (depending on the cardiac lesion). Thus the ductus remains open for infants with ductal-dependent lesions (see the following table) until surgery is performed. This great advance has allowed many infants to survive to surgery and eventually into adulthood.

Common Ductal-Dependent Lesions	Likelihood of Living Into Adulthood
Critical coarctation of aorta	Yes
Pulmonary atresia	Yes
Transposition of great arteries	Yes
Tetralogy of Fallot (with severe pulmonary stenosis or pulmonary atresia)	Yes
Tricuspid atresia	Yes
Hypoplastic left heart syndrome	Currently 20s at best
Interrupted aortic arch	Yes

All lesions may need further interventions, and some may need medical management of hypertension and atrial arrhythmias.

3. Which patients are most likely to survive into adulthood?

This question is currently a popular research topic. With more than 50 years of advances in the field, more and more infants and children with CHD are surviving into adulthood. More than 85% of patients are estimated to be likely to reach adulthood. Naturally those numbers depend on the complexity of the defect.

4. What are the most common types of heart defects?

Heart defects can be generally classified into the following three categories: obstruction to systemic blood flow, increased pulmonary blood flow, and decreased pulmonary blood flow. (See the table in Question 7.)

5. What does obstruction to systemic blood flow mean?

Obstruction to systemic blood flow is the inability of enough blood to reach the body because of a physical obstruction that prevents blood from ejecting from the heart. The condition results in low cardiac output.

6. What does increased pulmonary blood flow mean?

This condition is the most common physiologic effect. Blood flow is shunted from the left side of the heart to the right side (left to right shunt) in most cases, thus increasing the blood flow returning to the lungs. This is evidenced by signs of congestive heart failure (CHF).

7. What is meant by decreased pulmonary blood flow?

This condition is just the opposite of that described in the previous question. Blood flow is anatomically obstructed and reaches the lungs in smaller amounts or not at all. This is demonstrated by desaturation (mild to severe) of the blood. See the following table.

Obstruction to Systemic Blood Flow	Increased Pulmonary Blood Flow	Decreased Pulmonary Blood Flow
Aortic stenosis: narrowing of aorta at, below, or above valve	Patent ductus arteriosus: communication between aorta and pulmonary artery	Pulmonary stenosis: narrowing of pulmonary artery at, below, or above valve
Coarctation of aorta: narrowing of portion of descending aorta aorta	Atrial septal defect: communication between right and left atrium	Pulmonary atresia: absence of main pulmonary artery
Interrupted aortic arch (uncommon): lack of connection between ascending and descending aorta outflow tract	Ventricular septal defect (VSD): communication between right and left ventricle	Tetralogy of Fallot: malalignment of ventricular septum that leaves VSD and right ventricular obstruction

continued		
Obstruction to Systemic Blood Flow	**Increased Pulmonary Blood Flow**	**Decreased Pulmonary Blood Flow**
Hypoplastic left heart syndrome (uncommon): failure of left ventricle to develop	Atrioventricular canal (complete AV canal; 80% have Down syndrome): large communication between upper and lower chambers consisting of common atrioventricular valves Total anomalous pulmonary venous return (uncommon): absence of normal pulmonary venous connection to left atrium Truncus arteriosus (uncommon): one common systemic and pulmonary great vessel	Transposition of great arteries: abnormal origin of great vessels; they arise from inappropriate ventricle Tricuspid atresia: absence of tricuspid valve and portion of right ventricle

8. What is aortic stenosis?

Aortic stenosis is narrowing of the left ventricular outflow tract or the ascending aorta. It can occur at any level of the aorta but is most commonly found at the valve. Aortic stenosis can range from mild to severe and may not need any type of intervention (other than endocarditis prophylaxis) in a lifetime. Patients with moderate to severe stenosis may need a balloon valvotomy (children/young adults), surgical valvotomy, aortic valve replacement, or Ross procedure to relieve the stenosis and burden on the left ventricle.

9. What is the preferred surgery for correction of aortic stenosis?

A Ross procedure is the preferred surgery. This is a surgical procedure that requires cardiopulmonary bypass and aortic cross clamping. Essentially the aortic root and the pulmonary root are both excised. The pulmonary autograft is placed in the aortic position, and the coronary arteries are implanted. Then a cryopreserved pulmonary homograft is inserted in the position of the original pulmonary root.

10. What is coarctation of the aorta?

A portion of the aorta is constricted, impairing blood flow to the lower part of the body (usually descending). Eighty percent of patients with this defect also have a bicuspid aortic valve (valve with two leaflets instead of three).

Presentation depends on the degree of narrowing, but upper extremity hypertension and decreased pulses in the lower extremities are two of the hallmarks. The primary treatment of choice is currently surgical repair.

11. What are some of the most commonly encountered lesions that cause increased pulmonary blood flow?

- Patent ductus arterious. This is a connection between the pulmonary artery and the aorta that is supposed to close after fetal life. The size of the ductus determines how much extra blood flow is shunted to the lungs. Hence, a large persistent ductus would cause symptoms of CHF. One of the greatest dangers of these persistent connections is endocarditis. Treatment beyond the newborn period (indomethacin [Indocin] may be tried in the newborn) is catheter embolization with a coil or surgical ligation. However, the newest approach with great promise is video-assisted thorascopic surgery (VATS). The ductus is clipped during thorascopic visualization, and the patient is sent home the same day.
- Atrial septal defect (ASD). Three types of ASDs exist, but in essence an ASD is communication between the right atrium and the left atrium. Because the right side of the heart has lower pressures, blood that enters the left atrium goes through the defect and into the right side of the heart, increasing the volume and work load on that side of the heart. These defects are corrected either via surgical closure or device closure (performed in the catheterization lab).
- Ventricular septal defect (VSD). Several types of VSDs exist, but essentially a VSD is a communication between the right ventricle and the left ventricle. VSDs vary in size and hence presentation. Small VSDs may allow a patient to be asymptomatic, whereas moderate to large defects cause delayed growth, exercise intolerance, repeated pulmonary infections, and pulmonary hypertension if left untreated over time.

Surgical closure is the treatment of choice for moderate to large defects in patients with low pulmonary artery pressures. Catheter devices for closure are under investigation.

12. What is the most common defect found in adulthood?

Bicuspid aortic valve is the most common. The two leaflet valve is often unnoticed until aortic insufficiency or aortic stenosis develops in an adult.

13. What is the most common lesion seen that causes decreased pulmonary blood flow?

Tetralogy of Fallot (TOF) is the most common lesion seen that causes decreased pulmonary blood flow. This defect is actually a combination of defects that include right ventricular outflow tract obstruction (obstruction of the great vessel that directs blood flow to the lungs), VSD, right ventricular hypertrophy, and an aorta that overrides a VSD. The severity of the defect depends on the degree of stenosis at the pulmonary artery and the size of the VSD. These patients usually undergo diagnosis and repair in infancy. Regardless, complete correction is indicated when found even if the patient has a Blalock-Taussig shunt (an aorta to pulmonary shunt is used to provide blood flow to the lungs).

14. Why do patients with chronic cyanosis have high hematocrit levels?

Polycythemia in these patients is the body's response to prolonged tissue hypoxia. Adolescents and young adults who remain cyanotic may have symptoms related to hyperviscosity of the blood. Symptoms include headache, dizziness, blurred vision, fatigue, weakness, and chest or abdominal pain.

15. Why is it important that some patients not receive oxygen despite the fact that saturations may be no greater than 85%?

Individuals with palliated congenital heart defects may still have residual intra-cardiac shunting; thus, they are expected to have desaturated blood. Oxygen, which is a potent pulmonary vasodilator, may not increase PaO_2 levels but may lead to pulmonary overcirculation.

16. What defects are most likely to cause CHF?

Lesions that cause a left to right shunt (VSD, arteriovenous [AV] canal, PDA) are more likely to cause right heart failure. The remaining lesions that cause left heart obstruction (critical aortic stenosis, severe coarctation of the aorta) are more likely to cause left heart failure.

17. What is meant by a left to right shunt?

Blood takes the path of least resistance, so in the heart the blood flow will do the same. When blood enters the left side of the heart (the high pressure side) and an open communication exists to the right side (the low pressure side), then the blood will flow in that direction across the communication.

18. What is meant by the terms acyanotic and cyanotic in reference to CHD?

Acyanotic lesions are those defects in which the patients have normal oxygen saturations (96% to 100%). These are typically lesions that involve no right ventricular outflow tract obstruction or increased pulmonary blood flow. Cyanotic lesions are those that have right ventricular outflow tract obstruction or decreased pulmonary blood flow, which causes a bluish discoloration.

19. What are the surgical interventions for the most common defects, and should the nurse anticipate a patient who is acyanotic or cyanotic after repair?

Defect	Surgical Procedure(s)	Palliation or Repair	Acyanotic or Cyanotic after Repair
Aortic stenosis	Balloon valvuloplasty (catheterization lab), valvotomy, or Ross procedure	Valvotomy *may* only be palliation; Ross procedure is final repair	Acyanotic

continued

Defect	Surgical Procedure(s)	Palliation or Repair	Acyanotic or Cyanotic after Repair
Coarctation of aorta	Balloon dilation (catheterization lab), subclavian flap, end-to-end anastomosis or patch repair	Repair	Acyanotic
Interrupted aortic arch	Reconstruction of arch, ventricular septal defect (VSD) closure	Repair	Acyanotic
Patent ductus arteriosus	Coil (catheterization lab), ligate or clip via video-assisted thorascopic surgery	Repair	Acyanotic
Atrial septal defect	Device closure (catheterization lab), patch closure	Repair	Acyanotic
VSD	Patch closure	Repair	Acyanotic
Complete atrio-ventricular canal	Pulmonary atresia (PA) band (not first choice), patch closure	PA band is palliation	Acyanotic with primary repair
Pulmonary stenosis	Balloon valvuloplasty (catheterization lab), valvotomy	Repair	Acyanotic
Pulmonary atresia	Homograft placement	Repair (may require further surgeries as child grows)	Acyanotic
Tetralogy of Fallot	Blalock-Taussig (BT) shunt Pulmonary artery correction and VSD closure	Palliation Repair	Cyanotic Acyanotic
Transposition of great arteries	Arterial switch	Repair	Acyanotic
Tricuspid atresia	Shunt Bidirectional Glenn shunt Fontan	All are palliations	Cyanotic Cyanotic Acyanotic
Truncus arteriosus	Placement of homograft conduit and VSD closure	Repair, but children will need further surgeries as they outgrow homograft	Acyanotic
Hypoplastic left heart syndrome	Norwood procedure Bidirectional Glenn shunt Fontan	All are palliations	Cyanotic Cyanotic Acyanotic

Repair represents surgical correction that leaves patient with anatomically correct heart. *Palliation* refers to patients who will never have two ventricle repair/structurally normal heart.

20. **What are some of the most common findings after surgery in adulthood?**

At times residual problems remain after a surgery that may or may not be results of complications. These may include rhythm disturbances, valvular problems, ventricular function changes or size, pressure/resistance changes (either systemic or pulmonic), and developmental abnormalities.

The current belief is that children who have undergone surgical intervention may function slightly lower cognitively than their peer counterparts. The risk for delay increases with the complexity of the defect and the number of interventions. Some adolescents/young adults who have been interviewed believe they are excluded or discriminated against by their peers either based on the patient's lack of physical stamina or the peers' lack of knowledge. All patients and families should know that no intervention is without risk.

21. **What is the likelihood that the family or patient will have a child with CHD?**

The chance of a sibling having a defect is thought to be less than 2%. The chances increase if the mother has CHD. The likelihood of a patient with CHD having a child with CHD is believed to be 2.5% to as high as 18% (about 6.7%) if the mother has CHD and less than 3% if the father has CHD.

22. **What are four educational needs of adults with CHD?**

Clear consistent information about the defect and its treatment, measures to prevent endocarditis (if needed), physical capacity, and reproductive issues need to be addressed.

23. **Which patients are recommended to have bacterial endocarditis prophylaxis?**

Those patients with prosthetic valves, complex congenital heart physiology, surgically constructed shunts, thickened or abnormal valves, hypertrophic cardiomyopathy, or unrepaired septal defects or PDA are recommended to have bacterial endocarditis prophylaxis.

24. **Should patients with CHD see a CHD specialist?**

Specialist care is the most desirable, but this is often not feasible because of geographic constraints, cost, and the fact that very few cardiologists are trained in adult CHD (ACHD). Nurses can encourage patients with complex disease to seek a center with doctors who specialize in ACHD. Patients should be referred for the following conditions: change in functional status, changing murmur, pregnancy, pending noncardiac surgery, arrhythmias, neurological changes, decompensated polycythemia, and endocarditis, or when the patient feels it is necessary.

25. What does the future look like for adults with CHD?

By the end of the decade, more adults will have CHD than will children because the number of infants with CHD is not changing but the advancements in medicine are allowing these infants to grow into adulthood.

This situation already has created the need for specialists both on the medicine side and on the nursing side. Time and experience are necessary to take care of these often complicated cases. This is bringing about new adult cardiologists who specialize in CHD and advanced practice nurses to help bridge the gap between pediatric and adult medicine.

Key Points

- Eighty percent of children with CHD will live to be adults.
- The key to understanding the patient with CHD is obtaining a good history.
- Not all congenital heart defects can be repaired, but most can be at least palliated.
- Patients with congenital heart defects with left to right shunts have "too much blood flow" and experience CHF.
- Patients with congenital heart defects with right to left shunts or obstructions typically have "too little blood flow."

Internet Resources

American Heart Association:
www.AHA.org

Yale University School of Medicine: Congenital Heart Disease:
http://info.med.yale.edu/intmed/cardio/chd/

Congenital Heart Information Network:
www.tchin.org

Children's Healthcare of Atlanta:
www.choa.org

Cincinnati Children's Hospital Medical Center
www.cincinnatichildrens.org

Bibliography

Borowitz S: Alprostadil (PGE_1) for maintaining ductal patency, *Pediatr Pharmacother* 6:9, 2000.

Brickner EM, Hillis DL, Lange RA: Medical progress: congenital heart disease in adults (part 2 of 2), *N Engl J Med* 342:334-342, 2000.

Dajani AS et al: Prevention of bacterial endocarditis, *JAMA* 277:1794-1801, 1997.

Freedom R, Lock J, Bricker T: Pediatric cardiology and cardiovascular surgery, *Circulation* 102:IV58-IV68, 2000.

Harris G: Heart disease in children: primary care, *Clin Office Pract* 27:2, 2000.

Kay J, Colan S, Graham T: Congestive heart failure in pediatric patients, *Am Heart J* 142:923-928, 2001.

Kovach JA: Preventive and primary care of the adult with congenital heart disease, *ACC Curr J Rev* 10(4):94-98, 2001.

McMurray R et al: A life less ordinary: growing up and coping with congenital heart disease, *Coron Health Care* 5(1):51-57, 2001.

Moons P et al: What do adult patients with congenital heart disease know about their disease, treatment, and prevention of complications? A call for structured patient education, *Heart* 86:74-80, 2001.

Nettina S: Pediatric cardiovascular disorders. In *Lippincott manual of nursing,* ed 7, Philadelphia, 2001, Williams & Wilkins.

Perloff J, Warnes C: Challenges posed by adults with repaired congenital heart disease, *Circulation* 103:2637-2643, 2001.

Suddaby E: Contemporary thinking for congenital heart disease, *Pediatr Nurs* 27:233-238, 270, 2001.

Thorne S: Management of polycythaemia in adults with cyanotic congenital heart disease, *Heart* 79:315-316, 1998.

Chapter 17

Peripheral Vascular Disease

Penelope Ann Crisp

1. Define peripheral vascular disease (PVD).

Atherosclerosis of the abdominal aorta, iliac arteries, and arteries of the lower extremity is referred to as PVD. Patients with PVD most commonly have intermittent claudication and less often ischemic rest pain. PVD is a manifestation of systemic atherosclerosis and a predictor of cardiovascular and cerebrovascular disease and has thus generated a need for enhanced understanding of PVD.

2. What are the risk factors for PVD?

- Tobacco use is the single most common cause and most strongly associated risk factor of PVD
- Diabetes mellitus (DM)
- Hematologic factors
- Dyslipidemia
- Hyperhomocystinemia
- Hypertension

3. What is the relationship between tobacco and PVD risks?

- Tobacco use causes PVD by damaging the arterial wall. Plaque adheres to the vessel wall and causes a stenosis or blockage, disrupting the flow of blood.
- Even a half pack of cigarettes per day may increase the risk of development of PVD by 30% to 50%.
- Tobacco use is a common cause of myocardial infarction (MI), stroke, and death in as many as 5% to 15% of patients with PVD per year. Thus 50% of patients with PVD who smoke may have one of these severe events develop within 5 years after diagnosis.
- Tobacco use causes PVD to progress much more rapidly; one in five patients with claudication who smokes will have leg pain at rest develop, requiring a limb procedure, such as artery bypass surgery, angioplasty, or amputation.
- Vascular surgery or an interventional procedure such as angioplasty to repair blood vessels is much less likely to be successful or remain patent in patients who smoke.
- Amputation is much more likely to occur in patients who smoke.

4. What is the significance of DM and PVD?

Diabetes is thought to affect the vascular structure in several ways. Changes in glucose levels, particularly hyperglycemia, interfere with the platelet phases of coagulation. Hyperglycemia also increases the production of abnormal lipid metabolism. The arterial wall becomes calcified as a result of changes in blood glucose.

The risk of development of PVD is four times greater in patients with diabetes. DM is a contributing factor in about half of limb amputations unrelated to trauma because of the severity of associated PVD and the rapid progression to critical limb ischemia. The relative risk for limb amputation is 40 times greater for patients with diabetes than for patients without diabetes.

5. What is the relationship between hypertension and PVD?

Hypertension has been implicated as a factor of plaque pathogenesis, causing endothelial injury to vessel walls. Recent studies, including the Framingham study, have shown that hypertension is probably both a cause and an effect of PVD. Hypertension may delay the onset of symptoms of PVD by elevating the central perfusion pressure. Development of claudication symptoms after high blood pressure (BP) is treated is not uncommon for a patient with hypertension.

6. What is the relationship between dyslipidemia and PVD?

In PVD, several lipid fractions determine the presence and progression of disease. As part of the Physician's Health Study, risk factors for development of symptomatic arterial disease were assessed during a 9-year follow-up. Baseline C-reactive protein (CRP) levels and cholesterol–low-density lipoprotein cholesterol (LDLC) ratios were the strongest independent predictors of subsequent development of PVD. An elevated lipoprotein (a) level is a significant independent risk factor for PVD. CRP levels are indicative of injury to the vessel wall over time. Hyperhomocysteinemia is a significant risk factor in the development of PVD. Patients with high levels of homocysteine have increased morbidity and mortality rates from atherosclerotic disease and venous thromboembolism. Dietary supplements of folic acid and vitamins B_6 and B_{12} can normalize serum homocysteine. Whether normalization changes atherosclerotic risk remains unknown.

7. What are the signs and symptoms of PVD?

Claudication is a type of pain often described as cramping or tiredness in the lower extremities. The pain is brought on by exercise and relieved with rest. Claudication is the symptom most likely to bring a patient to a health care provider. With aortoiliac disease, the patient is most likely to have hip, buttock, or thigh claudication. Claudication that occurs in the calf is most likely superior femoral artery (SFA) stenosis or occlusion. Patients with PVD often have dependent rubor; in a sitting position, the feet appear red, and if the feet are raised, they become normal or pale in appearance. The pale appearance is from a lack of blood flow because of stenosis. The redness is caused by blood pooling in the foot by gravity.

8. **What is the difference between rest pain and claudication?**

Pain at rest, not induced by exercise, is most often a symptom of occlusion or a more severe stenosis. This pain typically occurs in the forefoot at night when the patient is lying flat. The pain may sometimes be relieved by hanging the foot over the edge of the bed or by getting out of bed.

9. **What is the most common diagnostic test used in evaluation of PVD?**

The Doppler ankle-brachial index (ABI) test is a simple vascular lab test for assessment of lower extremity circulation. The ABI is the lower extremity systolic pressure divided by the brachial artery systolic pressure.

10. **What is the significance of the values obtained in ABI testing?**

Ankle-Brachial Index	Severity of Disease
0.90-1.30	Normal
0.70-0.89	Mild
0.40-0.69	Moderate
<0.40	Severe

ABI testing along with the Doppler waveform is helpful in determination of the levels of arterial occlusive disease, whether aortoiliac, infrainguinal, or multilevel. Patients in the mild category are often helped with an exercise program and medication. Patients in the moderate category usually need intervention either surgically or with angioplasty. Patients in the severe category are typically in a limb-threatening situation and need surgical intervention and possibly amputation.

11. **How is the ABI test performed?**

This test can be performed at the bedside with a BP cuff and a handheld Doppler ultrasonic velocity detector. A BP cuff is placed over the upper arm and inflated above the systolic BP (SBP). Resumption of blood flow is detected with the Doppler probe over the brachial artery. If a discrepancy is found in the readings between the two arms, the higher of the two arm SBPs is used to calculate the ABI. The BP cuff is then moved to the ankle and inflated above the SBP. The Doppler ultrasonic velocity detector is first placed over the posterior tibial artery at the ankle and then over the dorsalis pedis artery. The higher of the two readings between the posterior tibial and the dorsalis pedis arteries should be used in calculation of the ABI. The ABI is then calculated with dividing the tibial or pedis SBP by the brachial SBP. The ABI should be measured in each leg.

12. **Who should have an ABI?**

All patients with claudication, rest pain, or tissue loss (gangrene) should have an ABI checked. This information is also helpful in patients with exercise-induced leg pain or foot pain with an unclear history. A low ABI is a marker for future cardiovascular disease.

13. What are treatment options for patients with PVD?

Treatment of PVD involves two major objectives. The first is prevention of atherosclerosis, reducing the risk of cardiovascular ischemic events, such as an MI or cardiovascular accident (CVA), and decreasing the progression of PVD, preventing limb loss. The second goal is to provide relief of symptoms and improve functional disability and quality of life.

Surgery is considered the first-line therapy for patients with PVD if the patient has lifestyle-limiting claudication, rest pain, nonhealing wound, or tissue loss. Consideration should be given to the patient's functional status.

14. When is PVD treated medically?

Claudication without rest pain or intermittent claudication that is moderately lifestyle limiting is generally treated nonoperatively. Patients need to stop smoking, begin a regular exercise program, and control diabetes, hypertension, and cholesterol. Today only two drugs have been approved by the US Food and Drug Administration (FDA) for claudication: pentoxifylline and cilostazol. Cilostazol appears more likely to provide a clinically significant increase in walking distance in most patients.

15. Are there options other than surgery?

Angioplasty with or without stenting is an option for some patients, dependent on the length and location of the stenosis or blockage. Aortoiliac disease is often focal and can be treated with endovascular procedures.

Infrainguinal disease, meaning below the inguinal ligament (involving the femoral arteries, the popliteal artery, and infrapopliteal arteries), is often not amenable to endovascular procedures. These lesions are typically long, and occlusive percutaneous intervention is unlikely to be durable. However, some short segment SFA lesions can be successfully treated with angioplasty and stenting.

16. What are the nursing considerations with PVD?

Nurses should emphasize a healthy lifestyle to these patients. They should encourage them to stop smoking, exercise, eat a heart healthy diet, and control diabetes and hypertension. After surgery or angioplasty, frequent pulse checks are necessary for assessment of graft or stent patency. Most patients with PVD also have a history of heart disease or stroke; therefore cardiac status should be closely watched. Respiratory status, pain control, fluid and electrolyte balance, and the risk of infection are all monitored by nursing.

17. What is an abdominal aneurysm (AAA)?

An aneurysm is a focal dilation of an artery more than 50% larger than the normal artery diameter. The average diameter of the abdominal aorta is 2 cm.

18. **What are risk factors for development of an AAA?**

The incidence rate of AAA is 3% to 10% for patients over 50 years old. Incidence rate is increased by a positive family history, older age, male gender, and smoking.

19. **What are the signs and symptoms of AAA?**

Most AAAs are asymptomatic until they rupture. AAAs are typically found as an incidental finding on physical exam by palpation or through testing for another medical problem (i.e., ultrasound for gallbladder, computed tomography [CT] of the chest and abdomen for any reason).

20. **What tests are used to define the size of an AAA?**

Ultrasound and CT may be used to define the extent and size of the aneurysm. Arteriography is not helpful in defining the size of an aneurysm but is helpful in defining the location and the condition of the surrounding vessels.

21. **What are complications of an AAA?**

Complications of aneurysms depend on the location of the aneurysm. Suprarenal AAAs extend above the renal arteries but not above the diaphragm. This type of aneurysm requires use of supraceliac clamp placement, causing an increase in renal and mesenteric ischemia time. The increase in ischemia time may lead to postoperative complications of ileus, acid-base imbalances, pulmonary complications, or acute tubular necrosis (ATN). Operative risk is less with infrarenal AAAs. A straight tube graft is used; this is a much less complicated procedure that requires less clamp time. Obviously death from rupture is the most serious complication.

22. **What are treatment options for AAA?**

Treatment options are based on the diameter of the AAA and patients age and comorbidities. Factors that contribute to the risk of rupture include: larger diameter, rapid expansion determined with serial ultrasounds or CT scans, smoking, chronic obstructive pulmonary disease (COPD), hypertension, strong positive family history, and eccentric shape of the aneurysm. There is no precise formula for calculation of rupture risk. Patients with small aneurysms are considered to be at low risk and are managed conservatively with ultrasound surveillance. However, in the event that the patient at low risk person is very young (i.e., has a long life expectancy), an eventual AAA repair may be considered because expansion of the AAA is almost certain. Likewise, some younger patients may prefer more aggressive management in the form of early surgical repair. If AAA rupture risk is average or high, the patient's life expectancy is considered in making treatment decisions. Would a prophylactic repair yield long-term benefit? Patients with comorbid diseases are less likely to die of AAA rupture and more likely to die of the comorbid disease itself and are therefore less likely to benefit from repair.

Estimated Risk of Aneurysm Rupture Related to Diameter	
Diameter (cm)	Rupture Risk (%/y)
<4	0
4-5	0.5-5
5-6	3-15
6-7	10-20
7-8	20-40
>8	30-50

The most recent development in the treatment of AAAs is endovascular stent graft repair. This procedure offers the possibility of reduction of perioperative risk of aneurysm repair. The first of these procedures was done in 1991; since that time, numerous devices and strategies have been developed and evaluated in clinical trials. In 1999, the FDA approved the use of an endograft inserted through a surgically exposed femoral artery. The advantages of the stent graft repair include less blood loss, reduced hospital stay, and fewer medical complications (i.e., MI, renal failure, pneumonia, or other respiratory complications).

23. What are operative risks of AAA repair?

The surgical mortality rate for open elective AAA repair ranges from 3.5% to 7.5%. In a large population-based study of 16,500 patients undergoing open AAA repair in the United States, mortality rates were independently affected by age, gender, race, and the presence of medical comorbidities, including COPD, preoperative renal insufficiency and carotid occlusive disease. The most common complications are listed in order of frequency: cardiac events including arrhythmias, prolonged ileus, congestive heart failure (CHF), respiratory failure, MI, graft thrombosis, limb ischemia, intraoperative emboli, postoperative bleeding requiring transfusions, wound infection, stroke, and dialysis dependence.

Complications for endograft repair include endoleaks. Endoleaks have been reported at a rate of 1.3% to 20% in the first year. Large aneurysms can change their lengths after endovascular repair; typically these aneurysms shrink in diameter, which has the potential of causing graft migration and limb dislodgement of the stent itself. Sometimes this condition can fixed with another endograft procedure, or conversion to an open procedure may be needed.

24. What are the signs and symptoms of a ruptured AAA?

Ruptured AAAs are serious surgical emergencies. About 15% to 20 % of AAA repairs are done emergently. Patients are seen with excruciating back or flank pain. The pain is sudden in onset associated with hypotension, tachycardia, and dyspnea.

25. What are nursing considerations for patients with AAAs?

Nurses should talk to these patients about modifying risk factors that the patient can control. The importance of smoking cessation, regular exercise, a heart-healthy diet, and control of hypertension with prescribed medications should be explained. Nurses should emphasize to the patient the importance of keeping scheduled appointments for serial ultrasounds.

After surgery, these patients will need intensive care unit (ICU) care for the first 24 to 36 hours. Monitoring these patients for cardiac status, respiratory status, renal function, bowel ischemia, and fluid and electrolyte balance is important in this period because of the large fluid volume shifts. Patients who have had a rupture need the same monitoring; these patients are in shock, with unstable and labile conditions with hypertension that is controlled with vasoactive drugs. Patients who have had endograft repairs typically go to the general nursing unit and should be monitored for bleeding in the groin (the incision site) and pain in the abdomen, indicative of an endoleak.

Key Points

- Risk factors for PVD include tobacco use, diabetes, dyslipidemia, hypertension, and hypercoagulable states.
- Claudication for the most part requires lifestyle modification and possibly percutaneous intervention.
- Rest pain most always requires an intervention—either surgery or percutaneous intervention.

Internet Resources

Peripheral Vascular Surgery Society:
www.pvss.org

Interventional and Vascular Medicine Forum:
www.endovascular.org

VascularWeb: One Source for Vascular Health Information:
www.vascularweb.org

Society for Vascular Medicine and Biology:
www.svmb.org

Society for Vascular Ultrasound:
www.svunet.org

Bibliography

Boersma E, Poldermans D, Bax J et al: Predictors of cardiac events after major vascular surgery, *JAMA* 285(14):1865-1873, 2001.

Clagett G: What's new in vascular surgery, *J Am Coll Surg* 194(2):165-200, 2002.

Dillavou E, Navyash G, Makaroun M: Endoleak following AAA repair, *Endovascular Today* 1(2):44-49, 2002.

Finlayson S, Birkmeyer J, Fillinger M, Cronenwett J: Should endovascular surgery lower the threshold for repair of abdominal aortic aneurysm? *J Vasc Surg* 29:973-985, 1999.

Jean-Claude J, Reilly L, Stoney R, Messina L: Pararenal aneurysms: the future of open aortic aneurysm repair, *J Vasc Surg* 29:902-912, 1999.

Money S, Herd J, Isaason J et al: Effect of cilostazol on walking distances in patients with intermittent claudication, *J Vasc Surg* 7:356-362, 1998.

Moore W: Concept of endovascular surgery. In Moore W, Ahn S, editors: *Endovascular surgery,* ed 3, Philadelphia, 2001, WB Saunders.

O'Reilly E: Abdominal aortic aneurysm, *Nurs Spectrum* 2(2):33-36, 2001.

Powell J, Greenhalgh R: Small abdominal aortic aneurysms, *N Engl J Med* 384(19):1895-1901, 2003.

Schwartz L: Basic principles of aortic surgery. In Gerwertz B, editor: *Surgery of the aorta and its branches,* Philadelphia, 2000, WB Saunders.

Tan W, Yadav JS, Wholey MH, Wholey MH: Endovascular options for peripheral arterial occlusive and aneurysmal disease. In Topol E, editor: *Textbook of interventional cardiology,* Philadelphia, 2003, WB Saunders.

TASC TransAtlantic Inter-Society Consensus: Management of peripheral arterial disease, *J Vasc Surg* 31(suppl part 2):1, 2000.

Zarins C, White R, Schwarten D et al: AneuRx stent graft versus open surgical repair of abdominal aortic aneurysms: multicenter prospective clinical trial, *J Vasc Surg* 29:292-308, 1999.

Pulmonary Hypertension

Susan K. Frazier

1. Define pulmonary hypertension.

Pulmonary hypertension indicates that an individual exhibits a mean pulmonary arterial blood pressure greater than 25 mm Hg during rest or a mean pulmonary artery pressure greater than 30 mm Hg during physical exercise.

2. Is there more than one type of pulmonary hypertension?

Yes. In 1998, the World Health Organization established a descriptive classification system that uses the pathophysiological processes to categorize pulmonary hypertension (see the following table).

Classification System For Pulmonary Hypertension

Classification of Pulmonary Hypertension	Common Associated Disorders
Pulmonary arterial hypertension	HIV Collagen vascular disease Drug/toxin ingestion Examples: fenfluramine hydrochloride, rapeseed oil
Pulmonary venous hypertension	Left ventricular failure Mitral valve disease
Pulmonary hypertension associated with pulmonary disorders or hypoxemia	Chronic obstructive lung disease Obstructive sleep apnea Alveolar hypoventilation Interstitial lung disease
Pulmonary hypertension associated with thrombotic/embolic disorders	Sickle cell disease Pulmonary embolus
Pulmonary hypertension associated with miscellaneous pathologies	Inflammation: sarcoidosis Compression of central pulmonary veins: tumor compression

3. Describe the pathological causes of pulmonary hypertension.

Increased pulmonary artery pressure may be induced by a number of mechanisms (see the following table). These mechanisms result in a change in vessel lumen diameter and an elevation in pulmonary arterial blood pressure. Several mechanisms produce an elevation in pulmonary vascular resistance (PVR) or resistance to forward blood flow.

Mechanisms That Produce Elevated Pulmonary Blood Pressure

Mechanism	Etiology
Structural alterations in pulmonary vessels	Pulmonary vessel remodeling Imbalance between mitogenic and antimitogenic mediators producing smooth muscle hypertrophy
Hypoxia-induced vasoconstriction	Rapid depolarization of smooth muscle cells mediated by Ca^{++} channels Increased pulmonary vascular resistance
Pulmonary vessel obstruction	Partial or complete obstruction by vessel lumen by thrombus with elevation in pressure proximal to obstruction External compression of pulmonary vessels producing partial or total occlusion of blood flow with increased pressure proximal to obstruction
Reduced ejection of blood from left atrium or ventricle	Increase in pulmonary blood volume with subsequent increase in pulmonary vessel pressure

4. Describe the clinical presentation of an individual with pulmonary hypertension.

The development of signs and symptoms that arise from pulmonary hypertension is subtle. Progressive dyspnea and fatigue are the most common symptoms. Syncope or near syncope and exercise intolerance are also common. Peripheral edema, hepatomegaly, and splenomegaly may be detected once cardiac involvement occurs, and the patient may report palpitations. Chest pain similar to angina may be reported as cardiovascular involvement becomes more severe. Hoarseness may also develop with advanced pulmonary hypertension. Cardiac auscultation may detect a narrow split of S2 with accentuation of P2, the presence of a systolic ejection murmur consistent with tricuspid regurgitation, and a pulmonary ejection click and ejection murmur (see Chapter 2, Physical Examination of the Cardiovascular Patient, for further explanation of heart sounds).

5. What causes this clinical presentation?

Dyspnea is likely produced by a number of factors. Hypoxemia and stimulation of receptors in pulmonary vessels particularly contribute to this subjective sensation. Fatigue is produced by hypoxemia and reduced oxygen delivery. Syncope or near syncopal episodes occur when cardiac output is significantly decreased. Cardiac output reductions are the result of two mechanisms: (1), a reduction in left ventricular end-diastolic volume from a decrease in blood volume ejection from the right ventricle into the pulmonary vessels; and (2), right ventricular dilation with a shift of the interventricular septum into the left ventricular chamber. Peripheral edema, hepatomegaly, and splenomegaly are a result of elevated systemic venous pressure produced with inadequate right ventricular ejection. Chest pain is produced with right ventricular dilation, an increase in right ventricular wall stress, and reduction of coronary artery blood flow with subsequent myocardial ischemia. Hoarseness occurs when an enlarged pulmonary artery compresses the left laryngeal nerve.

6. Is there a system to classify the severity of pulmonary hypertension?

Severity of pulmonary hypertension can be described with a ranking system similar to the American Heart Association classifications for heart failure (see the following table).

World Health Organization Classifications of Pulmonary Hypertension Severity	
Classification	**Description of Signs/Symptoms**
Class I	No limitation of physical activity No signs/symptoms with activity/exercise
Class II	Asymptomatic at rest Slight limitation of physical activity Signs/symptoms occur with activities of daily living
Class III	Comfortable at rest Pronounced limitation in physical activity Signs/symptoms with any activity
Class IV	Signs/symptoms present at rest Severe limitation in physical activity Right heart failure present

7. How is pulmonary hypertension diagnosed?

Diagnostic testing for patients with the previous presentation includes tests that evaluate pulmonary and cardiac function. These tests are detailed in the following table.

Common Diagnostic Tests and Findings

Diagnostic Test	Findings Related to Pulmonary Hypertension
Chest radiograph	Early findings: normal radiograph Later findings: enlarged pulmonary artery and hilar vessels, peripheral pulmonary vessels pruned (abrupt loss of vessel), enlarged cardiac silhouette
Echocardiogram with Doppler flow studies	Dilation of right atrium and ventricle and main pulmonary artery, presence of right ventricular systolic dysfunction, tricuspid regurgitation, flattened interventricular septum, right ventricular hypertrophy Pulmonary artery systolic pressure may be reliably estimated from regurgitant flow velocity
Electrocardiogram	P pulmonale (tall peaked P wave) in inferior leads (leads II, III, AVF) Right axis deviation (QRS axis >90 degrees) Incomplete right bundle branch block in presence of right ventricular hypertrophy ST depression, T wave inversion in inferior leads or right precordial leads (from reduction in myocardial blood flow)
Arterial blood gas	Respiratory alkalosis (pH >7.45; $PaCO_2$ <35 mm Hg) Hypoxemia
Pulmonary function test	Dependent on underlying mechanism of pulmonary hypertension For example: with structural vessel alterations, reduction in diffusion capacity (DLco performed with pulmonary function testing); with chronic obstructive lung disease, reduction in air flow, abnormal flow volume curves
Ventilation perfusion scan or pulmonary angiogram	Assists in differential diagnosis In presence of thromboembolic disorders: high probability scan With pulmonary hypertension from other mechanisms: low probability scan is likely Pulmonary angiogram will identify presence and location of thrombus or embolus
Right heart catheterization	Reduction in cardiac output/cardiac index Elevations of pulmonary artery systolic, diastolic, and mean pressure; right atrial and ventricular pressure Significant elevations in pulmonary vascular resistance Test vascular response to vasodilators.

8. What are common therapeutic methods used to manage pulmonary hypertension?

Management is directed at the underlying mechanism that produces the elevated pulmonary pressure. The intent of effective management is reduction of pulmonary artery pressure and vascular resistance to preserve right ventricular function and to increase cardiac output and improve oxygen delivery. The following table provides common management strategies.

Management of Pulmonary Hypertension

Management Strategy	Rationale	Special Considerations
Oxygen therapy	To reduce hypoxic pulmonary vasoconstriction	May require continuous low flow oxygen Maintain SpO_2 >90%
Anticoagulation therapy (warfarin)	To reduce likelihood of venous thrombus formation	International Normalized Ratio (INR) goal, 2-3
Diuretic therapy	To reduce fluid volume overload and venous congestion	Right ventricle is preload dependent, so significant reduction in volume may decrease cardiac output and blood pressure; electrolyte imbalances possible
Thrombolysis Thromboendarterectomy Vena caval filter	To dissolve or remove thromboses or emboli, to prevent further embolism	Reduction in pulmonary pressure should occur within 48 h of surgical intervention
Calcium channel antagonists Nifedipine Nicardipine hydrochloride Diltiazem hydrochloride	To reduce influx of calcium into pulmonary vascular smooth muscle and produce vascular relaxation and dilation	Doses required to produce vasodilation may be up to twice maximum normal dose Common adverse effects include systemic and orthostatic hypotension, tachycardia, and fluid retention
Prostaglandin therapy Epoprostenol (Flolan; prostacyclin)	To produce pulmonary vasodilation, inhibit platelet aggregation, and reduce proliferation of pulmonary vascular smooth muscle	Must be administered as continuous intravenous infusion through central venous catheter until transplantation Tolerance develops over time, thus dose requires adjustment at intervals Abrupt cessation of drug can result in sudden death from acute right heart failure Cost of drug may be >$10,000/yr
Lung, heart-lung transplantation	To improve pulmonary and cardiovascular function and increase systemic oxygen delivery	In 1998, nearly 25% of heart-lung transplants in United States for pulmonary hypertension Survival after lung transplant reported to be 83% at 1 yr, 70% at 3 yr, and 54% at 5 yr

9. Describe important patient education responsibilities for nurse clinicians.

Timely diagnosis and effective management can improve quality of life and prolong survival. Appropriate patient education tailored to the individual's ability to understand and counseling empowers the patient and significant others to actively participate in patient care and decision making. The issues that must be addressed are detailed in the following table.

Topics for Education and Counseling

Classification of Information	Specific Topics
General Information	Tailored information about underlying condition
	Prognosis, life expectancy
	Expected signs/symptoms and cause of these
	Treatment plan
	Patient/significant other responsibilities in care
	Sexuality, coping with sexual difficulty
	Advance directives for health care
Pharmacological interventions	Expected effects of drugs, instructions for preparation and administration
	Required lab evaluation of efficacy (i.e., INR for warfarin administration)
	Central venous catheter care (for continuous administration of prostacyclin)
	Use of intravenous infusion pump for prostacyclin infusion
	Potential adverse effects
	Suggested actions for adverse effects
	Financial aid for high-cost drugs (epoprostenol)
Nonpharmacological interventions	Activity prescription: may receive at completion of pulmonary rehabilitation program
	Dietary prescription (depends on underlying pathology)
	Smoking cessation
	Vaccination for influenza and pneumococcal pneumonia
Surgical interventions	Standard preoperative education specific to procedure
	Transplant wait list procedure
	Care requirements after transplant (i.e., antirejection drug regimen); see Chapter 26, Heart Transplantation

Key Points

- Pulmonary hypertension indicates that an individual exhibits a mean pulmonary arterial blood pressure greater than 25 mm Hg during rest or a mean pulmonary artery pressure greater than 30 mm Hg during physical exercise.
- Increased pulmonary artery pressure may be induced by a number of mechanisms that result in a change in vessel lumen diameter and an elevation in pulmonary arterial blood pressure.
- Severity of pulmonary hypertension can be described with a ranking system similar to the American Heart Association classifications for heart failure.
- The intent of effective management is to reduce pulmonary artery pressure and vascular resistance, to preserve right ventricular function, and to increase cardiac output and improve oxygen delivery.

Internet Resources

Pulmonary Hypertension Association:
http://www.phassociation.org/

Pulmonary Hypertension: The Complete Resource:
http://www.phcentral.org/

Primary Pulmonary Hypertension Cure Foundation:
http://www.pphcure.org/

Bibliography

Califf RM, Adams KF, McKenna WJ et al: A randomized controlled trial of epoprostenol therapy for severe congestive heart failure: the Flolan International Randomized Survival Trial (FIRST), *Am Heart J* 134:44-54, 1997.

Frazier SK: Diagnosing and treating primary pulmonary hypertension, *Nurs Pract* 24:18-41, 1999.

Gibbs JS, Higenbottam TW: Recommendations on the management of pulmonary hypertension in clinical practice, *Heart* 86:i1-i13, 2001.

Gomez A, Bialostozky D, Zajarias A et al: Right ventricular ischemia in patients with primary pulmonary hypertension, *J Am Coll Cardiol* 38:1137-1142, 2001.

Keck BM, Bennett LE, Fiol BS et al: Worldwide thoracic organ transplantation: a report from the UNOS/ISHLT International Registry for Thoracic Organ Transplantation, *Clin Transpl* 39-52, 1998.

Kessler R, Faller M, Weitzenblum E et al: "Natural history" of pulmonary hypertension in a series of 131 patients with chronic obstructive lung disease, *Am J Respir Crit Care Med* 164:219-224, 2001.

Meyers BF, Lynch J, Trulock EP et al: Lung transplantation: a decade of experience, *Ann Surg* 230:362-370, 1999.

Morrell NW, Wilkins MR: Genetic and molecular mechanisms of pulmonary hypertension, *Clin Med* 1:138-145, 2001.

Chapter 19

Shock

Susan K. Frazier

1. What is shock?

Shock is defined as impairment of cellular metabolism associated with inadequate perfusion. Shock reduces the delivery of oxygen and nutrients like glucose or alters the ability of cells to properly use oxygen and nutrients that are necessary for aerobic metabolism. Anaerobic metabolism results.

2. Is there more than one kind of shock?

Yes. Types of shock may be categorized by the underlying cause of the shock state as described in the following table.

Classifications of Shock

Type of Shock	Typical Causes	Oxygen and Nutrient Delivery Impairment
Hypovolemic	Hemorrhage Burn trauma Dehydration Excessive diuresis	Significant loss of intravascular volume or interstitial fluid
Cardiogenic	Heart failure from any cause Acute myocardial infarction Cardiac dysrhythmias	Significant reduction in cardiac output
Anaphylactic	Exposure to antigen to which individual is sensitized (i.e., food, drugs, dyes, latex)	Release of histamine and histamine-like mediators that causes massive vasodilation and relative hypovolemia; loss of fluid from vascular compartment into interstitial spaces from capillary leak
Neurogenic	Spinal cord injury Spinal anesthesia	Loss of vasomotor tone that produces generalized vasodilation and relative hypovolemia
Septic	Gram-negative bacteria Gram-positive bacteria Viruses Fungi	Massive vasodilation, pooling of blood in periphery and relative hypovolemia

3. Are there typical stages as shock develops?

If not detected and managed effectively, shock may progress through three stages. The earliest stage, compensated or reversible shock, is that period of time when the body uses compensatory mechanisms to maintain homeostasis in response to a reduction in tissue perfusion. A transient decrease in cardiac output occurs and stimulates the sympathetic nervous system, the renin-angiotensin-aldosterone system, and the hypothalamic pituitary axis. Vasoconstriction and sodium and fluid retention return cardiac output and blood pressure to normal values. Shock progresses to the intermediate or progressive phase when these compensatory mechanisms can no longer maintain a homeostatic state. Cardiac output and blood pressure decrease, anaerobic metabolism occurs to a greater degree, and cellular wastes like lactic acid accumulate and stimulate coagulation abnormalities and thrombus formation, particularly in the microcirculation. Cellular death and necrosis occurs, and organ system dysfunction becomes obvious. The final stage of shock, irreversible shock, is the consequence of continued hypoperfusion and cellular destruction. The pancreas releases a myocardial depressant factor that further reduces oxygen delivery. Failure of the vasomotor system causes massive vasodilation and an increase in capillary permeability with movement of vascular volume into the interstitial spaces. Although some improvement in condition may be obtained with aggressive therapy, at this stage multisystem organ failure occurs and death is inevitable.

4. What signs and symptoms are evident in patients with shock?

Signs and symptoms vary by the type of shock and the stage of shock. These signs and symptoms are detailed in the following table.

Signs and Symptoms of Shock by Stage and Organ System

Organ System	Compensated	Progressive	Irreversible
Neuro-psychological	All types: difficulty with concentration, restlessness, anxiety, and feeling of impending doom, with pupils normal and reactive and thirst evident	All types: agitation, anxiety, and confusion to lethargy, with pupils dilated and reactive and marked thirst	All types: lethargy to nonresponsiveness, with pupils dilated with sluggish reaction and severe thirst reported if individual is conscious
Cardiovascular	Heart rate: all types except neurogenic: tachycardia; neurogenic: bradycardia Cardiac output: initially, transient decrease in CO; then maintained for all but septic; with septic, is increased: hyperdynamic (increased cardiac output)	Heart rate: tachycardia with some dysrhythmias for all types except neurogenic; with neurogenic: serious bradycardia with dysrhythmias Cardiac output: reduced for all types	All types: cardiac output and blood pressure significantly reduced; hemodynamic instability with position change; systemic vascular resistance decreased for all: vasomotor center failure

Signs and Symptoms of Shock by Stage and Organ System *continued*

Organ System	Compensated	Progressive	Irreversible
	Systemic vascular resistance: increased with hypovolemic and cardiogenic; reduced with neurogenic, anaphylactic, and septic Blood pressure: maintained for all	Systemic vascular resistance: increased with hypovolemic and cardiogenic; reduced with septic, anaphylactic, and neurogenic Blood pressure: reduced with all types, orthostatic blood pressure changes obvious	
Respiratory	Rapid, deep respirations Arterial blood gas: mild respiratory alkalosis	Rapid, shallow respirations Cardiogenic: bilateral crackles Anaphylactic: severe bronchoconstriction Arterial blood gas: mixed acid base disturbance: respiratory alkalosis, metabolic acidosis	Rapid, shallow, irregular respirations to apnea Anaphylactic: airway obstruction All other types: bilateral pulmonary infiltrates, crackles Arterial blood gas: severe metabolic and respiratory acidosis in presence of hypoventilation
Renal	Urinary output decreased but remains within normal limits	Oliguria <20 mL/h	Renal failure, anuria
Gastrointestinal	Hypoactive bowel sounds	Hypoactive to absent bowel sounds; possible gastrointestinal bleed from stress-induced gastritis or ulcer	Absent bowel sounds: probable paralytic ileus; gastrointestinal bleed from stress-induced gastritis or ulcer
Integumentary	Skin temperature: cool with hypovolemic and; cardiogenic warm with septic, neurogenic, and anaphylactic Skin color and condition: pale and diaphoretic with hypovolemic and cardiogenic; flushed and dry with septic and neurogenic; warm and flushed with angioedema in anaphylactic Neurogenic: skin warm and flushed	Skin temperature: cold with hypovolemic and cardiogenic; warm with septic, neurogenic, and anaphylactic Skin color and condition: pale, diaphoretic, and cyanotic with hypovolemic and cardiogenic; pale and warm with all others; cyanotic when ≥5 g of hemoglobin is desaturated	Skin temperature: cool to cold in all types of shock Skin color and condition: pale, cyanotic, and diaphoretic in all types of shock

5. Who is at risk for the development of shock?

Individuals at risk for the development of shock include:
- Individuals who have experienced any type of trauma
- Individuals with reduction in fluid intake (reduced thirst, confusion) or increase in fluid loss (vomiting, diarrhea)
- Individuals with significant fluid shifts, third spacing (burns)
- Individuals with acute insult to the myocardium (acute myocardial infarction)
- Individuals with dysrhythmias that influence cardiac filling and ejection
- Individuals exposed to antigens after sensitization (common: insect stings, shellfish, peanuts, drugs)
- Individuals with a known infection (gram-negative or gram-positive bacteria, fungus, virus, rickettsiae)
- Individuals with signs of undetected infection (fever, elevated white blood cell count, fatigue, anorexia)
- Individuals with invasive catheters (Foley catheter, central venous catheter) or those after instrumentation (endotracheal tube, cystoscopy)
- Individuals with a compromised immune system

6. Can shock be prevented? How?

Yes. Anaphylactic shock may be avoided by ensuring that an individual with a known hypersensitivity to an antigen is not exposed to this antigen. Thus careful assessment of allergies by the clinician is essential. The early recognition and effective management of infection may prevent the development of septic shock. In broad terms, lifestyle alterations that influence the development of coronary artery disease and acute myocardial infarction may prevent cardiogenic shock. Hypovolemic and neurogenic shock that result from trauma may be prevented with comprehensive safety educational programs during primary and secondary education that focus on risky behaviors like alcohol and drug use in combination with operation of a motor vehicle. For individuals already in the hospital, meticulous nursing evaluation for those at risk for the development of shock is vital. With early detection and intervention, development of progressive shock may be prevented.

7. What assessments enable the clinician to detect shock?

Necessary assessments are described in the following table.

Assessments for Those at Risk for Development of Shock

Body System	Assessments	Important Early Observations
Neurological	Neurological assessment, Glasgow Coma Scale, pain and anxiety assessments with 0 to 10 scale (0 = no pain, no anxiety; 10 = worst possible pain, worst possible anxiety), subjective report of impending death	Any change in level of consciousness or orientation, presence of new or increasing anxiety or "feeling of doom"

Assessments for Those at Risk for Development of Shock *continued*

Body System	Assessments	Important Early Observations
Cardiovascular	Heart rate and rhythm, heart sounds, blood pressure, capillary refill, peripheral pulses, cardiac output, and systemic vascular resistance when available	Increase in heart rate, alteration in capillary refill (increased or decreased)
Respiratory	Respiratory rate and depth, oxygen saturation, arterial blood gases, breath sounds, subjective reports of dyspnea with 0 to 10 scale (0 = no dyspnea; 10 = worst possible dyspnea)	Increased rate and depth of ventilation, respiratory alkalosis, change in breath sounds from baseline
Renal	Intake and output from all sources, hourly urinary output, serum creatinine level, daily weight	Decrease in urinary output, alteration in balance of intake and output
Integumentary	Skin temperature, skin color, presence of edema, presence of diaphoresis, core body temperature (especially during resuscitation with large volumes of cold blood products or room temperature intravenous solutions)	Skin pale, temperature change to cool or to warm / Presence of flushing, angioedema
Gastrointestinal	Bowel sounds, appetite, bowel function, evaluation of all stool and emesis for presence of obvious or occult blood	Decreased bowel sounds, anorexia, thirst
General	Evaluation for hyperkalemia/hypokalemia, hyperglycemia, hypocalcemia/hypercalcemia, serum	Hyperglycemia, hypokalemia

8. Are there diagnostic tests that are useful in patients with shock?

Yes. A number of diagnostic tests may be useful in the diagnosis and ongoing management of patients with shock. These tests are detailed in the following table.

Diagnostic Tests for Patients with Signs of Shock

Diagnostic Test	Abnormalities Found
Complete blood cell count	Hemoglobin and hematocrit reduced with hypovolemia from hemorrhage; increased with dehydration and hemoconcentration; normal in other types of shock / White count normal in all types except septic shock; may be elevated or seriously decreased with abnormal differential in septic shock

Diagnostic Tests for Patients with Signs of Shock *continued*

Diagnostic Test	Abnormalities Found
Arterial blood gas	Early shock: respiratory alkalosis (pH >7.45; PaCO$_2$ <35 mm Hg) Progressive shock: respiratory alkalosis and metabolic acidosis Irreversible shock: respiratory and metabolic acidosis
Serum chemistry panel	Increased serum glucose and sodium with early shock Decreased serum potassium in early shock; increased serum potassium in progressive and irreversible shock Increased blood urea nitrogen and creatinine in irreversible shock Decreased serum calcium with early shock and with multiple transfusions; increased serum calcium with lactic acidosis
Serum lactate	Increased in all types of progressive and irreversible shock
Urinalysis	Increased urine specific gravity with all types of progressive shock
Creatine kinase–myocardial band (CK-MB) and troponin levels	Increased in presence of acute myocardial infarction
Culture and sensitivity: blood, urine, sputum, wound	Positive culture results
Electrocardiogram	Electrical changes indicative of myocardial ischemia and infarction
Right heart catheterization	Cardiac output reduced in all types of shock except initial stage of septic shock (hyperdynamic) Pulmonary artery occlusion pressure (wedge pressure) reduced in all types of shock except cardiogenic; increased with cardiogenic shock Systemic vascular resistance increased with hypovolemic and cardiogenic shock; reduced with neurogenic, anaphylactic, and septic shock
Diagnostic peritoneal lavage	Positive for blood in peritoneal lavage solution

9. What is the overall goal of shock management?

The goal of shock management is the return to normal cellular metabolism. This goal is accomplished with improving tissue oxygen delivery.

10. How is shock treated?

The management of shock is focused on the identification and effective correction of the underlying cause of the shock state. Common therapies are detailed for each type of shock in the following table.

Management of Shock

Type of Shock	Therapies
Hypovolemic	Administer oxygen, ensure patent airway Control hemorrhage or fluid loss Expand plasma volume: replace blood, plasma, or fluid deficit; common fluids: normal saline solution, lactated Ringer's solution Replace calcium if large volumes of blood transfused
Cardiogenic	Administer oxygen, ensure patent airway Thrombolytic therapy or percutaneous transluminal coronary angioplasty for acute myocardial infarction in appropriate patients for early reperfusion Optimize preload with fluid bolus, diuretics, and vasodilators (guide with hemodynamic measures) Reduce systemic vascular resistance or afterload and myocardial oxygen demand with vasodilators, intraaortic balloon counterpulsation, ventricular assist devices Carefully augment myocardial contractility with positive inotropic agents Monitor and treat dysrhythmias, restore sinus rhythm
Anaphylactic	Administer oxygen, ensure patent airway Remove antigen Epinephrine to promote vasoconstriction and bronchodilation Bronchodilators to reduce bronchoconstriction Corticosteroids to stabilize cell membranes and reduce fluid shifts
Neurogenic	Administer oxygen, ensure patent airway Stabilize cervical spine if spinal cord injury possible Vagolytic drug (atropine sulfate) to increase heart rate Cautious fluid administration to increase preload
Septic	Administer oxygen, ensure patent airway Appropriate antibiotic/antifungal therapy ideally tailored to causative agent Aggressive fluid resuscitation and cautious use of vasopressor agents (guided by hemodynamic measures) to increase cardiac output and blood pressure With gram-negative sepsis, administration of monoclonal antibodies to endotoxins may reduce mortality With severe sepsis (APACHE score >25), administration of Xigris, a recombinant form of human activated protein C with antithrombotic and potentially antiinflammatory actions, may reduce mortality

11. What vasoactive drugs are used to manage patients with shock?

Specific vasoactive drugs that are commonly used to manage patients with shock are described in the following table.

Vasoactive Pharmacological Therapies Used with Shock

Drug	Drug Class	Action
Epinephrine	Sympathomimetic	Stimulates $\alpha 1$ adrenergic receptors: vasoconstriction; $\beta 1$ adrenergic receptors: increased heart rate and contractility; $\beta 2$ adrenergic receptors: bronchodilation
Dobutamine hydrochloride	Sympathomimetic	Stimulates $\beta 1$ adrenergic receptors: augments myocardial contractility and cardiac output
Dopamine hydrochloride	Sympathomimetic	Stimulates α and $\beta 1$ adrenergic and dopaminergic receptors: dose-dependent effects include renal vasodilation at low doses; at low to moderate doses, increased contractility, heart rate. and cardiac output; at high doses, vasoconstriction
Norepinephrine bitartrate	Sympathomimetic	Stimulates $\beta 1$ receptors: increased myocardial contractility, heart rate, and cardiac output; stimulates α adrenergic receptors: vasoconstriction
Phenylephrine hydrochloride	Sympathomimetic	Stimulates α adrenergic receptors: vasoconstriction
Isoproterenol hydrochloride	Sympathomimetic	Stimulates $\beta 1$ adrenergic receptors: increased myocardial contractility, heart rate, and cardiac output; stimulates $\beta 2$ adrenergic receptors: bronchodilation
Nitroglycerin	Nitrate	When administered intravenously: peripheral vasodilation; coronary artery dilation; reduced preload, afterload, and myocardial oxygen demand
Nitroprusside sodium	Vasodilator	Relaxes arterial and venous smooth muscle; dilates coronary arteries; reduces preload, afterload, and myocardial oxygen demand
Atropine sulfate	Anticholinergic	Increases heart rate

12. What determines whether fluid or vasoactive drugs should be given?

As a general rule, vasoactive drugs should not be administered to individuals with hypovolemia. Volume should be replaced initially, and hemodynamics reevaluated. If hypoperfusion persists with adequate fluid volume, then vasoactive drugs should be initiated to improve tissue perfusion. For example, in individuals with reduced systemic vascular resistance, fluid resuscitation is often necessary because third spacing of fluid has occurred (as with anaphylactic and septic shock). Then if systemic vascular resistance is significantly reduced and hypoperfusion persists, vasoactive drugs may be titrated to increase vascular resistance and improve preload, cardiac output, and organ perfusion. If afterload is significantly increased as with cardiogenic shock, then afterload reduction with vasodilator drugs should be initiated. If blood volume is lost with hemorrhage after trauma, then when available, blood should be replaced and plasma expanders considered. If fluid is lost as with dehydration, fluid replacement is the appropriate therapy.

13. What determines whether colloids or crystalloids should be given during fluid resuscitation?

Although this topic has been a point of discussion for nearly 3 decades, no consensus has been reached as yet. Both colloids and crystalloids have advantages and disadvantages. Colloids like albumin are held within the vascular system significantly longer and exert a pressure that helps maintain intravascular fluid volume. Much less colloid must be infused in comparison with crystalloid; however, colloid is more expensive. In those patients with increased capillary permeability, colloid escapes into the interstitial space, exerts a pressure in that area, and produces edema. Crystalloid solution like normal saline solution is readily available and less expensive, but about 80% of the infused volume is out of the vascular space within a short time period. The selection of the most appropriate fluid is based on the electrolyte composition and the tonicity of the solution. With hypotonic solutions like dextrose in water, little solution (~10%) remains in the vascular system within 30 minutes and administration of this type of fluid may promote cellular edema. Balanced solutions (similar to osmolality of plasma) like normal saline solution and Ringer's lactate solution are preferred for large volume fluid resuscitation, particularly with the loss of considerable blood volume. Hypertonic solutions (3% saline solution) increase the tonicity of plasma and move fluid from the interstitial space to the vascular space. Transient hypernatremia may occur with the use of hypertonic saline solution.

Understanding the cause of the fluid volume deficit should assist with this choice. For replacement fluid for the extracellular space, crystalloids should be administered. The choice of crystalloid solutions (saline solution versus Ringer's lactate solution) is most often based on individual clinician preference. Colloids are useful to expand the existing plasma volume when capillary integrity is present.

14. Are there specific complications that may occur with shock?

Yes. Complications related to shock are life threatening and most likely arise from disruption in organ microcirculation. These complications include acute renal failure from acute tubular necrosis, acute respiratory distress syndrome, disseminated intravascular coagulopathy, acute gastrointestinal bleeding, and multiple organ dysfunction syndrome. In acute renal failure, ischemia of the renal tubules results in necrosis and sloughing of the tubular epithelial cells, tubule obstruction, and cessation of urine formation. Acute respiratory distress syndrome is the consequence of increased capillary permeability in the lung and is likely the result of a systemic inflammatory response. Movement of fluid out of the vascular space produces a noncardiogenic pulmonary edema and shunt that is refractory to oxygen therapy. Disseminated intravascular coagulopathy is a complication of shock that produces microvascular coagulation. Platelets, fibrinogen, and other clotting factors are depleted in the microcirculation and are not available for clotting. The result is abnormal bleeding or hemorrhage. Acute gastrointestinal bleeding is the consequence of superficial gastrointestinal mucosal lesions that develop as a result of reduced organ perfusion. These lesions commonly develop soon after the trauma or shock episode, and bleeding is evident within 2 to 10 days. Multiple organ dysfunction syndrome or multiple organ failure is a particularly serious complication of shock. Organ dysfunction arises initially as a result of inadequate organ perfusion and then continues and worsens from a secondary insult from a severe inflammatory reaction. Mortality rates associated with multiple organ dysfunction syndrome are reported to be as high as 100%.

15. Should the patient with shock receive nutrition?

Yes. These patients should receive either enteral or parenteral nutrition to prevent or manage the negative nitrogen balance that results from protein catabolism. The enteral route of feeding is preferred when bowel function permits. Enteral or parenteral nutrients should be determined with comprehensive examination of organ system function and evaluation of daily caloric requirements. Malnutrition is associated with immunosuppression, reduced ventilatory drive, prolonged wound healing, reduced colloid osmotic pressure, and edema.

16. What patient and family teaching is appropriate with a patient who experiences shock?

The patient and family should be regularly apprised of the following:
- Physical condition (cause of shock)
- Prognosis
- Current therapies used for patient management, with explanation of each
- Expected outcome or goal of each therapy
- Change in condition for better or worse

Appropriate information must be tailored to the individual's ability to understand and provided in a supportive manner. Visiting time for the patient experiencing shock should be maximized.

 Key Points

- Shock is defined as impairment of cellular metabolism associated with inadequate perfusion.
- The goal of shock management is the return to normal cellular metabolism.
- If not detected and managed effectively, shock may progress through three stages: compensated, progressive, and irreversible.
- The management of shock is focused on the identification and effective correction of the underlying cause of the shock state.
- Complications related to shock are life threatening and most likely arise from disruption in organ microcirculation.

Internet Resources

Postgraduate Medicine Online article: Optimal Management of Septic Shock:
http://www.postgradmed.com/issues/2002/03_02/fitch2.htm

EMedicine Article: Anaphylaxis:
http://www.emedicine.com/aaem/topic15.htm

Bibliography

Dark PM, Delooz HH, Hillier V et al: Monitoring the circulatory responses of shocked patients during fluid resuscitation in the emergency department, *Intensive Care Med* 26:173-179, 2000.

Deakin CD, Low JL: Accuracy of the advanced trauma life support guidelines for predicting systolic blood pressure using carotid, femoral, and radial pulses: observational study, *Br Med J* 321:673-674, 2000.

De Jonghe B, Cheval C, Misset B et al: Relationship between blood lactate and early hepatic dysfunction in acute circulatory failure, *J Crit Care* 14:7-11, 1999.

Kaplan LJ, McPartland K, Santora TA, Trooskin SZ: Start with a subjective assessment of skin temperature to identify hypoperfusion in intensive care unit patients, *J Trauma* 50:620-628, 2001.

Landry DW, Oliver JA: The pathogenesis of vasodilatory shock, *N Engl J Med* 345:588-595, 2001.

Mikhail J: Resuscitation endpoints in trauma, *AACN Clin Issues* 10:10-21, 1999.

Miller PR, Meredith JW, Chang MC: Randomized, prospective comparison of increased preload versus inotropes in the resuscitation of trauma patients: effects on cardiopulmonary function and visceral perfusion, *J Trauma* 44:107-113, 1998.

Section IV

Therapeutic Options

C h a p t e r 20

Percutaneous Coronary Interventions

Lisa A. Kiger and Monty Yoder

1. What procedures are inclusive of percutaneous coronary interventions (PCIs)?

- Percutaneous transluminal coronary angioplasty (PTCA)
- Intracoronary stent implantation
- Directional coronary atherectomy (DCA)
- Percutaneous transluminal coronary rotational ablation (PTCRA)
- Excimer laser coronary angioplasty (ELCA)
- Cutting balloon angioplasty (CBA)
- Intravascular brachytherapy (IVBT)
- Thrombectomy procedures

2. What are the clinical indications for PCIs?

- Inducible ischemia on stress testing
- Angina refractory to medical therapy
- Recurrent ischemia after myocardial infarction
- Acute myocardial infarction (AMI) with obstructed infarct-related coronary artery (IRA)
- Patients with AMI who are not candidates for fibrinolysis or surgery

3. What are the essential components of preprocedure care for patients undergoing PCI?

- A complete history including review of previous lab data, diagnostic studies, and results of previous cardiac catheterizations or PCI.
- A complete physical exam including assessment of vital signs, heart and lung sounds, and carotid and peripheral pulses.
- Recent 12-lead electrocardiogram (ECG), chest radiograph, complete blood count, complete metabolic panel, and coagulation studies. A serum pregnancy test is recommended for all menstruating female patients.
- Target preprocedure lab studies include prothrombin time (PT) <15 seconds, international normalized ratio (INR) <1.5 seconds, serum creatinine level <1.4 mg/dL, serum potassium >4.0 or <5.0 mEq/L, hemoglobin (Hgb) >9g/dL, hematocrit (Hct) >30%, and platelet count >130,000 mm^3.
- Verify allergic reactions to dyes used in previous tests or procedures: iodine, shellfish (i.e., crab or shrimp), and strawberries. Antihistamines, corticosteroids,

and H1 and H2 histamine blockers may be administered prophylactically to decrease allergic and anaphylactic reactions to contrast agent.
- Patient and family teaching regarding procedure, medications, diet, and activity.
- Informed consent is obtained after explanation of the procedure, its purpose, potential benefits, and possible risks and all questions are answered.
- Patients should be NPO, except for medications, after midnight the day of the scheduled procedure. Patients whose PCI procedures are not scheduled until the afternoon may have a light liquid breakfast.
- Certain medications may need to be discontinued or the dosage reduced. Insulin and food intake should be adjusted if patient has diabetes. Patients usually receive half of their insulin dosage the morning of the procedure. Oral hypoglycemic agents, such as metformin (Glucophage), should be held 24 to 48 hours before PCI and for 48 hours afterwards. Renal function tests should be assessed, and results should be in the normal range before reinstitution.
- Anticoagulants, such as warfarin (Coumadin), should be discontinued at least 48 hours before the elective percutaneous transluminal angioplasty. Subcutaneous low–molecular-weight heparin should be discontinued at least 6 to 12 hours before the procedure. Intravenous unfractionated heparin therapy may be continued.
- Antiplatelet agents and antithrombotic agents, such as aspirin and clopidogrel bisulfate (Plavix), should be administered. An empiric dose of aspirin 80 to 325 mg given at least 2 hours before the PCI procedure is generally recommended. Clopidogrel bisulfate 300 mg loading dose followed by 75 mg daily may be used in patients in whom intracoronary stenting is likely. In elective settings, clopidogrel bisulfate should be given at least 72 hours before the procedure to achieve maximum platelet inhibition.
- Catheter insertion sites (i.e., femoral, radial, or brachial artery and femoral or jugular vein) should be shaved and cleansed.
- An intravenous line is necessary for administration of fluids, medications, and conscious sedation.
- Continuous cardiac monitoring is necessary for myocardial ischemia, injury, infarction, arrhythmias, or hemodynamic instability.

4. What happens during the PTCA procedure?

- Percutaneous transluminal coronary angioplasty is performed in the catheterization lab, which is supplied with a variety of monitoring devices, video monitors, and radiograph equipment. The preparation is similar to that of angiography (see Question 5 in Chapter 7, Invasive Cardiovascular Testing).
- Intravenous unfractionated heparin therapy (100 to 150 U/kg initial bolus with additional boluses adjusted to maintain the activated clotting time [ACT] around 300 seconds) is given to prevent platelet deposition and fibrin formation at the PTCA site. The ACT is checked within 5 to 10 minutes of heparin administration. The ACT goal with unfractionated heparin in combination with glycoprotein (GP) IIb-IIIa receptor agonist is around 200 to 250 seconds.
- A guide catheter is inserted through the sheath and advanced to the coronary artery. The guide catheter acts as a pathway to the coronary artery in which the balloon catheter follows.

- The balloon catheter (with a deflated balloon on the tip) is advanced to the narrowing of the artery over an intracoronary guidewire. This intracoronary guidewire acts as a safety wire and stays in the coronary artery until the procedure is complete. The balloon is inflated for 1 to 2 minutes and deflated several times to break the plaque deposits and compress these against the arterial wall. This improves blood flow through the coronary artery.
- During balloon inflation, the coronary blood flow is occluded and anginal symptoms are often provoked. However, symptoms usually resolve spontaneously after balloon deflation and blood flow is restored. Intracoronary nitroglycerin may be administered during the procedure to dilate coronary arteries and prevent reactive vasospasm after balloon inflation.

5. What symptoms may the patient experience during the procedure?

Symptoms that the patient may have are similar to those listed in Question 7 of the Angiography section of Chapter 7, Invasive Cardiovascular Testing. In addition, the patient may experience chest pain as the balloon catheter is inflated.

6. What happens after a PCI?

- After the procedure is completed, the intracoronary guidewire, interventional device, and guide catheter are removed.
- Sheath management and removal are guided with institutional protocols. The sheath may be removed, and hemostasis may be obtained with manual compression or percutaneous vascular closure devices. The sheath may be left in place until the effects of anticoagulation therapy are reversed and the ACT has returned to normal.
- When the sheath is removed, firm pressure is applied to the insertion site for 15 to 30 minutes until hemostasis is obtained. A band aid–type dressing may be applied.
- Post–sheath removal activity guidelines vary with institutional protocol. Typically after 2 to 6 hours of bed rest, the patient may resume normal activity. Patients incurring percutaneous vascular closure devices may return to normal activity within 2 to 3 hours. Times may be prolonged if bleeding complications occur or if patients receive unfractionated heparin, low–molecular-weight heparin, or GP IIb-IIIa inhibitors.
- Patients may be admitted to a short-stay unit or cardiac unit where they should be closely monitored.
- Postprocedural assessments include assessment for presence of ischemic symptoms (i.e., chest pain), frequent monitoring of vital signs, pulses distal from insertion site, and insertion site for presence of localized tenderness, hematoma, femoral bruit, or pulsatile mass.
- Continuous cardiac monitoring and monitoring of any new onset ST segment elevation or T wave changes (acute restenosis) in the lead directly related to the revascularized coronary artery should be initiated. This may be determined by looking at the ECG wave tracing during balloon inflation to see which lead

most prominently displays ST segment changes. Myocardial ischemia, injury, infarction, arrhythmias, or hemodynamic instability should be monitored. Reperfusion arrhythmias are common.
- One should obtain and monitor 12-lead ECG, complete blood counts, coagulation studies, serial cardiac enzymes, and troponin levels.
- Adequate hydration through intravenous fluids and oral intake should be maintained to minimize renal insufficiency.
- The patient should advance to a prudent diet.
- Intravenous nitroglycerin (usually up to 12 hours after the procedure), unfractionated heparin, and GP IIb-IIIa platelet aggregator infusions should be maintained as prescribed.
- The need for the patient to report chest pain immediately should be reinforced. Any symptom of chest pain should be evaluated.

7. What closure techniques are used to achieve hemostasis after sheath removal?

Refer to Question 9 in the Angiography section of Chapter 7, Invasive Cardiovascular Testing).

8. What activity guidelines* are recommended after sheath removal for manual compression and vascular closure devices?

	Bed Rest With Head of Bed Elevated	Dangle Legs	Ambulate
Perclose	45 degrees for 1 hr		2 hr
AngioSeal	45 degrees for 1 hr		2 hr
VasoSeal	30 degrees for 1 hr		1 hr
Duett	30 degrees for 1 hr, 90 degrees for 2nd hr		2 hr
4F Sheath	45 degrees for 2 hr	3 hr	3.5-4 hr
5F Sheath	45 degrees for 2 hr	4 hr	4.5-5 hr
6F Sheath	15 degrees for 1 hr, 30 degrees for 2nd and 3rd hr	5 hr	6 hr
7F Sheath	15 degrees for 2 hr, 30 degrees for 3rd hr, 90 degrees for 4th hr	6 hr	7 hr
8-10F Sheath	15 degrees for 3 hr, 30 degrees for 4th and 5th hr, 90 degrees for 6th hr	7 hr	8 hr

*Activity levels may vary according to manufacturer guidelines, institution policy, physician preference, and individualized needs of patient. Times may be prolonged if bleeding complications occur or if patient receives unfractionated heparin, low–molecular-weight heparin, or GP IIb-IIIa inhibitors.

9. What are the complications of PCIs?

- Acute closure or vasospasm of coronary artery manifested by chest pain
- Cardiac arrhythmias, bradycardia, conduction disturbances
- Bleeding or hematoma at insertion site
- Retroperitoneal bleed, pseudoaneurysm, arteriovenous fistula
- Arterial perforation, thrombosis, embolus, dissection
- Fracture of intracoronary guidewire
- Allergic reaction to contrast agent
- Renal insult from contrast agent
- Hypovolemia or hypotension
- Vascular compromise of catheterized extremity
- Myocardial infarction, stroke, death

10. What precautions should be observed after the procedure to monitor and prevent complications?

- Removal of the sheaths or the application of manual or mechanical pressure on the insertion site can cause bradycardia and hypotension. A bolus of intravenous fluid and atropine may be given to correct these symptoms.
- Patients should keep leg straight and avoid bending at the hip for 2 to 8 hours after the sheath is removed.
- Patients should be instructed to hold the dressing firmly if they need to cough or sneeze.
- Patients should be instructed to immediately report discomfort or sudden pain at the insertion site.
- Swelling, a warm moist sticky feeling, or bleeding at the insertion site may occur.
- Any discomfort in chest, neck, jaw, arms or upper back may be seen.
- Shortness of breath, nausea, weakness, or dizziness may occur.

11. What are the most common signs and symptoms of retroperitoneal bleeding?

- Back or flank pain
- Hypotension
- Tachycardia
- Decreased Hgb and Hct
- Restlessness and agitation

12. When should the nurse alert the physician or nurse practitioner/physician assistant (NP/PA) for patients undergoing PCI?

A physician or NP/PA should be notified if the patient has oozing or bleeding at the insertion site or with development of a hematoma or pain/tenderness at the insertion site, a decrease in peripheral pulses, affected extremity pain or numbness, hemodynamic instability, and chest pain (or anginal equivalent).

13. What necessary actions does a nurse perform if a patient has a hematoma develop at the femoral insertion site?

For overt bleeding or hematoma, the nurse should apply continuous direct pressure with a gloved hand ¹/₂ to 1 inch above the insertion site for a minimum of 15 minutes without release. Once hemostasis is obtained, the site is cleaned and observed for bleeding and Band-Aid–type or clear dressing is applied. Vital signs, insertion site, extremity pulses, and activity precautions should be monitored. The area of hematoma is marked for later comparison.

14. Describe the various types of interventional procedures that are performed in adjunct to PTCA.

Intracoronary stents are used to reduce closure of the coronary artery and can be deployed after any percutaneous interventional procedure. Stents are expandable metal coils or wire mesh mounted on a balloon catheter. Balloon-expanded stents are mounted on a balloon catheter and on inflation of the balloon are expanded. Self-expanding stents are mounted or loaded on a catheter with a protective covering. When the cover is slid back, the stent pops open or self expands. The intracoronary stent is deployed to the area of stenosis. The balloon is inflated, and the stent expands against the wall of the artery. The balloon is deflated and removed, leaving the stent permanently in place to keep the artery open. Stents reduce the rate of restenosis in primary angioplasty and achieve a TIMI III (normal or brisk flow through the coronary artery) flow in 96% of patients. After 4 to 6 weeks, the stent becomes covered with a thin layer of arterial tissue to help keep the stent in place. To reduce the risk of restenosis at the site of stent placement, medications such as aspirin and antiplatelet agents (such as clopidogrel bisulfate) may be prescribed. Stents may be coated with antiinflammatory agents (such as dexamethasone), antithrombotics (such as heparin), antiproliferative agents (such as paclitaxel), or antibiotics that inhibit cell growth (such as sirolimus [Rapamune], or actinomycin D). These drug-coated stents may reduce in-stent restenosis.

Directional coronary atherectomy is a procedure that removes atheromatous plaque from the artery (debulking). The DCA catheter tip has a cutting chamber on one side and a balloon on the other. The chamber is positioned at the lesion, the balloon is inflated, and a rotating cutter cuts the plaque. The device traps the shavings in the nose cone and removes them from the artery when the catheter is withdrawn. The DCA device may require balloon dilation before, during, and after PCI for optimal results.

Percutaneous transluminal coronary rotational ablation is a procedure that reduces plaque with minimal stretching of the vessel. The Rotablator is a flexible catheter with a high-speed, rotating burr covered with microscopic diamond crystals. The tip is driven at speeds of up to 140 to 190,000 rpm. The burr cuts the plaque into tiny particles, which are smaller than a red blood cell (RBC). As the plaque is cut, it is dispersed into the bloodstream and removed from the circulation by the reticuloendothelial system, especially in the lung, liver, and spleen. A series of different sized burrs is used to achieve the size of the lumen necessary. An adjunctive balloon angioplasty is completed after PTCRA to smooth out the vessel wall and reduce restenosis. PTCRA is efficacious in highly calcified lesions resistant to balloon angioplasty, plaque debulking before intracoronary stent implantation, and plaque debulking when stents restenose (in-stent restenosis).

In ELCA, the laser-tipped catheter is inserted at the site of plaque obstruction. The laser is activated and emits pulsating bursts of ultraviolet light that vaporize obstructing plaque. As a result, the blocked artery is opened and blood flow is improved. Frequently laser angioplasty is used to create an opening in the plaque so that balloon angioplasty or intracoronary stent implantation can be successfully performed.

Cutting balloon angioplasty (Cutting Balloon) is a balloon catheter with micro-surgical blades (atherotomes) on the balloon. When the balloon is inflated, the microsurgical blades incise the plaque, creating a more controlled cut and minimizing vessel wall trauma. It is ideal for small vessels, bifurcations, ostial side branches, and distal lesions and is used to predilate fibrotic lesions before intracoronary stent implantation or IVBT.

Intravascular brachytherapy is an approach used to treat in-stent restenosis. A catheter is positioned at the treatment site, and a wire (also referred to as a seed train or ribbon) containing the radiation is placed within the catheter. A calculated dose of radiation is delivered to the treatment site. Once the dose has been delivered, the wire and catheter are withdrawn. Radiation affects the proliferation of smooth muscle cells responsible for restenosis, thereby potentially minimizing the incidence of recurrent stenosis.

Thrombectomy procedures are also performed. AngioJet is indicated for coronary thrombus. Its powerful high-velocity saline jets create suction at the catheter tip, causing rapid clot lysis and removal through the catheter lumen. The X-Sizer is also a thrombectomy device that both cuts and extracts material from the coronary artery or saphenous vein grafts.

15. What are the discharge instructions for patients undergoing PCI procedures?

Discharge instructions are similar to that of angiography (see Question 22 in Chapter 7, Invasive Cardiovascular Testing). In addition, patients should be educated regarding the benefits of cardiac rehabilitation and restenosis potential. If a stent is placed, a patient identification card, a stent booklet, and education regarding antiplatelet medications should be provided.

16. When should patients contact their physician or NP/PA?

Patients should contact their physician or NP/PA if they notice any of the following symptoms:
- Bleeding, swelling, redness, or drainage at the insertion site
- Dizziness, shortness of breath, chest pain, or pressure

- Numbness; change in color, temperature, or sensation in the arm or leg in which the catheter was inserted
- Fever

17. What adjunctive technology can be used to improve PCIs?

Intracoronary ultrasound (ICUS) is a catheter with a tiny ultrasound transducer on the tip that is advanced into the coronary arteries to provide a cross-sectional view of the vessel wall. It is used during interventional procedures for assessment of lumen size, degree of stenosis, structure of arterial wall, and proper stent placement.

Distal protection devices aim to capture atherosclerotic material and thrombus that is released from the treated lesion in saphenous vein grafts, thus reducing distal embolization. The Angioguard system consists of a polyurethane filter basket attached to a guidewire that allows continuous perfusion with ensuring effective capture of microemboli. The filter is deployed, the lesion is treated, and the basket is recaptured with the embolic material. The PercuSurge device consists of a guidewire that incorporates a balloon on its distal tip. The balloon is inflated distal to the lesion, the lesion is treated, and an aspiration catheter is advanced over the wire; particulate debris is aspirated, and the balloon deflated.

18. What pharmacologic agents are frequently used in adjunct to PCIs?

- Glycoprotein IIb/IIIa inhibitors (see Chapter 28, Antiplatelet and Antithrombotic Agents) may be administered before the procedure and continued after the procedure to prevent platelet aggregation and thrombus formation. Duration of therapy for dual antiplatelet therapy (acetylsalicylic acid [ASA] plus clopidogrel bisulfate) is discussed in Chapter 28.
- Thrombin inhibitors such as unfractionated heparin are maintained throughout the PCI procedure to prevent thrombus formation. Anticoagulation therapy with unfractionated heparin is routinely discontinued after PCI for sheath removal. The therapy may be restarted in patients considered at high risk for acute thrombus formation. Low–molecular-weight heparins (i.e., enoxaparin, dalteparin sodium) may be administered before the procedure and may be continued after the procedure at the discretion of the prescribing physician. In patients in whom unfractionated heparin, GP IIb-IIIa inhibitors, or low–molecular-weight heparins are not appropriate, direct thrombin inhibitors (i.e., Angiomax, Refludan, Argatroban) may be administered before the procedure and may be continued after the procedure at the discretion of the prescribing physician.
- Antiplatelet agents such as aspirin are administered before the procedure and continued indefinitely to prevent platelet aggregation. If the patient is aspirin intolerant, clopidogrel bisulfate (Plavix) may be administered. Clopidogrel bisulfate 300 mg PO should be given before the procedure, and 75 mg PO daily may be administered after the procedure up to 1 month after intracoronary stent implant and up to 3 months after IVBT.

- Nitrates may be administered before the procedure to control angina and may be continued up to 24 hours after PCI to prevent coronary spasm. Intracoronary nitroglycerin may be administered during the procedure to dilate coronary arteries and prevent reactive vasospasm after balloon inflation.
- Beta-blockers, such as metoprolol or atenolol, may be administered to decrease both the myocardial oxygen demand and the risk of ventricular arrhythmias.
- Angiotensin-converting enzyme (ACE) inhibitors may be administered to decrease mortality and prevent progression of heart failure.
- Lipid-lowering agents are administered to achieve a total cholesterol of <200 mg/dL, LDL <100 mg/dL, HDL >40 mg/dL, and triglycerides <200 mg/dL.

19. What lies in the future for PCI?

Angiogenesis. Angiogenesis is an experimental treatment that promotes the creation of new blood vessels. Growth factors, such as basic fibroblast growth factor (bFGF) and vascular endothelial growth factor (VEGF), are delivered directly to the myocardium to stimulate growth of collateral blood vessels. Chemicals that stimulate the production of growth factors, genes that directly manufacture growth factors, and medications that mimic the effects of growth factors are also being investigated.

Sonotherapy. Sonotherapy is a catheter-based technology that uses ultrasound energy to reduce intimal hyperplasia for in-stent stenosis. Therapeutic ultrasound energy is emitted from the catheter to treat the stented area. It is hypothesized that the ultrasound will have antirestenotic effects on the vascular smooth muscle cell.

Key Points

- PCI is inclusive of a number of procedures including PTCA, ICS, DCA, PTCRA, ECLA, CBA, IVBT, and thrombectomy procedures. Read further to understand the "alphabet soup."
- Understanding the preprocedure, intraprocedure, and postprocedure care for patients undergoing PCI is imperative.
- Various closure techniques, such as Perclose, Angioseal, and Vasoseal, among others, are used to achieve hemostasis after sheath removal.
- Postsheath activity levels may vary according to manufacture guidelines, institutional policies, physician preference, and individualized patient needs.
- Pharmacologic agents, such as thrombin inhibitors, GP IIb/IIa inhibitors, antiplatelet agents, nitrates, beta-blockers, ACE inhibitors, and lipid-lowering agents, are used in adduct to PCI. Understanding the indications, contraindications, dosage and administration, and side effects of these agents is imperative.

Internet Resources

American Heart Association:
www.americanheart.org

American College of Cardiology:
www.acc.org

Angioplasty.org:
www.ptca.org

Interventional Cardiology and Vascular Medicine Community:
www.tctmd.com

The Heart.org:
www.theheart.org

Bibliography

Apple S, Lindsay J, editors: *Principles and practice of interventional cardiology*, Baltimore, 2000, Lippincott Williams & Wilkins.

Axelberg A, Mayer D: Arterial closure method: pull, plug, or close, *Am J Nurs* (suppl):11-4, 2000.

Fasseas, P, Orford J, Denktas A, Berger P: Distal protection devices during percutaneous coronary and carotid interventions, *Curr Control Trials Cardiovasc Med* 2(6):286-291, 2001.

Gentz CA: Perceived learning needs of the patient undergoing coronary angioplasty: an integrative review of the literature, *Heart Lung J Acute Crit Care* 29(3):161-172, 2000.

Lowe HC, Oesterle SN, Khachigian LM: Coronary in-stent restenosis: current status and future strategies, *J Am Coll Cardiol* 39(2):183-193, 2002.

Nicholaus MJ, Chambers CE, Ettinger SM et al: Advances in interventional cardiology: beyond the balloon, *Nurs Clin North Am* 35:897-912, 2000.

Norell MS, Perrins EJ, editors: *Essential interventional cardiology*, London, 2001, Harcourt.

Reynolds S, Waterhouse K, Miller K: Patient care after percutaneous transluminal coronary angioplasty, *Nurs Manage* 32:51-54, 56, 2001.

Schwertz D, Vaitkus P: Drug eluting stents to prevent blockage of coronary arteries, *J Cardiovasc Nurs* 18:11-16, 2002.

Smith SC Jr, Dove JT, Jacobs AK et al: ACC/AHA guidelines for percutaneous coronary intervention: a report of the American College of Cardiology/American Heart Association Task Force on Practice Guidelines (Committee to Revise the 1993 Guidelines for Percutaneous Transluminal Coronary Angioplasty), *J Am Coll Cardiol* 37:2239, i-lxvi, 2001.

Thorbs N, Barbiere C, Wayland R, Morgan P: Coronary rotational atherectomy: a nursing perspective, *Crit Care Nurse* 20:77-84, 2000.

Chapter 21

Cardiovascular Surgery

Sharron Rushton and Penny Kay Kalpin

This chapter focuses on adult surgical treatments for coronary artery disease and valvular disease. Treatments for congenital heart disease and heart failure and aspects of cardiac transplantation are covered in other chapters.

1. What are some categories of cardiovascular (CV) surgery?

There are five major groupings of cardiac surgery. The most common group of CV surgery is for treatment of coronary artery disease and includes traditional and minimally invasive coronary artery bypass grafting (CABG) and transmyocardial laser revascularization (TMR). A second kind of CV surgery includes surgeries for the treatment of valvular disorders and typically involves the valve being repaired or replaced. A third category of CV surgery consists of treatments for the repair of structural defects, repair of septal defects (atrial and ventricular), repair of patent ductus arteriosus, Fontan procedure, repair of ventricular aneurysm, and dissections. A fourth combination of CV surgery includes procedures to correct arrhythmias (e.g., the maze procedure), ablation therapy, skeletonization, insertion of an automatic internal cardiac defibrillator, and surgical interruption of the conduction pathway. The final class includes CV surgery for the treatment of left ventricular (LV) failure, like cardiac transplantation, insertion of ventricular assist devices, and dynamic cardiomyoplasty.

2. What are the indications for the previously mentioned categories of CV surgeries?

Surgery	Indications
Coronary artery bypass grafting	Significant left main stenosis (or left main equivalent [left anterior descending artery + circumflex artery]), coronary artery disease (three-vessel), unstable angina, myocardial infarction
Valve replacement/repair	Severe aortic stenosis or regurgitation, mitral stenosis or regurgitation, tricuspid stenosis or regurgitation, Ebstein's anomaly, endocarditis

continued

Surgery	Indications
Congenital heart surgery	Patent foramen ovale, atrial septal defect, ventricular septal defect
Cardiac transplantation	Inoperable coronary artery disease, end-stage cardiomyopathy
Ablation or surgical interruption of dysrhythmias	Sinus tachycardia, atrial fibrillation, Wolff-Parkinson-White syndrome, ventricular tachycardia (refractory to medication)

3. What are the preoperative needs for patients undergoing CV surgery?

Before surgery, a preoperative evaluation is completed. The first step is a history, physical, allergy review, and anesthesia evaluation. Also before surgery, the patient undergoes a 12-lead electrocardiogram (ECG), posteroanterior (PA)/lateral chest radiograph, and laboratory tests that include a chemistry panel, complete blood cell count (with platelet count), bleeding times (prothrombin time [PT], international normalized ratio [INR], and an activated partial thromboplastin time [PTT]), type and cross for blood, liver function tests, and urine analysis. The patient may have also undergone a stress test (either pharmacological or exercise), a coronary angiogram, an echocardiogram, pulmonary function tests, and carotid Doppler study. Patients with valvular disease may also have a dental exam to decrease the risk of endocarditis. A nursing assessment should also occur before surgery and should include a head-to-toe exam. The patient's social situation should be carefully evaluated to identify those individuals who may need additional assistance after discharge. The nursing assessment should also include baseline functional data, educational needs assessment, cultural/religious needs, nutrition screen, identification of baseline pain scale rating, and a review of advanced directives.

In addition, preparation of the body is necessary to decrease the risk of infection. The physician orders the type of preoperative cleansing need. An example might be two showers with chlorhexidine gluconate solution before surgery. The patients are shaved or clipped by either the nursing or the operating room staff depending on the institution.

After a discussion with the attending physician, the consent forms need to be signed and witnessed by a member of the team. Verification of the consent signed before the premedication administration is important; otherwise, surgery may be delayed.

Some institutions administer medications on call to the operating room. These medications may include sedation and intravenous (IV) antibiotics. In addition, in some facilities patients receive mupirocin intranasally before surgery. The current recommendation is that the patient receive the mupirocin for 5 days before surgery. However, because of emergent or next-day surgeries, this early administration frequently does not happen. The physician may elect to continue the mupirocin for 3 days after surgery to ensure that a patient receives a 5-day course. Limited research suggests that this reduces the incidence of sternal infections with *Staphylococcus aureus*.

The night before surgery the patient may be offered a medication to assist with relaxation and sleep, such as lorazepam (Ativan) or zolpidem tartrate (Ambien). The patient needs to be NPO after midnight, which reduces the risk of aspiration as in other general anesthesia cases. In addition, changes are made to the patient's home regime before surgery that are discussed subsequently.

4. What changes may be made in the patient's home medication regime before admission for CV surgery?

Aspirin and nonsteroidal antiinflammatory medications should be stopped 7 days before surgery if possible. Dipyridamole should be discontinued at least 3 days before surgery. Warfarin also needs to be stopped before surgery to allow for normalization of INR. The INR falls within normal limits in an average of 96 to 115 hours. Patients may be brought into the hospital a few days before surgery if they are on warfarin therapy for a heparin drip. This allows the maintenance of safe anticoagulation therapy until surgery but also allows the surgical team to have better control of clotting cascade. Clopidogrel bisulfate (Plavix) may also need to be stopped before surgery because of increased risk of bleeding; however, the surgeon may opt to continue it until the day before surgery. In addition, vitamin E, herbal therapies, and cox-2 inhibitors should also be stopped before surgery because they may increase the risk of bleeding.

Cardiac and antihypertensive medications are generally continued until surgery. Diabetic regimes are continued until the morning of surgery when oral agents are held and insulin is generally given as a half dose. Thyroid agents are generally continued until the morning of surgery. Other medications are evaluated based on patient condition.

5. What should be included in the preoperative teaching?

The preoperative teaching should include an overview of the entire procedure. A brief review of the anatomy and physiology is helpful. This gives the patient a reference point for later discussions of the surgical process. The teaching should include an explanation of the preoperative testing, the need for showering to decrease risk of infection before surgery, which medications should be taken the morning of surgery as dictated by the physician, and the need to be NPO after midnight.

In addition to general preoperative teaching for all patients undergoing general anesthesia, a few requirements are specific to CV treatment. The patient needs to know about the respiratory work that is necessary after surgery, and the patient should be taught how to splint the chest with a pillow or bath blanket before coughing and deep breathing. In addition, the correct technique for the use of the incentive spirometer should be explained. The patient should also receive a detailed explanation of the benefits before the day of surgery. This allows the patient to be comfortable with the new equipment and be prepared after surgery. Talking with the patient about the need for pain control in the postoperative period is also important. Patients need to understand that they play a role in the pain control and that they need to let their health care providers know about their pain level.

Furthermore, the patient and patient's family may be offered a tour of the intensive care unit (ICU) as a possible way to decrease anxiety. In addition, although the discharge instructions are repeated at a later time, initiation of the discharge instruction process before surgery is imperative because the more times the patient hears the information, the more information is retained. The family should be informed as to how it will receive information during surgery and immediately after surgery. This should help alleviate some of the anxiety and also acknowledges the needs of the family.

6. How is the decision made to undergo a percutaneous transluminal coronary angioplasty (PTCA) versus CABG?

If coronary artery disease is suspected, the patient usually undergoes a coronary angiogram. An interventional cardiologist then reviews the results, and a decision is made as to whether the lesion can be corrected interventionally or whether it requires surgical correction. Some of the factors in this decision are:
- The number of vessels involved
- The location of plaques (branch, proximally or distally)
- The overall health of the patient (age, CV risk factors, symptoms, etc)
- A history of cardiac surgery (which may limit the number of available conduits)

7. What is CABG?

Coronary artery bypass grafting is a surgical procedure for the treatment of coronary artery disease. CABG is generally the best option when medical therapy and angioplasty with or without a coronary stent have failed. During the CABG, an alternative pathway for the blood is created, bypassing the blockage and leading to coronary revascularization. A conduit or graft is attached proximally to the aorta with the distal anastomosis site located beyond the atherosclerotic plaque on the affected vessel. The blood is essentially rerouted and then can freely flow from the aorta to the cardiac muscle. A person may have multiple grafts depending on the number of plaques.

8. What are conduits or grafts?

Conduits, grafts, or bypasses are the blood vessels that are used to reroute the blood around the blockage. They are used to connect the aorta to the distal portion of the coronary artery as a means of rerouting the blood supply around the blockage in the native vessel. Certain arteries and veins generally are chosen based on multiple criteria (see Question 9).

9. How are the conduits chosen for CABG?

The surgeon chooses the type of graft based on characteristics of the patient (comorbidities and clinical presentation), condition of the native vessels, and the potential grafts. The internal mammary artery (IMA) is the conduit of choice because it has a greater patency rate at 10 years (83%) compared with saphenous vein grafts (41%). Arterial grafts are thought to make better conduits than vein grafts because they are accustomed to the higher pressures systems on the arterial side and therefore are less likely to have atherosclerotic plaques develop over time. However, some arteries, particularly the radial arteries, are prone to spasm and need prophylactic treatment (with nitrates or calcium channel blockers) to prevent the spasm.

The location can also determine the choice of conduit. For example, the left internal mammary artery (LIMA) is frequently used for grafting to the left anterior descending artery (LAD). If the patient has previously undergone bypass surgery, the choice of conduit may be limited. In those circumstances, the surgeon may chose to use cephalic/basilic veins, gastroepiploic artery, inferior gastric artery, and radial artery.

10. What are some systemic responses that may result from the cardiopulmonary bypass machine?

- Pulmonary hypertension
- Bleeding
- Thrombocytopenia
- Hemoglobinemia
- Stroke
- Air emboli
- Hypotension
- Hypertension
- Tachycardia
- Fluid retention
- Hypokalemia
- Hyperglycemia
- Hypothermia
- Myocardial depression

11. What are the three most common postoperative morbidities associated with coronary artery bypass surgery?

The most common morbidity is renal dysfunction, which occurs in approximately 8% of the patients. Renal dysfunction is defined as a creatinine level greater than 2.0 mg/dL or a rise in baseline by 0.7 mg/dL. The second most common morbidity is neurological impairment, which occurs in approximately

6% of patients undergoing CABG. The neurological changes can stem from hypoxia, emboli, hemorrhage, ischemia, or metabolic dysfunction. The third most common morbidity is mediastinitis, which is a sternal wound infection that occurs in up to 4% of patients undergoing CABG.

12. What is TMR?

Transmyocardial laser revascularization is the latest development in the treatment of refractory angina. Patients whose conditions are declared unsuitable for revascularization via CABG or percutaneous transluminal coronary intervention (PCI) with continuing chronic debilitating angina may be candidates for TMR. TMR has been shown to decrease angina, decrease physical limitations, and improve quality of life. In this surgery, a laser is used to insert channels in the myocardium in the area of ischemia. This procedure is believed to lead to angiogenesis, which increases blood supply to the previously starved myocardium. It may be performed in conjunction with CABG in certain situations to maximize therapy.

13. What types of tests are commonly ordered for patients who undergo valve repair or replacement?

- Radiograph
- ECG
- Holter monitor
- Echocardiogram (transthoracic or transesophageal)
- Exercise tests
- Cardiac catheterization

14. What types of surgical procedures are available for patients with valvular disease?

Chapter 14 (Valvular Heart Disease) includes an explanation of the different types of valvular disease and their pathophysiology. Patients may undergo a repair or replacement of the malfunctioning valve in an invasive procedure. Patients may undergo valvuloplasty, which is an intervention done to avoid surgical valve replacement for a few years. Cannulas are placed in bilateral femoral sites, and catheters are advanced to the stenotic valve. A balloon catheter is placed and inflated within the valve. In addition, the heart valve may be repaired or replaced. Patients with mitral valve stenosis can also undergo balloon valvuloplasty and commissurotomy, which is a surgical incision in which the adhesions that cause the leaves of the valve to adhere to each other are incised.

15. What are the types of valves seen in valve replacement surgery?

The three main types of valves used in valve replacement surgery are as follows:
- **Mechanical valves.** These valves generally are made of metal, and the greatest advantage is the long life of the valve. However, these valves require anticoagulation therapy.

- **Bioprosthetic valves.** These valves are made of a combination of animal tissue and metal/polyester support. The main advantage is the lack of need for long-term anticoagulation therapy, but the valves may require short-term anticoagulation therapy.
- **Homograft valves.** These are tissue valves that have good functional results after surgery and do not require anticoagulation therapy. However, they can only be used in the aortic or pulmonic valve location.

16. Why is anticoagulation therapy used after valve surgery?

Anticoagulation therapy is required for surgery with mechanical valves. These artificial valves are recognized as foreign entities and elicit the response of the immune system, which leads to the activation of the coagulation cascade. Because the coagulation cascade is activated chronically, the anticoagulation therapy may be required for a lifetime. The bioprosthetic valves may require anticoagulation therapy for the short term as determined by the surgeon.

17. Are there any additional considerations for patients who have undergone aortic valve replacement in addition to those generally described for patients undergoing any CV surgery in the early phase of recovery?

- Avoidance of postoperative hypertension is important in this patient population. Generally, systolic blood pressure should be less than 120 mm Hg. Hypertension avoidance is essential to decrease the strain on the suture line of the new/repaired valve.
- Patients may also have more difficulty with dysrhythmias early in the course, such as heart block or ventricular tachycardia. Symptomatic heart block can be managed with a pacemaker, and ventricular tachycardia with antiarrhythmics and potassium and magnesium replacement.
- Another potential complication is the development of atrial fibrillation (A fib) (see Question 33 for treatment methods).
- This patient population is also at risk for ventricular failure, even with a normal ejection fraction before surgery. This condition must be managed with afterload reduction, diuresis, inotropes, and intraaortic balloon pump.
- These patients are at a high risk for bleeding because anticoagulation therapy is needed almost immediately to decrease the risk of emboli formation.

18. What are some additional risks in the early recovery period for patients undergoing mitral valve surgery that are different from traditional CV surgery?

Although most care is similar to that described previously, some additional risks exist in this patient population. Patients are more likely to have left ventricular (LV) failure, with or without ventricular dysrhythmias and pulmonary dysfunction. The LV failure can be corrected with afterload reduction and inotropes. The ventricular tachycardia is managed with antiarrhythmics, potassium replacement, and magnesium replacement. Pulmonary hypertension can also occur. For decrease in pulmonary artery pressures, a pulmonary vascular bed vasodilator like nitroglycerin may be used. A fib is also frequently seen after surgery (see Question 33 for its management).

19. What is the usual sequence of events for patients after CV surgery?

Following is an example of a care plan for a patient who has undergone open-heart surgery. Significant variations may be seen based on individual progress and physician and institute policies. An "X" in the table indicates that the activity should be performed.

Intervention	Day 0	Day 1	Day 2	Day 3	Day 4	Day 5	Day 6	Day 7
Respiratory								
Assessment	X	X	X	X	X	X	X	X
Extubation	X							
Oxygen at 2-4 L/min to keep saturations >92%	X	X	X	prn	prn	prn	prn	prn
Pulmonary toilet (coughing, deep breathing, incentive spirometry)	X	X	X	X	X	X	X	X
Chest physiotherapy			X					
Oxygen saturations	X	X	X	prn	prn	prn	prn	prn
Chest tube removal			X					
Chest radiograph	X	X	X	prn	prn	prn	prn	prn
Activity								
Dangling	X							
Ambulation		X	X	X	X	X	X	X
Physical therapy consult		X	prn	prn	prn	prn	prn	prn
Laboratory (may include the following)								
Arterial blood gas	X	X	prn	prn	prn	prn	prn	prn
Complete blood cell count	X	X	X	X	prn	prn	prn	prn
Electrolyte panel	X	X	X	X	prn	prn	prn	prn
Activated partial thromboplastin time/ international normalized ratio/prothrombin time	X	X	X	X*	X*	X*	X*	X*

continued

Intervention	Day 0	Day 1	Day 2	Day 3	Day 4	Day 5	Day 6	Day 7
Laboratory (may include the following)								
Electrocardiogram	X	X	X	prn	prn	prn	prn	prn
Echocardiogram (status after valve surgery)						X		
Cardiovascular								
Assessment	X	X	X	X	X	X	X	X
Telemetry	X	X	X	X	X	X	X	X
Hemodynamic monitoring (Swan-Ganz or central venous pressure)	X	X	X	X	X	X	X	X
Fluid status balance	X	X	X	X	X	X	X	X
Epicardial wire removal				X				
Wounds								
Monitor incisions	X	X	X	X	X	X	X	X
Dressing changes per hospital protocol		X	X					
Gastrointestinal								
Assessment	X	X	X	X	X	X	X	X
Nutrition								
NPO to ice chips	X							
Clear liquids		X						
Low-sodium, low-cholesterol diet			X	X	X	X	X	X
Weights	X	X	X	X	X	X	X	X
Initiation of bowel protocol		X	X	X	X	X	X	X
Discharge								
Education		X	X	X	X	X	X	X
Planning	X	X	prn	prn	prn	prn	prn	prn
Social work consult		prn						

*Coagulation level tests are done more frequently for those who are undergoing anticoagulation for postmechanical valve placement or for chronic atrial fibrillation.

prn, As required.

20. What complications may occur in the postoperative period for patients undergoing CV surgery?

Early complications can include such problems as low cardiac output from postoperative bleeding, cardiac tamponade, myocardial stunning, perioperative myocardial infarction, arrhythmias, acute graft closure, hypotension, and hypertension. In addition, acute complications can occur in the pulmonary system, including pulmonary edema, atelectasis, pneumonia, and aspirations. Additional complications include acute renal failure (occurs infrequently but has a high mortality rate) and gastrointestinal (GI) problems (abdominal distention, ileus, gastroduodenal bleeding, cholecystitis, and potentially lethal pancreatitis).

Complications can also occur in the later phases of the postoperative course. Some of the later complications include pneumonia, postpericardiotomy syndrome, cardiac tamponade, and wound infection. Some of these can occur even after discharge. Remembering to educate the patient about signs and symptoms of these conditions is important. In addition, patients should have contact numbers for the on-call physician and outpatient clinic contact numbers should questions arise after discharge.

21. What are key nursing considerations in the care of patients who have undergone CV surgery and are being transferred from the ICU to a progressive care or step-down unit?

- **Cardiac assessment.** Arrhythmias, monitoring of vasoactive drips, temporary pacemakers, heart sounds, and peripheral pulses should all be monitored frequently according to hospital policy.
- **Pain control.** Continued pain control is imperative as the patient makes the transition from IV to oral medication, and continuous monitoring is needed.
- **Respiratory management.** Frequent respiratory assessments are needed, as are proactive efforts to prevent respiratory complications, which can be accomplished with coughing/deep breathing and incentive spirometry.
- **Early ambulation.** Early ambulation is important to decrease the risk of deep vein thrombosis and pneumonia. The goal is to have patients out of bed and to a progressive care unit within 24 hours of surgery.
- **Need for sleep.** Patients undergo an enormous amount of stress and potential sleep deprivation in the ICU, all of which contribute to fatigue. They need to get plenty of rest to promote healing and general well-being.
- **Nutrition.** Providing enough calories and protein is critical to good wound healing and can be a problem in that patients may have a decreased appetite after surgery.
- **Intake and output.** Urinary output, chest tube output, and oral/IV intake need frequent assessment.

22. What can nurses do to support the rapid return of bowel function after surgery?

Several techniques are used to help patients return to their regular bowel routine after surgery. The first step is assessment of the last bowel movement and the patient's regular pattern. These patients may have a routine used at home that works for them and needs to be restarted early. Because general anesthesia and opioid use for pain management cause decreased GI motility, some patients have difficulty with the resumption of normal bowel pattern. Common techniques generally include: ambulation, increased intake of oral fluids (if not contraindicated), prune juice, laxative per provider order, or enemas as ordered. Some institutions have a bowel protocol to facilitate return of function. It is frequently the nurse who identifies these problems early. The nurse needs to work with the physician early on to obtain those items that require a physician's order if the facility does not have standing orders.

23. What can nurses do to facilitate "pulmonary toilet" particularly after open-heart surgery?

Nursing can prevent or minimize respiratory complications with frequent respiratory assessments. The nurse may be the first to identify the impending problem. Respiratory assessments should include respiratory rate, respiratory effort, lung sounds, oxygen saturation, and patient's subjective symptoms of shortness of breath and dyspnea. For prevention of respiratory complications, pulmonary toilet must be done on a frequent basis. Pulmonary toilet is a term used to describe aggressive interventions related to pulmonary mobilization of secretions. Encouragement of the frequent use of coughing/deep breathing, the use of incentive spirometer, and ambulation is important. In addition, pain control is critical in these patients. If the patient has pain, he or she does not want to take deep breaths, which in turn may lead to atelectasis. In addition, encouragement of the use of chest splinting can facilitate the respiratory process and decrease the discomfort.

24. Are there any special considerations when caring for patients with diabetes after open-heart surgery?

Patients with diabetics are at an increased risk for wound infection. The main consideration in care for patients with diabetes is to help them maintain blood glucose levels less than 140 mg/dL. Frequent monitoring of the glucose level, followed by administration of oral agents or insulin as soon as possible, helps keep blood glucose levels at a desirable level. An insulin drip may be initiated as soon as the first blood glucose level exceeds 140 mg/dL. Patients may also benefit if an insulin drip is maintained until postoperative day 3 before subcutaneous insulin is started to keep blood glucose levels less than 180 mg/dL. One should remember that patients without diabetes can actually have high blood sugars from epinephrine and norepinephrine or phenylepinephrine use in the ICU. These patients still need to be treated as diabetic during the time frame to keep blood sugars down. Control of blood sugars is critical in the promotion of proper wound healing and prevention of long-term complications of diabetes.

25. What is meant by the term "pump head?"

"Pump head" is medical slang that refers to a syndrome that is sometimes seen after CV surgery with patients who appear to have a neurological deficit. The term is used to refer to patients who appear confused or have decreased cognitive functioning in the postoperative period. Some additional symptoms include fatigue, restlessness, anxiety, hallucinations, and distraction, among others. The condition appears to be a multifactorial issue that involves both medical (patient history) and surgical (effects of anesthesia, length of surgery, and use of cardiopulmonary bypass machine) issues. The degree and length of time patients are affected varies. More research is needed to sort out the causes in the hopes of prevention.

26. How are epicardial wires used?

Epicardial wires are temporary pacing wires connected directly to the surface of the heart and pulled through the chest wall. They are most commonly inserted at the end of the operation. Generally two sets of wires are used: one set for the atrium and one for the ventricle. The wires provide a means to connect a temporary pacemaker to maintain heart rate, atrial-ventricular synchrony, and cardiac output. The wires may be connected to a temporary pacing box and used to increase the heart rate in cases of severe bradycardia, complete heart block, or A fib with a slowed ventricular response.

27. Are there any special considerations health care providers must be aware of when caring for patients with epicardial wires?

Health care providers must remember to wear gloves when handling the wires. The wires should be secured to the chest when not in use. Some institutions have advocated the wires be "capped off" in addition to being contained in a dressing.

28. When are epicardial wires discontinued, and what is done during discontinuation of the wires?

The epicardial wires are generally discontinued during the fourth postoperative day. Removal of the wires as soon as the physician feels it is safe from a rhythm standpoint is important to help prevent infection and to prevent the wires from becoming permanently imbedded in the heart muscle. At this time, the INR should be within normal range before the wires are discontinued to minimize bleeding. The patient should be kept on bed rest for a least an hour after removal of the wires, with frequent vital sign tests and frequent checks of the removal site, because the patient is at risk for cardiac tamponade (see Question 29).

29. What are the signs and symptoms of cardiac tamponade?

Cardiac tamponade is the accumulation of fluid/blood in the pericardial space that leads to an increase in pericardial pressure, which decreases the ability of the ventricles to fill during diastole. A decrease in systolic blood pressure, a narrowing of the pulse pressure (systolic blood pressure-diastolic blood pressure), tachycardia, presence of pulsus paradoxus (a pulse that changes with intensity based on the respiratory cycle), distension of the neck veins, symptoms of shortness of breath, and dyspnea may indicate cardiac tamponade.

30. What is the mechanism for A fib in the postoperative patient?

Approximately 30% of patients undergoing open heart surgery are estimated to have developed postoperative A fib, which most commonly occurs on the second or third postoperative day but may occur at any time. The exact mechanism for A fib has not been determined. Some potential mechanisms are mechanical (trauma to electrical conduction pathways and pericardial irritation) or metabolic (ischemia, electrolyte disturbances, and stress-released catecholamines).

31. What are the consequences of postoperative A fib?

Patients in whom postoperative A fib develops are at an increased risk for complications compared with nonsurgical patients with new onset A fib. These complications of A fib may include cerebral vascular accident, hypotension, decreased cardiac output (from loss of atrial kick and a worsening heart failure), and pulmonary edema.

32. Which patients are most likely to have A fib develop after CV surgery?

Which patients have A fib develop is not known exactly. However, increasing age, intraatrial conduction delay, hypertension, male gender, history of A fib, and history of congestive heart failure before surgery have been suggested to lead to A fib in the postoperative period. Length of aortic cross-clamp time, location of venous cannulation, need for postoperative atrial pacing, and altered respiratory status may also all lead to postoperative A fib.

33. How is postoperative A fib typically treated?

Although some patients may have spontaneous conversion to sinus rhythm, others need immediate treatment. As with other patients with A fib, the two main strategies for treatment include restoration of sinus rhythm and ventricular rate control. Rate control can be achieved with beta-blockers, digoxin, and calcium channel blockers. Rhythm conversion can be achieved with electrolyte replacement; antiarrhythmic drugs (types IA and IC), sotalol hydrochloride, amiodarone, ibutilide acetate, and dofetilide (see Chapter 34, Antiarrhythmic Agents). Patients generally are on the medication for some time after discharge.

Given the potential complications and cost of postoperative A fib, some investigation has begun into the benefit of prophylactic treatment. On the basis of a metaanalysis, beta-blockers, sotalol hydrochloride, and amiodarone have all been shown to decrease postoperative A fib, with no significant differences among them. In addition, biventricular pacing has shown promise as a potential treatment.

34. What should be included in discharge teaching for patients and their families?

Patients are generally discharged from the hospital at postoperative day 5 to 7. However, total recovery can take up to 6 to 12 weeks. A good time to reinforce the importance of risk factor modification is as the patient nears release from the hospital. Patients need to be aware of all risk factors so that they do not continue to engage or begin to engage in behaviors that increase risk of advancement of the valve or coronary artery disease. Discharge topics should include: incisional care, diet, exercise, smoking cessation, pain management, rest, driving, use of antiembolism stockings, airplane flights, wound care, and sexual intercourse. Medications are also an important topic to cover. The patient must understand the reasons for the medications and how and when to take them. The offer to create a medication schedule may be helpful, especially with a large number of new medications. The patient may also be referred to cardiac rehabilitation at the request of the physician and can be included in the discharge teaching if ordered.

Discharge teaching should begin early in the hospital course. At the time of admission, assessment of the patient's barriers to learning is important so that an educational plan can be put into action that accounts for those barriers. Repeated teaching is often necessary to ensure the patient gets all the possible information. The presence of family members or caretakers is helpful so they have the information as well and for frequent opportunities to ask questions. The patient should also be given written materials to take home for reference, which may alleviate anxiety.

35. What is the difference between traditional and minimally invasive cardiac surgery?

Traditional cardiac surgery refers to a procedure in which surgery is performed with sternotomy incision, a nonbeating heart, and cardiopulmonary bypass. Minimally invasive surgery actually refers to a set of surgical procedures that tend to decrease the invasiveness of the surgery by eliminating one of the procedures necessary for traditional surgery. In minimally invasive surgeries, some of the following combinations are used: hearts are not stopped and not put on the bypass machine or no sternotomy incision is used but a more lateral incision or a port incision is used. Some of these surgeries include: off-pump coronary artery bypass, minimally invasive CABG via thoracotomy approach, port access CABG, and valve/bypass surgeries done with port access on pump.

36. What is off-pump bypass and why is it used?

Off-pump bypass is the performance of CABG without the use of the cardiopulmonary bypass machine or the arresting of the heart for the surgery. Instead, the heart is allowed to continue beating during the harvesting of conduits and completion of the vessel's proximal and distal anastomoses.

Off-pump or beating heart procedures were developed in a select group of patients as a means of decreasing the risks of traditional CV surgery associated with the bypass machine. Potential off-pump candidates are evaluated on the basis of coronary anatomy, hemodynamic status, and the comfort level of the surgeon. In particular, the need to avoid blood loss, renal insult, cognitive dysfunction, myocardial dysfunction, and initiation of inflammatory cascade may lead to the use of beating heart techniques.

37. Are any new promising CV surgeries on the horizon?

As the number of patients diagnosed with heart failure increases a quest to explore surgical options for these patients has begun. Myosplint is also showing promise as a new treatment for cardiomyopathy. The device essentially uses three splints to support the heart, decrease the size of the LV, and correct the shape. These changes are believed to improve LV function.

The Acorn Cardiac Support Device is also in clinical trials as a treatment for heart failure. This device is a "jacket" for the LV. The concept is to decrease the myocardial stretch and wall strain. The belief is that the signals for LV hypertrophy are avoided, which thus prevents the subsequent heart failure.

The use of robotics in surgery may be a promising technique for CV surgery. Robotics are currently used for the repair of the mitral valve and are under investigation for use in CABG surgery. This new technique is being introduced into training institutions.

One of the latest techniques currently under investigation is the combination of surgical ventricular restoration (SVR) with CABG for the treatment of ischemic dilated cardiomyopathy. For this procedure, the akinetic wall is surgically removed from the LV in an attempt to restore a normal shape to the LV. The CABG portion increases blood flow to the heart muscle. This combination of return to normal shape and blood flow is hoped to reverse the effects of ischemic cardiomyopathy.

Because a limited number of hearts are available for transplantation, there has been an ongoing quest to identify alternatives. One possibility is the use of artificial hearts, which is currently under investigation.

38. What controversies exist in CV surgery?

One of the biggest controversies in CV surgery is the benefit of off-pump CABG compared with conventional CABG. Larger studies are needed to definitively answer that question. A second controversy is the use of gene therapy. An example of this is the injection of vascular endothelial growth factor (VEGF) into the myocardium with the hope of inducing angiogenesis during CV surgery.

Key Points

- A nursing assessment should also occur before surgery and should include a head-to-toe exam. The patient's social situation should be carefully evaluated to identify those individuals who may need additional assistance after discharge.

Key Points   *continued*

- Thorough preoperative teaching for both the patient and the family helps decrease the anxiety before surgery and while the patient is in the ICU and assists in an easier transition to progressive care units and to home.
- Patients with diabetes are at an increased risk for wound infection. The main consideration in care for patients with diabetes is to help them maintain blood glucose levels less than 140 mg/dL.
- A decrease in systolic blood pressure, a narrowing of the pulse pressure (systolic blood pressure–diastolic blood pressure), tachycardia, presence of pulsus paradoxus (a pulse that changes with intensity based on the respiratory cycle), distension of the neck veins, symptoms of shortness of breath, and dyspnea may indicate cardiac tamponade.
- Approximately 30% of the patients undergoing open heart surgery have postoperative A fib develop.

Internet Resources

Frontiers in Bioscience: Heart Sounds Tutorial:
http://www.bioscience.org/atlases/heart/sound/sound.htm

Society of Thoracic Surgeons:
www.sts.org

Coronary Artery Bypass Graft Surgery Guidelines:
http://www.acc.org/clinical/guidelines/bypass/dirIndex.htm

ACC/AHA Guidelines for the Management of Patients With Valvular Heart Disease:
http://www.acc.org/clinical/guidelines/valvular/dirIndex.htm

Bibliography

Chitwood W, Nifong L, Chapman W et al: Robotic surgical training in an academic institution, *Ann Surg* 234:4, 2001; available online: http://www.MDconsult.com/.

Cimochowski G, Harostock M, Brown R et al: Intranasal mupirocin reduces sternal wound infection after open-heart surgery in diabetics and non-diabetics, *Ann Thorac Surg* 71(5):1572-1578, 2001.

Crystal E, Connolly S, Sleik K et al: Interventions on prevention of postoperative atrial fibrillation in patients undergoing heart surgery: a meta-analysis, *Circulation* 106(1):75-80, 2002.

Eagle K, Guyton R, Davidoff R et al: ACC/AHA guidelines for coronary artery bypass graft surgery: executive summary and recommendations: a report of the American College of Cardiology/American Heart Association Task Force on Practice Guidelines, *Circulation* 100:1464-1480, 1999.

Franco K, Verrier E: *Advanced therapy in cardiac surgery*, Hamilton, Ontario, 1999, BC Decker.

Heorcher K, Vacha C, McCarthy P: Left ventricular splints and wraps for end stage heart failure: a new approach in the new millennium, *J Cardiovasc Nurs* 16(3):82-86, 2002.

Inwood H: *Adult cardiac surgery: nursing care & management*, London, 2002, Whurr Publishers.

Irwin R, Cerra F, Rippe J: *Intensive care medicine*, ed 4, Philadelphia, 1999, Lippincott-Raven.

Jacobs L, Nusbaum N: Perioperative management and reversal of antithrombotic therapy, *Clin Geriatr Med* 17:189-202, 2001.

Kim M, Kini A, Sharma S: Refractory angina pectoris: therapeutic options, *J Am Coll Cardiol* 39(6):923-934, 2002.

Kluytmans JA, Mouton JW, VandenBergh MF et al: Reduction of surgical-site infections in cardiothoracic surgery by elimination of nasal carriage of *Staphylococcus aureus* [comment], *Infect Control Hosp Epidemiol* 17(12):780-785, 1996.

Lorenz B, Coyte K: Cardiopulmonary artery bypass graft surgery without cardiopulmonary bypass: a review and nursing implications, *Crit Care Nurs* 22:51-60, 2002.

Mack M: Coronary surgery: off-pump and port access, *Surg Clin North Am* 80:1575-1591, 2000; available online: http://www.mdconsult.com.

Maisel W, Raen J, Stevenson W: Atrial fibrillation after cardiac surgery, *Ann Intern Med* 135(12):1061-1073, 2001.

Markovitz LJ: Description and evaluation of a glycemic management protocol for patients with diabetes undergoing heart surgery, *Endocr Pract* 8(1):10-18, 2002.

Mooss A, Wurdeman R, Mohiuddin S et al: Esmolol versus diltiazem in the treatment of postoperative atrial fibrillation/atrial flutter after open heart surgery, *Am Heart J* 140:1, 2000; available online: http://www.mdconsult.com/.

Passman R, Beshai J, Pavri B, Kimmel S: Predicting post-coronary bypass surgery atrial arrhythmias from the preoperative electrogram, *Am Heart J* 142:806-810, 2001.

Selnes O, Goldsborough M, Borowicz L et al: Determinants of cognitive change after coronary artery bypass surgery: a multifactorial problem, *Ann Thorac Surg* 67(6):1669-1676, 1999.

Spell N: Stopping and restarting medications in the perioperative period, *Med Clin North Am* 85:1117-1128, 2001.

Spertus J, Jones P, Coen M et al: Transmyocardial CO_2 laser revascularization improves symptoms, function, and quality of life: 12-month results from a randomized controlled trial, *Am J Med* 111:341-348, 2001.

Usry G, Johnson L, Weems J, Blackhurst D: Process improvement plan for the reduction of sternal surgical site infection among patients undergoing coronary artery bypass graft surgery, *Am J Infect Control* 30(7):434-436, 2002.

Van den Berghe G, Wouters P, Weekers F et al: Outcome benefit of intensive insulin therapy in the critically ill: insulin dose versus glycemic control, *Crit Care Med* 31(2):359-366, 2003.

VandenBergh MF, Kluytmans JA, van Hout BA et al: Cost-effectiveness of perioperative mupirocin nasal ointment in cardiothoracic surgery, *Infect Control Hosp Epidemiol* 17(12):786-792, 1996.

Woods S, Froelicher E, Motzer S: *Cardiac nursing*, ed 4, Philadelphia, 2000, Lippincott Williams & Wilkins.

Zerr K, Furnary A, Grunkemeier G et al: Glucose control lowers the risk of wound infection in diabetics after open heart operations, *Ann Thorac Surg* 63(2):356-361, 1997.

Zevola D, Raffa M, Brown K: Using clinical pathways in patients undergoing cardiac valve surgery, *Crit Care Nurse* 22:31-50, 2002.

Temporary Pacing, Cardioversion, and Defibrillation

Margaret C. Herbst and Vickie Strang

1. What is the purpose of temporary pacing?

Temporary pacing is most commonly used to provide transient heart rate support and subsequent improvement in cardiac output for the patient with hemodynamically significant bradycardia. It is used until the condition causing the bradycardia resolves or the patient undergoes implantation of a permanent pacemaker. Alternatively, temporary pacing can be used to provide "overdrive" pacing to convert tachyarrhythmias and is also routinely used during diagnostic electrophysiologic studies. Indications for temporary pacing can be elective or emergent. Emergent reasons include acute hemodynamic decompensation from bradycardia or asystole caused by acute myocardial infarction or the occurrence of serious ventricular arrhythmias induced by profound bradycardia.

2. What methods of temporary pacing exist and how do these vary?

Temporary pacing can be performed by the following routes:
- Transcutaneous
- Epicardial
- Transvenous
- Transesophageal

In each type of temporary pacing, the electrode or lead wire is attached to an external pulse generator capable of providing sufficient energy to pace the heart at the desired rate.

Transcutaneous pacing is the oldest form of temporary pacing and was first introduced by Zoll in 1952. Currently transcutaneous pacing is performed via placement of cutaneous electrodes on the chest wall that are connected to an external pacing pulse generator.

Epicardial pacing is most commonly seen in the patient undergoing cardiac surgery, such as cardiac bypass or valve replacement surgery. This mode of pacing provides heart rate support during the postoperative period. The electrodes are loosely sewn to the epicardium and threaded through to the skin during the operative procedure. These wires can be attached to an external generator and can also be used for diagnostic purposes or to overdrive pace the heart in an attempt to terminate tachyarrhythmias (see the following figure).

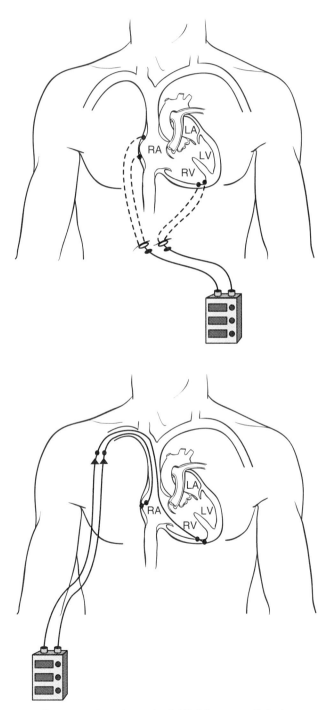

Temporary pacing systems: epicardial (*top*), transvenous (*bottom*).

Transvenous pacing entails passage of a temporary pacing wire through a central vein (most commonly the internal jugular, subclavian, antecubital, or femoral vein) to the endocardial surface of the right atrium or ventricle (see the figure in Question 2).

Transesophageal pacing is more rarely used and is performed to help with diagnosis and overdrive pacing of atrial tachyarrhythmias. The patient swallows a pill electrode, or an electrode is positioned via transesophageal visualization into the esophagus adjacent to the atrium. This is more commonly used with children than adults.

3. When is transcutaneous pacing used, and what is the nurse's role?

Transcutaneous pacing is predominantly limited to emergency use and is used as a short term "bridge therapy" until a temporary transvenous pacemaker can be placed. Two large adhesive electrodes are applied to the anterior chest or in the anterior-posterior position and are connected to an external generator. If time allows, the chest should be shaved and prepped before electrode placement because poor contact may result in inadequate pacing. The nurse should explain the need for transcutaneous pacing to the patient and family and sedate the patient before pacing because this procedure can be quite painful. After application of the surface leads, the nurse should verify that a clear QRS complex, without noise or interference, is displayed on the monitor. After the chest is prepped, the defibrillation patches are placed in the anterior-posterior position. The anterior patch is positioned approximately at the location of lead V3, and the posterior patch is positioned beneath the left scapula. Lead V3 is located between lead V2 (slightly left of the sternum at the fourth intercostal space) and lead V4 (left mid clavicular line at the fifth intercostal space; see the following figure). The electrodes are attached to the connection cables, and the external pacemaker is set to the desired rate. The nurse then turns on the pacemaker power and gradually increases the output (energy delivered to the heart) until capture is evident on the electrocardiogram (ECG) screen and is confirmed with palpation of the carotid or femoral pulse. The pacing rate then is set as ordered, and the procedure is documented in the medical record. See the figure on page 244.

4. Are there any contraindications for application of a transcutaneous pacemaker?

Contraindications for transcutaneous pacing include the patient with a C-spine injury or with a flail chest.

5. What type of nursing care is necessary for the patient with epicardial pacing wires?

The specific details for care of epicardial pacing wires may vary according to institutional policy. The exit sites for the wire should be cleaned every 24 to 48 hours with an iodine solution and covered with an occlusive dressing. During dressing changes, the nurse should wear sterile gloves and a mask, examine

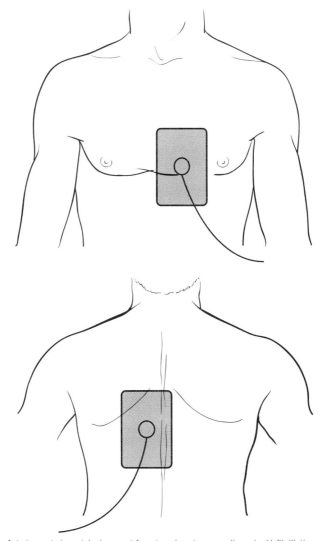

Anterior-posterior patch placement for external pacing or cardioversion/defibrillation.

for any signs of infection at the site, and avoid using scissors, which could inadvertently cut the wires. If epicardial wires are being intentionally disconnected from an external pulse generator, they should be capped, labeled "atrium" or "ventricle" as appropriate, coiled, and secured under dry gauze.

6. What are the components of transvenous and epicardial systems?

Each system has lead wires connected to the heart, the tips of which are inserted into one end of the connecting cable. The other end of the cable has pins that plug into the temporary pacemaker pulse generator. The generator for the temporary pacing system has dials for control of rate, output (expressed in milliamperes), and sensitivity (measured in millivolts).

7. How is a temporary pacing wire inserted, and what is the nurse's role in assisting with the procedure?

The nurse may be asked to assist with placement of a temporary transvenous pacemaker and should confirm that the patient is on a monitor and that emergency medications and a defibrillator are easily accessible. Lead placement may, on occasion, stimulate arrhythmias. Fluoroscopy may be requested to assist in visualization during lead positioning, and the nurse should assist in explaining the procedure to the patient and family and be available to answer questions. The pulse generator must be checked before use by turning it to the asynchronous (not sensing) mode and confirming that the pacing indicator is flashing. Extra batteries should be readily available. The nurse assists the physician in placing the patient in the supine position and in prepping and draping the appropriate area. After the lead has been positioned by the physician, the nurse attaches the lead pins to the proper connection terminals and secures the pins. The pacemaker is turned on, and threshold and sensitivity tests are performed. The nurse positions the pacemaker settings as ordered and covers the dials with a protective cover to prevent inadvertent reprogramming. The generator then is placed in a plastic bag and secured to the patient or the bed. Assistance with placement of the site dressing is provided by the nurse, and a postprocedure chest radiograph is obtained to document lead position.

8. How does the nurse perform sensitivity and threshold testing of the temporary pacemaker?

In some institutions, evaluation of temporary pacing efficacy is performed by nurses as established by hospital policy. For evaluation of the pacing threshold, the patient needs to be in a paced rhythm or the rate of the pacemaker should be increased to greater than the patient's own (intrinsic) rate. Threshold is evaluated with closely watching the cardiac monitor while gradually decreasing the output dial until capture (successful response of the heart muscle to the pacing stimulus) is lost and then increasing the output until capture is regained. The threshold is the minimum value at which consistent capture is detected. The output of the generator is programmed to two to three times the threshold value to provide an adequate safety margin. If a substantial increase in threshold is noted at the time of testing, the nurse should notify the physician because this may indicate potential lead dislodgement. The frequency of threshold testing varies according to institutional policy but should be at least twice daily. Sensitivity is a measure of the pacing system's ability to detect intrinsic electrical activity and can only be evaluated if the patient has a stable intrinsic rhythm. Sensitivity cannot be evaluated in the patient who is pacemaker dependent. For evaluation of sensitivity:

- The nurse sets the pacemaker rate to approximately 10 beats below the intrinsic rate and confirms that the patient's condition is hemodynamically stable.

- Gradually the sensitivity dial is turned to the least sensitive setting by increasing the sensitivity number (see Chapter 24, Permanent Pacemakers, for a more detailed discussion of sensitivity). This usually results in the inability of the pacemaker to "see" the intrinsic complexes, and fixed rate pacing is observed. The sensitivity dial is gradually decreased, and thus the sensitivity increases until the device is able to sense the intrinsic rhythm accurately. Most systems have a sense indicator light that flashes when intrinsic activity is sensed.
- The point at which the pacemaker consistently senses intrinsic activity is the threshold, and the sensitivity setting is programmed to approximately one half the threshold value.
- After testing sensitivity, the pacemaker rate setting is returned to the pretest value (see the following figure).

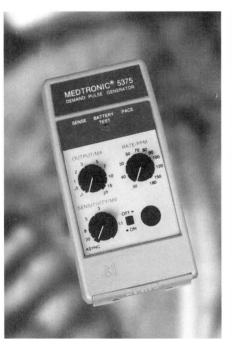 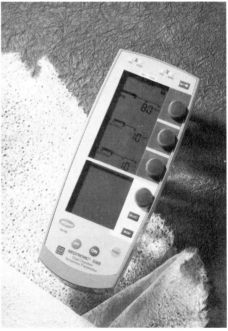

Temporary pacemaker generators used with temporary pacing leads for impulse generation and testing of both sensitivity and threshold. *(Medtronic models 5375 [left] and 5388 [right], © Medtronic, Inc, 1998.)*

9. What complications can occur with temporary pacing, and how do these possibilities impact postprocedure nursing care?

Complications can occur in up to 20% of patients during and after insertion of a temporary pacing wire and most commonly include pneumothorax (collapsed lung), myocardial perforation, postpericardiotomy syndrome, occurrence of ectopy or nonsustained ventricular tachycardia, bleeding, and infection.

Patients with a temporary pacing wire should have continuous ECG monitoring and regular postprocedure monitoring of vital signs. Any increase in shortness of breath, dyspnea, decrease in oxygen saturation, onset of new chest or pleural pain, hypotension, development of a new pericardial friction rub on cardiac exam, evidence of diaphragmatic pacing, or occurrence of hiccups at a frequency consistent with the pacing rate should be promptly reported. Any of these findings may indicate one of the previously mentioned complications. The nurse should monitor for any signs of increased bleeding or infection at the pacemaker site and for evidence of fever or an increase in white blood cell count. Care of the lead insertion site should be performed according to hospital policy.

10. What additional nursing procedures should be incorporated into the care of patients with a temporary pacemaker?

Proper care of the pacing system itself is important and includes securing the lead cable and generator in a manner that prevents dislodgement of the lead and regularly inspecting the system for loose connections. These steps are especially important if any evidence of pacemaker malfunction is noted during continuous ECG monitoring. Replacement batteries, cables, and pulse generators should always be readily available. The temporary pacemaker wire can act as a direct electrical conductor to the heart, and the nurse should be careful to avoid allowing the lead to come into contact with any external electrical noise or interference. Rubber gloves should be worn when handling the lead wire, and any unused terminal pins on the lead should be insulated with caps, needle covers, or finger cots. All electrical equipment in the room should be properly grounded, and the nurse should avoid conducting static electricity to the lead pins such as with use of a slide board. Assuring tight connections in the system helps prevent conduction of stray electricity. In addition, the dressing over the insertion site should be kept dry because a damp dressing may act as an unwanted conductor of electricity.

11. What patient education issues should be addressed?

Education of the patient undergoing temporary lead placement and associated family members should be performed before insertion or as soon as possible if the procedure is performed emergently. The patient should be instructed not to touch the exposed part of the system or manipulate the lead or dressing to prevent infection or lead dislodgement. The patient should not use any unapproved electrical device (such as an electrical shaver from home) and should be informed about any limitation in movement. The patient with a pacemaker placed in the femoral vein is not able to get out of bed to sit or walk and needs assistance with activities of daily living.

12. What is the purpose of electrical cardioversion?

Cardioversion is used to terminate a tachyarrhythmia by delivering a synchronized electrical shock in an attempt to restore a normal rhythm. Cardioversion is most commonly used for treatment of atrial fibrillation, atrial flutter, and stable ventricular tachycardia. The defibrillator in this instance tracks the intrinsic R wave, and the shock delivery is thereby synchronized at a preset time in the cardiac cycle. Synchronization of the shock prevents shocking on the T wave, which can induce ventricular fibrillation (VF).

13. What is the difference between cardioversion and defibrillation?

Cardioversion is more often elective and uses a synchronized shock, and defibrillation is usually performed emergently with an unsynchronized shock and higher energy levels. Defibrillation is indicated for life-threatening arrhythmias such as VF or pulseless ventricular tachycardia. The delivery of the shock causes depolarization of the heart muscle cells, which hopefully stops the arrhythmia and allows normal conduction to resume.

14. What is the nurse's role in cardioversion or defibrillation?

Cardioversion is usually elective, and defibrillation is emergent. In case of elective cardioversion, the nurse should help the patient and family understand the purpose and procedure and be available to answer questions. Adequate sedation before the procedure is essential. In some institutions, the nurse provides conscious sedation for the procedure, and in other settings, a member of the anesthesia department may assist with sedation.

The skin should be shaved and prepped so that adequate contact of the paddles or adhesive electrodes can be assured. If adhesive pads are used, they are placed

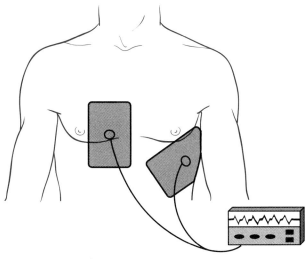

Proper placement of anterior patches for external pacing or cardioversion/defibrillation. This placement is also used for automatic external defibrillators.

either in the anterior-posterior position (left precordium and left infrascapular region) or on the anterior chest at the apex and base of the heart (see the figures on pages 244 and 248). Anterior-posterior placement is usually preferred, which is more easily accomplished with adhesive electrodes than paddles. Transdermal medication patches should be removed and the skin wiped dry before application of electrode pads or paddles. Alcohol application should be avoided because alcohol can be ignited with shock delivery. The patient's dentures and jewelry should be removed before the procedure.

The nurse assisting with the procedure should confirm that the following supplies are available:
- Sources of oxygen and suction
- Defibrillator with continuous ECG (with monitoring, synchronizing, and recording capabilities)
- Pulse oximeter, bag-valve mask, airway management supplies, and intubation equipment
- A fully stocked code cart

That the patient have adequate intravenous (IV) access for administration of sedatives or emergency drugs if needed is essential. The nurse should be sure that the "synch" button is pushed if cardioversion is intended and confirm that the synchronization marker on the rhythm recorder is properly aligned with the R wave. The defibrillator on the nursing unit should be checked regularly so that it is always in optimal operating condition.

15. What are the essential components of postprocedure nursing care for the patient who has undergone cardioversion?

The patient should be closely monitored until fully awake with a satisfactory oxygen saturation and spontaneous respiration. A 12-lead ECG should be obtained and reviewed after the procedure. Any postprocedure change in mental status or neurologic function should be promptly reported to the physician or nurse practitioner.

16. What complications can occur with a cardioversion?

If the shock is not properly synchronized during a cardioversion it is possible to induce VF. In this event, the patient should undergo immediate defibrillation with turning off the "synch" button and charging the defibrillator to 200 J with immediate delivery to the patient. Postconversion bradycardia can occur after cardioversion, and the transcutaneous pacing capability should be readily available. Many of the hands-free adhesive electrode systems currently in use allow for cardioversion, defibrillation, and transcutaneous pacing through the same set of pads. Electrical burns to the chest are a complication of cardioversion and defibrillation, and the nurse should obtain a postprocedure order for silver sulfadiazine or hydrocortisone cream application to ease discomfort if the skin surface has sustained burns.

17. What factors play a role in the efficacy of cardioversion and defibrillation?

In the elective situations, confirmation that the patient has normal electrolytes (especially potassium level) and a therapeutic digoxin level is important. Factors that affect transthoracic impedance should be considered, including: the energy level selected, the size of both the electrodes and the patient's chest, the electrode position, and the quality of contact between the electrode pad or paddle and the skin. Good contact with adequately prepped skin is not only important to the efficacy of cardioversion but also prevents the rare complication of "arcing" of the electricity between the electrodes. Firm pressure should be applied if paddles are used, or a sandbag can be placed on top of the anterior adhesive electrode to improve electrode contact. Transthoracic impedance is also decreased if shock delivery is performed at end expiration, which minimizes the area through which the current must pass to reach the heart.

18. What specific concerns should be addressed for the patient undergoing elective cardioversion for atrial fibrillation?

Patients with atrial fibrillation duration that is greater than 48 hours or of unknown duration are at increased risk for cerebral vascular accident (CVA) because the lack of normal atrial contraction encourages stagnation of blood in the atrium and possible clot formation. If cardioversion (electrical or pharmacological) is planned, care must be taken to reduce the risk of CVA with anticoagulation therapy with warfarin to a target international normalized ratio (INR) of 2 to 3 for 3 to 4 consecutive weeks before the procedure (see Chapter 29, Chronic Anticoagulation). Patients who undergo subsequent cardioversion to normal sinus rhythm should continue therapeutic anticoagulation for 4 weeks after the procedure during which the atrium gradually regains full mechanical function. Alternatively, for patients who are unable to undergo anticoagulation because of a history of bleeding disorders or for patients in whom a delay of 3 to 4 weeks is not desirable, a transesophageal echocardiogram (TEE) can be performed to rule out the presence of atrial thrombi before electrical cardioversion.

The energy level for cardioversion of atrial fibrillation is usually set to 100 to 200 J, and 50 to 100 J may be sufficient to convert atrial flutter or supraventricular tachycardia. Pretreatment with IV antiarrhythmics, such as ibutilide acetate, may improve the likelihood of conversion from atrial fibrillation to normal sinus rhythm, and postprocedure ECG monitoring for the occurrence of arrhythmias is imperative.

19. What is an AED?

An AED is an automatic external defibrillator. The most common cause of cardiac arrest is VF, and time to defibrillation is the most critical factor in determining survival in the patient with VF. Survival rates after cardiac arrest from VF decrease approximately 7% to 10% for each minute the defibrillation is delayed. Many emergency medical systems, nursing units, and public areas, such as airports, golf courses, restaurants, and malls, now have AEDs.

20. How does an AED work?

Health care providers should be familiar with the use of the AED, and such instruction is now included as part of Basic Life Support courses. Although device function varies somewhat based on the manufacturer, the basic steps for use are similar. The nurse should be familiar with the type of device in the department.

- In the event of apparent cardiac arrest, the nurse should assess the patient for the presence of an airway, breathing, and circulation.
- The AED should be applied only to the patient with no spontaneous respiration or pulse.
- The device is turned on, and the electrodes are attached to dry skin at the upper right sternal border below the clavicle and in the V4 to V6 region (between the midclavicular line and the left anterior axillary line along the fifth intercostal space), lateral to the left nipple with the top edge of the pad about 3 in below the axilla. Many AED systems have pictures detailing proper pad placement either on the device itself or on the electrode package (see the figure in Question 14).
- The device may analyze the rhythm spontaneously, or the nurse may be directed to push a button to activate the analysis.
- If the device determines the patient's rhythm needs a shock, it audibly or visibly advises a shock. After "all clear" is said aloud and after confirmation that no one is touching the patient, the AED shock button is pushed.
- After the shock, the rhythm is reanalyzed; this pattern continues until a maximum of three shocks are delivered.
- If a shock is not advised, the patient should be assessed for return of breathing and pulse. If the patient is apneic and pulseless, cardiopulmonary resuscitation (CPR) should be continued.

21. Are there any circumstances in which the nurse needs to modify AED use?

Various situations may require modification of AED use, including the following:

- If the patient with cardiac arrest is found in water (such as the shower), they should be removed from the area and dried off well before application of the AED pads.
- Transdermal medication patches located on the anterior chest or near the sites of intended electropad placement should be removed and the skin surface wiped clean before pad application.
- Patients with an implanted pacemaker or implantable cardioverter defibrillator (ICD) should not have the defibrillator pads placed directly on top of the implanted device. These devices appear as a hard lump in the region below the left or right clavicle or in the upper left abdominal region.

Key Points

- It is imperative that the nurse fully understand the operation of the external defibrillator/transcutaneous pacing system and the temporary transvenous pacemakers in his or her department the function of these devices varies among manufacturers and between institutions.
- Before cardioversion, the nurse should always confirm that the defibrillator is in the synchronized mode to prevent shocking on the T wave with subsequent VF.
- Any topical medication patches on the chest should be removed before cardioversion or defibrillation.
- Good contact is essential for successful cardioversion, so the chest should be shaved and prepped as needed.
- Temporary pacing can be performed in a variety of manners, including: transcutaneous, epicardial, transvenous, and transesophageal.

Internet Resources

NASPE Heart Rhythm Society:
www.naspe.org

American Heart Association:
www.americanheart.org

American Heart Association: Defibrillation:
http://www.americanheart.org/presenter.jhtml?identifier=30

American Heart Association: Ventricular Tachycardia:
http://www.americanheart.org/presenter.jhtml?identifier=64

American Heart Association: Treating Ventricular Rhythm Disturbances:
http://www.americanheart.org/presenter.jhtml?identifier=66

Bibliography

Beaumont E: Teaching colleagues and the general public about automatic external defibrillators, *Prog Cardiovasc Nurs* 16:26-29, 2000.

Cottle S: Temporary transvenous cardiac pacing, *Nurs Times* 93(48):48-50, 1997.

Dell'Orfano JT, Naccarelli GV: Update on external cardioversion and defibrillation, *Curr Opin Cardiol* 16:54-57, 2001.

ECC guidelines: part 6: advanced cardiovascular life support: section 2: defibrillation, *Circulation* 102(suppl I):I90-I94, 2000.

ECC guidelines: part 4: the automated external defibrillator: key link in the chain of survival, *Circulation* 102(suppl I):I60-I76, 2000.

Gammage MD: Temporary cardiac pacing, *Heart* 83(6):715-720, 2000.

Kaushik V, Leon AR, Forrester JS et al: Bradyarrhythmias, temporary and permanent pacing, *Crit Care Med* 28(10 suppl):N121-N128, 2000.

Mancini ME: AEDs: changing the way you respond to cardiac arrest, *Am J Nurs* 99(5):26-30, 1999.

Urden LD, Stacy KM, Lough ME, editors: Cardiovascular therapeutic management. In *Thelan's critical care nursing: diagnosis and management*, ed 4, Philadelphia, 2001, Mosby, pp 439-450.

Walker JR: Anesthesia for cardioversion, *J Perianesthesia Nurs* 14(1):35-38, 1999.

Ventricular Assist Devices and Intraaortic Balloon Pump

Scott Kowalczyk and Vickie Strang

1. **What are the basic facts nurses need to know about invasive treatments for shock?**

   Common devices used for the treatment of cardiogenic shock include artificial ventricles or pumps. The pump mechanics are located externally or implanted in an abdominal pocket. These devices are either mechanically, electro-mechanically, or pneumatically driven. Besides the pump, the system includes a driveline (that could be percutaneous if the pump is implanted), a portable control panel (or console), and a power source. Pumping systems designed for short-term use utilize centrifugal or roller pumps. These devices provide pulseless blood flow similar to the perfusion provided with heart-lung bypass machines. Ventricular assist devices (VADs) can be one-sided, such as the right ventricular assist device (RVAD) or left ventricular assist device (LVAD), or can support both ventricles, referred to as a biventricular device (BiVAD). Large cannulas attach to the native great vessels and heart to divert blood flow. This diversion bypasses ventricular function, unloading the failing chambers and causing decompression.

VENTRICULAR ASSIST DEVICES

2. **How is blood surgically routed when a VAD is used?**
   - **RVAD:** A cannula attaches to the right atrium; blood flows through that inflow cannula to the pump device and is then pumped out through an outflow cannula to an attachment on the pulmonary artery. One-way valves in the conduits prevent backflow.
   - **LVAD:** Blood is rerouted from the left atrium or through a hole created in the apex of the left ventricle into the inflow cannula. The pump then ejects blood through the outflow cannula into an attachment on the ascending aorta.
   - **BiVAD:** RVAD and LVAD are used simultaneously, taking over the entire function of the heart. See the following figures.

3. **What are the indications for VAD placement?**

   A VAD is indicated when clear failure of maximal medical therapy is evidenced by progressive deterioration of cardiac function. Maximal medical therapy includes use of pulmonary artery catheterization, angiotensin-converting

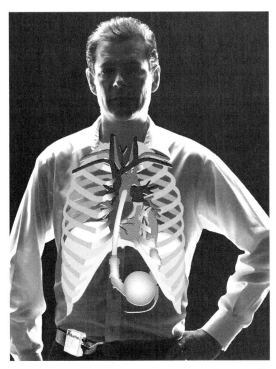

An implanted LVAD with blood being taken from the LV and pumped into the ascending aorta. *(Reprinted with permission from Thoratec Corporation.)*

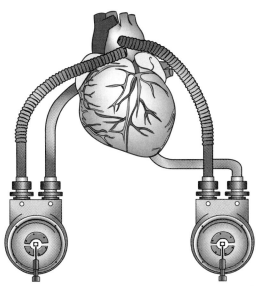

Cannula insertion sites when a biventricular device is in place. *(Reprinted with permission from Thoratec Corporation.)*

enzyme (ACE) inhibitors, intravenous diuretics, afterload reducers, inotropes, and intraaortic balloon pumps (IABPs). The following conditions are common hemodynamic criteria for a VAD:

- Cardiac index (cardiac output L/min ÷ body surface area) <2 L/min/m^2
- Pulmonary capillary wedge pressure >20 mm Hg
- Systolic blood pressure <80 to 90 mm Hg
- Systemic vascular resistance >2000 dynes/s/cm^{-5}
- Urine output <20 mL/h

4. What are common heart failure etiologies that lead to VAD support?

Common heart failure etiologies that lead to VAD support include: ischemic, viral, idiopathic, and postpartum cardiomyopathies and acute myocardial infarction. In the United States, VADs are approved for use as a bridge to transplant and for those who are active candidates and need temporary assistance for postcardiotomy shock or inability to be weaned from the heart-lung bypass machine. VADs are approved as destination therapy in Europe. In other words, implantable devices are used in nontransplant candidates as an alternative to transplant. Some patients are discharged home and occasionally return to work. VADs as destination therapy are under investigation in the United States.

5. What would exclude someone from being a VAD recipient?

General VAD Exclusions:
- Malignant disease
- Recent cerebral vascular damage
- Multiple end-organ failure
- Sepsis
- Mitral stenosis, severe aortic regurgitation, or mechanical aortic valve
- Systemic disease such as amyloidosis
- Psychosocial dysfunction

Left Ventricular Assist Device Exclusions:
- Severe, irreversible right ventricular (RV) failure
- Extremely high pulmonary vascular resistance
- Body surface area <1.5 m^2

6. What are the more commonly used VADs?

Temporary and Nonpulsatile Pumps
- **BioMedicus Biopump (Medtronic Corp):** RVAD, LVAD, or BiVAD. This electrical pump uses centrifugal force to propel blood. The blood flow output is controlled with adjustment of the revolutions per minute of an internal cone. The vortex creates an output of up to 8 L/min. The US Food and Drug Administration (FDA) has approved four models.
- **Nimbus Hemopump (Thoratec Corp):** This rotary pump contains a turbine inside a cannula. It is inserted intravascularly, requiring no sternotomy. The

pump then is positioned inside the left ventricular chamber. Rotation of blades provides flow from the left ventricle through the aortic valve. This pump creates a cardiac output of up to 5 L/min.

Temporary and Pulsatile Pumps
- **Abiomed BVS 5000 (Abiomed Corp):** Used for short-term assistance for postcardiotomy support or as a bridge to transplant. The device is able to support one or both ventricles. Dual pneumatically driven pumping chambers are attached to bedside poles. The stimulus to eject blood is derived from full pumping chambers. This pump provides up to 5 L/min.
- **Thoratec (Thoratec Corp):** RVAD, LVAD, or BiVAD. The inflow and outflow tubing passes through the abdominal wall attaching to the pumps. The pumps rest on the exterior of the abdomen. Blood sacs are contained in rigid plastic housings. Sensors detect when the sacs are full and send a signal to the console to eject. Ejection is accomplished with pneumatic pressure, and vacuum pressure assists filling. This pump provides up to 7 L/min. Because the pumps are located externally, they can accommodate various body sizes.

Pulsatile, Abdominally Implanted LVADs
- **Novacor (WorldHeart Corp):** This device has electrically driven dual pusher plates housed in a rigid case. Dual pressure plates compress the pump sac expelling the blood volume. Output is up to 10 L/min.
- **HeartMate (Thoratec Corp):** Provides a choice of pneumatic (for those patients who stay in the hospital until transplant) or electrical pump drivers. This is the only device approved by the FDA for long-term therapy. A single pusher plate compresses the blood-filled pump sac. The HeartMate has a specially textured pump sac. The sac's blood-compatible surface reduces the incidence of thromboembolism. When blood contacts these surfaces, it deposits blood components, creating a lining similar to that found inside blood vessels. This biologic surface decreases the requirement for anticoagulation therapy. Provides up to 12 L/min.
- Both the Novacor and HeartMate systems have drivelines that exit from the lower abdomen. This line houses an air vent and wiring. The line courses to a device such as a portable controller, console, or laptop computer. See the figure on p. 259.

7. What are common complications from a VAD?

- **Bleeding:** Associated events that contribute to bleeding are: repeat or redo sternotomy, oozing from an anastomosis site, postcardiopulmonary bypass coagulopathy, hepatic congestion from heart failure with deficient clotting factors, and preoperative anticoagulation use. Cardiac tamponade can result from bleeding as evidenced by signs of right heart failure and low LVAD outputs.
- **Infection:** Positive blood cultures can result from an infected device, abdominal pump pocket, driveline, or conduit. Other sites of infection are the sternal incision and the sternum itself, and catheter-related infections and pneumonia can result.

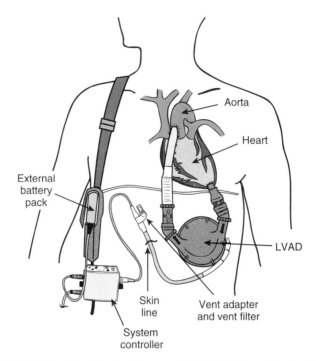

Diagram of the implanted device along with external components. *(Reprinted with permission from Thoratec Corporation.)*

- **Device problems:** Low battery, lack of redundant power source, sensor failure, console/controller malfunction, and damaged driveline cable are all possible device problems.
- **Low cardiac output:** RV failure, pulmonary hypertension, hypovolemia, systemic hypertension, kink in the outflow cannula from body position (such as bending forward), and ventricular dysrhythmias may be causes of low cardiac output.
- **Stroke:** Thromboembolism from a dislodged clot originating in the device or a hemorrhagic event related to the required anticoagulation therapy or preexisting coagulopathy may cause a stroke.
- **Hypoxia:** Fluid overload, pneumonia, prolonged cardiopulmonary bypass, or a patent foramen ovale may cause hypoxia.

8. Do patients with a VAD need intensive care unit (ICU) settings for care?

Patients are recovered after surgery and stay in the ICU until their medical status is stable and they are able to ambulate. When all continuous intravenous medications (such as inotropes, vasodilators, and vasoconstrictors) are discontinued, the fluid volume status is stable, no derangement lab values are seen, the patient is eating, and no evidence is found of bleeding, patients may be transferred to a regular nursing unit. The next step varies among institutions.

Some programs discharge patients home or to a hospital-sponsored facility nearby. Depending on the occupation, there are reports of patients actually returning to work.

9. What monitoring does a nurse perform when caring for a patient with a VAD?

The bedside nurse observes for changes in monitored lab or machine values, changes in physical assessment findings, and activation of a device alarm.

10. What lab and machine values are monitored when caring for a patient with a VAD?

Ventricular assist devices are volume-dependent machines. Nurses monitor and document machine outputs, volumes, and pressures according to the device in use. These values are documented in the nursing record as frequently as indicated in institutional nursing procedures/protocols. Documentation can be as frequent as every 15 minutes in the ICU to every 4 to 8 hours in the nursing unit. Pump filling difficulties could be the result of cardiac tamponade, increase in pulmonary hypertension, fluid volume deficit, or arrhythmias. Problems with emptying could arise from systemic hypertension (increased afterload), a kink in the pump outflow tubing or conduit (increased afterload), or loose connections. Coagulation studies, renal and hepatic function, and other monitored lab values are checked according to institutional protocol and patient condition.

11. What are key components of the nursing assessment in care for a patient with a VAD?

Nurses assess for changes in cardiac rhythm, blood pressure, lung sounds, mentation or other neurological change, urine output, arterial pulses, extremity pain or edema, signs of infection, and bleeding. Common problems (as detailed in Question 12) are related to infection, thromboembolism, bleeding, renal dysfunction, pulmonary changes, symptoms of right heart failure, and inadequate nutritional intake.

12. Describe the clinical manifestations of common problems in patients with VADs.

Local or systemic infections are suspected with any evidence of pain, tenderness, swelling, or exudate at the driveline exit site. Fever, chills, unexplained sweating, increase in white blood cell (WBC) count with shift, dysuria, and sputum production should all be suspect for signs/symptoms of infection. Device recipients undergo pan culture (blood, sputum, and urine) at any sign, regardless how small, of a possible infection.

A thromboembolic event should be suspected with a change in mental status, sensation, speech, vision, or motor function. Blood clots can form inside the pump pocket or on one of the conduit valves. Mobilization of a dislodged clot can cause a neurologic deficit. Use of devices other than the HeartMate with its blood compatible blood sac requires anticoagulation therapy and monitoring of coagulation values. Lower extremity pain and swelling or positive Homans' sign could indicate the presence of a deep vein thrombosis. Prolonged bed rest, edematous extremities, and pooling of blood from a previously poor cardiac output can contribute to clot formation. Antiembolism stockings/devices, passive range of motion, and early ambulation are essential nursing interventions.

Bleeding from an incision or catheter exit site, a decrease in hemoglobin, low blood pressure, or elevated coagulation studies can be signs of postoperative bleeding. Devices can be destructive to platelets.

A decrease in renal function can be evidenced by a fall in urine output or a rise in serum creatinine from poor pump flows, nephrotoxicity from intravenous antibiotics, or hemoglobinemia from the destruction of red blood cells (RBCs) and the release of plasma-free hemoglobin.

Atelectasis is a frequent complication of patients with devices. The use of bedside incentive spirometry, coughing, deep breathing, repositioning, and early ambulation is encouraged. Symptoms of pleuritic pain, cough with sputum production, or dyspnea are infectious concerns.

Right heart failure causes decreased VAD outputs. Other signs are distended neck veins, liver engorgement/right upper quadrant (RUQ) tenderness, nausea, anorexia, jaundice, rise in bilirubin, and peripheral edema.

Nutritional status is a concern because the low cardiac output with advanced heart failure causes a hypoperfused, edematous gut and resultant anorexia. Patients may be malnourished before surgery. The VAD may cause a unique problem with appetite. The location of the device in the left abdominal pocket can put pressure on abdominal organs, causing early satiety. Adequate caloric intake is essential. Small frequent meals or enteral feeds may be necessary.

13. What type of alarms do VADs generate?

Specific device alarms are referenced in abbreviated operator's manual note cards. These cards are typically kept next to the console or laptop. The reference material defines frequent causes for specific alarms and troubleshooting strategies.

14. How do staff learn how the VADs function?

Structured class time is provided to staff before these devices become part of the patient care routine. Hands-on time with the equipment is provided, and refresher courses are periodically offered on a revolving basis. A major responsibility is ensuring that back-up equipment is available nearby and fully functional.

INTRAAORTIC BALLOON PUMPS

1. What is the purpose of an IABP?

The IABP is a LVAD that primarily increases myocardial oxygen supply and decreases myocardial oxygen demand. The IABP system consists of a polyurethane balloon mounted on a polyurethane catheter inserted into the descending thoracic aorta just distal to the left subclavian artery and proximal to the renal arteries. It is connected to an IABP power console, which shuttles helium in and out of the balloon.

2. How does the IABP work?

The balloon is set or "timed" to inflate and deflate in synchronization with the mechanical cardiac cycle.
- Inflation of the intraaortic balloon (IAB) occurs at the onset of ventricular diastole, resulting in proximal and distal displacement of blood volume in the aorta. The proximal displacement of blood creates elevated pressures in the aorta during diastole. Coronary artery filling occurs during this diastolic phase of the cycle. The increased pressure in the aorta results in increased coronary artery perfusion or augmentation of the coronary artery blood flow, increasing myocardial oxygen supply.
- Deflation of the IAB occurs just before the onset of ventricular systole. As the balloon deflates (30 to 50 mL), it provides a significant decrease in aortic pressure for the next ventricular systole. The aortic valve opens at a lower pressure. This action decreases the heart's afterload or myocardial oxygen demand. See the figures at the top of p. 263.

3. How is the balloon timed to inflate and deflate?

Timing refers to inflation and deflation of the IAB in relation to the mechanical cardiac cycle. The balloon should be inflated during diastole and deflated during systole. Synchronization of IAB inflation and deflation with the cardiac cycle is called counterpulsation. The balloon pump requires a trigger signal from which it determines systole and diastole. The most commonly used trigger signal is the electrocardiogram (ECG). This signal is obtained from the ECG leads that are placed on the patient and connected directly to the IABP console. Fine tuning refers to the timing performed by the IABP operator, nurse, perfusionist, or physician, depending on institutional policy. The timing is manually adjusted with moving the inflation or deflation points on the console with the arterial waveform for reference. Most adult IABs have an arterial central lumen that continuously monitors the pressure of the aortic root. The inflation and deflation of the IAB changes the appearance of the arterial waveform, reflecting the effects of blood displacement. See the figure at the bottom of p. 263.

Inflation of the IAB is timed to occur during diastole when most of coronary artery perfusion occurs. The dicrotic notch on the arterial waveform signifies aortic valve closure or the onset of diastole. Therefore the balloon is timed to inflate on the dicrotic notch. As the balloon inflates, aortic diastolic pressure

Diastole: inflation
(Augmentation of
diastolic pressure)

Increased coronary perfusion

Systole: deflation
(Decreased afterload)

Decreased cardiac work
Decreased myocardial oxygen consumption
Increased cardiac output

Inflation ↑

Deflation ↓

Inflation of the intraaortic balloon during diastole and deflation of the balloon before systole.

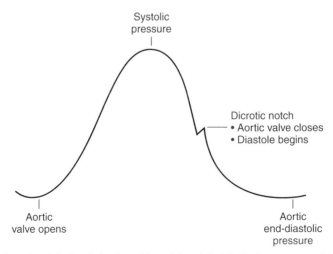

Systolic
pressure

Dicrotic notch
— • Aortic valve closes
  • Diastole begins

Aortic
valve opens

Aortic
end-diastolic
pressure

Normal arterial waveform indicating the locations of the systolic and diastolic blood pressures unassisted by the IABP.

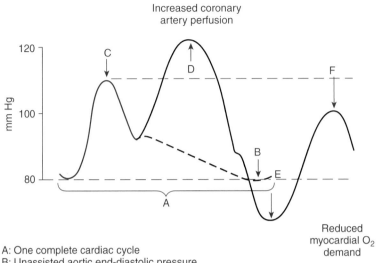

A: One complete cardiac cycle
B: Unassisted aortic end-diastolic pressure
C: Unassisted systolic pressure
D: Diastolic augmentation
E: Assisted aortic end-diastolic pressure
F: Reduced systolic pressure

Arterial waveform comparing an unassisted beat (dotted line) to an IABP assisted beat.

is augmented and a second peak is observed. This peak is called diastolic augmentation. Any condition that causes a decrease in stroke volume, such as tachycardia, arrhythmias, or a mean arterial pressure (MAP) less than 50 mm Hg, causes a decrease in augmentation.

Deflation of the IAB is timed to occur at the end of diastole or before the onset of the next systole. Precise timing of deflation uses the arterial waveform to assure deflation before the next systole. Optimal IAB deflation is selected to achieve the greatest reduction in the next systole. This valley on the arterial waveform is called assisted end diastole.

4. What are some common operator IABP timing errors?

Common IABP timing errors that could affect augmentation and afterload reduction are: early inflation, late inflation, early deflation, and late deflation.
- Early inflation occurs before the aortic valve closes, possibly causing an increase in myocardial oxygen demand.
- Late inflation could result in suboptimal coronary artery perfusion.
- Early deflation could result in suboptimal coronary artery perfusion and suboptimal afterload reduction.
- Late deflation could result in the absence of afterload reduction.

5. What are the clinical indications for an IABP?

IABP therapy is indicated in a variety of conditions that affect left ventricular oxygen supply and demand imbalance regardless of the cause. Examples include cardiogenic shock, refractory ventricular failure, myocardial infarction, unstable refractory angina or impending infarction, and ischemia related to intractable ventricular arrhythmias.

The IABP may be used alone or as an adjunct to other supportive measures, such as oxygen, inotropes, vasodilators, or diuretics, to improve hemodynamic recovery. Surgical indications for the IABP include assistance with weaning from cardiopulmonary bypass, low output syndrome after cardiac surgery, or generating intraoperative pulsatile flow. The IABP may also be inserted to stabilize mechanical complications from acute myocardial infarction, such as ventricular septal defects, mitral regurgitation, or papillary muscle rupture, until more definitive measures, usually surgical, are taken.

In addition, the IABP may be inserted prophylactically in an attempt to support and stabilize the cardiac patient at high risk during coronary angiography or a coronary intervention or in the cardiac patient at high risk undergoing general surgery.

6. What are contraindications for IABP placement?

Some common contraindications for IABP placement include the following conditions:
- Severe aortic insufficiency is a specific contraindication to IAB insertion. During balloon inflation, blood is displaced proximally into the aortic root. In severe aortic insufficiency, the incompetent aortic valve may allow the blood to be displaced backward into the left ventricle, thereby increasing myocardial stretch and increasing the myocardial workload.
- Severe calcific aortoiliac disease or peripheral vascular disease is usually evaluated because the most common insertion site is the femoral artery. If the vascular disease is too severe, the IAB may occlude the femoral artery and cause limb ischemia.
- Other contraindications that are evaluated before insertion are abdominal or aortic aneurysm and scarring of the groin.

7. How is balloon size determined?

Appropriate balloon sizing is important because a balloon that is too large may occlude the aorta and a balloon that is too small may not displace enough blood to benefit the myocardium. In the adult, the balloon size is based on the patient's height. For example, 25 mL for less than 60 inches, 34 mL for 60 to 64 inches, 40 mL for 64 to 72 inches, and 50 mL for greater than 72 inches. The 34-mL and 40-mL balloons are most common. Balloon sizes for the pediatric patient vary with the child's size.

8. How is an IABP placed?

The IAB is most often inserted percutaneously with fluoroscopy. It can be inserted with or without an introducer sheath. The physician maintaining strict sterile technique inserts the carefully prepped IAB into the aorta until it is properly placed. The IAB is then attached to the balloon pump console, and pumping is initiated. The IAB catheter has radiopaque tips on both ends of the catheter to allow for proper placement visibility on chest radiograph.

9. What are complications with IABP implantation?

Patients who need IABP therapy are often older and frequently female and have concomitant diseases, such as severe peripheral vascular disease, hypertension, or diabetes, that may lead to an increased risk of complications. The duration of IABP insertion has been shown to be an independent risk factor. The benefits of the IABP in these patients must be carefully balanced with the potential risks of complications. The nurse caring for the patient with an IABP must be aware of the potential complications so that he or she may carefully monitor for them and take appropriate action if a complication occurs. See the following table.

Complication	Cause	Signs and Symptoms	Treatment
Limb ischemia	Arterial or catheter thrombus	Poor capillary refill, decreased peripheral pulse, cool or painful extremity	Anticipate removal of catheter, reinsertion in other leg, possible embolectomy/thrombectomy
Bleeding from insertion site or development of retroperitoneal bleed	Anticoagulation, thrombocytopenia related to balloon's action on platelets, or mechanical trauma at insertion	Saturated dressing, hematoma, decrease in hematocrit/hemoglobin levels, increase in girth of thigh measurement, and pain in back, abdomen, or groin	Anticipate computed tomography/magnetic resonance imaging; mechanical pressure to stop bleed, monitor coagulation status (prothrombin time/international normalized ratio/partial thromboplastin time); surgical intervention
Local or systemic infection	Bacterial portal of entry through invasive device or site	Fever, chills, change in vital signs, drainage at insertion site	Meticulous sterile technique during insertion and insertion site dressing changes
Balloon leak causing clot inside balloon or gaseous embolic injury	Balloon inflating in aorta with calcified plaque or defective device	Flecks of blood or frank bleeding into intraaortic balloon pump tubing	Balloon removal or possible surgical intervention if intraluminal clot is large
Renal artery or left subclavian artery occlusion	Migration of balloon placement	Decreased or absent extremity pulse or sudden decrease in urine output	Daily chest radiographs to confirm position of balloon; immediate chest radiograph if migration is suspected

10. What is the typical duration for IABP use?

The length of time that the IAB stays in the patient depends on its indication. The time varies from a couple of days to weeks. Before discontinuation, the balloon is weaned to assess the patient's hemodynamic stability.

11. How is the IABP discontinued?

The patient must be weaned from the IABP. The patient's hemodynamic stability is evaluated during the weaning process. The weaning process is as follows:
- The assist frequency ratio is decreased. In other words, balloon inflation and deflation per every heartbeat are changed to one inflation and deflation for every other beat or balloon inflation and deflation for every third beat.
- The amount of augmentation is decreased. This entails decreasing the volume of helium used for balloon inflation.
- A combination of both of the previously mentioned procedures may be used during the weaning process.
- When indicated, the catheter is pulled out at the bedside and pressure is applied until hemostasis is achieved. The nurse then performs frequent assessments of the insertion site for bleeding or signs of compartment syndrome.

12. What would be an outline of nursing care for the patients with an IABP?

Nursing care involves intensive monitoring of the patient's hemodynamics, physical assessment, working knowledge of the functions of the IABP, and an awareness of potential complications of IABP therapy. See the following table.

System Involved	Potential Problem	Nursing Interventions
Cardiac	Left ventricular failure, low cardiac output, myocardial infarction, arrhythmia, pulmonary edema, and cardiac arrest	Monitor vital signs; record and analyze pulmonary artery catheter measurements; watch for dysrhythmias; maintain optimal diastolic augmentation and afterload reduction through appropriate timing of intraaortic balloon pump (IABP)
Respiratory	Atelectasis, pneumonia, and pulmonary emboli from immobility	Encourage patient to cough, deep breathe, and use incentive spirometer on scheduled basis; elevate head of bed to 30 degrees especially during eating; turn cautiously if hemodynamically stable
Renal	Renal insufficiency or renal failure from decreased cardiac output or possible malposition of intraaortic balloon (IAB)	Strict intake and output; monitor urinary output and report if <30 mL/h or sudden decline in urinary outputs; obtain daily weights; monitor blood laboratory values (potassium, blood urea nitrogen, creatinine); monitor position of IABP on chest radiograph

Continued

Continued

System Involved	Potential Problem	Nursing Interventions
Vascular	Vascular problems from balloon insertion site and anticoagulation therapy	Assess peripheral pulses every 2 h; assess color and temperature of involved leg every 2 h; avoid flexion of hip and knee of involved leg; maintain anticoagulation protocol; monitor coagulation studies; observe for internal or external bleeding
Neurological	Cerebral embolization as consequence of IAB catheter malfunction in aorta; complications such as balloon rupture or displacement of plaque resulting in embolism	Neurological assessments including pupillary response, level of consciousness, and sensory/motor function every 2 h and more frequently as required
Psychiatric	Psychosis is possibly related to anxiety, immobility, loss of control, and sensory overload in intensive care unit	Normalization of environment (television, radio, relaxation tapes, computer games, family visits); offer emotional support and pharmacologic sedation if indicated
Gastrointestinal	Nutritional deficits, stress ulcers, and paralytic ileus from anorexia, nausea, difficulty eating, decreased activity, and narcotic administration	Provide food choices from hospital menus and encourage family members to bring in favorite foods within prescribed diets; calorie counts; monitor for presence of bowel sounds; observe for abdominal distention; allow rest periods before and after meals; administer stool softeners as needed per prescription
Musculoskeletal	Foot drop and decubitus ulcer are possible complications from immobility	Turn patient (log roll) if hemodynamically stable every 2 h; use appropriate mattress or special bed; perform active range of motion to unaffected leg and dorsiflexion of foot on involved leg
Immunological	Wound infection or sepsis related to IAB, other invasive lines, or urinary drainage catheter	Monitor temperatures: use sterile technique when changing dressings or manipulating invasive lines; monitor appearance, color, and odor of urine; monitor appearance of insertion sites of invasive lines; monitor white blood cell counts
IABP	Inadequate balloon assistance or IABP complications from mechanical function.	Obtain optimal diastolic augmentation and afterload; monitor and adjust timing; maintain adequate electrocardiographic and arterial tracings; monitor for signs of IAB catheter leak; assure that IAB is not immobile for >30 min; flush arterial tubing every 2 h

13. **What essential components are to be included for patient and family teaching when an IABP is used?**

The patients and family members often have varied concerns and educational needs. A major concern for both the patient and family is that of death. The addition of the IABP often accelerates fears of impending death. Other fears concentrate around the IABP's function and possible complications. Prompt recognition of those fears and educational and emotional support may decrease anxiety. Nursing interventions include providing assurance that the pump is just an assist and that if the machine stops, the heart continues to beat; giving simple explanations of how the heart works and the IABP's action and encouraging questions; providing reassurance to the patient and family that the nurse will be conducting frequent assessments of the patient's condition and that continuous monitoring provides staff members with vital information and enables them to recognize small changes in the patient's condition; and of the utmost importance, establishing a clear agreement with the patient that he or she inform the nurse of any changes in condition.

 Key Points

Ventricular Assist Devices

- Indication for a VAD is continued cardiac deterioration as evidenced by no improvement in hemodynamics despite intensive care with maximal medical therapy.
- Implantable VADs require external pneumatic/electrical/air vent lines that exit the abdomen. Fully implantable devices are in development.
- Ventricular assist devices are used most commonly as a bridge to heart transplant but are used as destination therapy in some nontransplant candidates.
- Right ventricular function must be intact with a LVAD alone.
- Adequate ventricular assist function is volume dependent.
- The requirement for anticoagulation therapy after implantation depends on which device is used.

Intraaortic Balloon Pump

- The IABP inflates during diastole, displacing blood to augment coronary blood flow. Deflation decreases the aortic pressure, assisting the heart before it expels its volume in the next beat.
- The IABP is a percutaneous procedure used for temporary support until there is recovery or other measures of treating the heart failure are instituted.
- Common IABP complications include limb ischemia, bleeding, and infection.

Internet Resources

Datascope: Intra-Aortic Balloon Pump
www.datascope.com

Thoratec Left Ventricular Assist System and Ventricular Assist Devices:
www.thoratec.com

WorldHeart: Left Ventricular Assist System:
www.worldheart.com/section5/index.html

CHF Patients.com: Left Ventricular Assist Devices:
www.chfpatients.com/implants/lvads.htm

Bibliography

Bond E, Nelson K, Germany C, Smart A: The left ventricular assist device, *Am J Nurs* 103(1):32-41, 2003.

Christensen D: The ventricular assist device, *Nurs Clin North Am* 35(4):945-955, 2000.

Cianci P, Lonergan-Thomas, Slaughter M, Silver M: Current and potential applications of left ventricular assist devices, *J Cardiovas Nurs* 18(1):17-22, 2003.

Cook L, Pillar B, McCord G, Josephson R: Intra-aortic balloon pump complications: a five-year retrospective study of 283 patients, *Heart Lung* 28(3):195-202, 1999.

Datascope Clinical Support Services: Concepts of Counterpulsation Therapy System 98/System 98 XT, 2000, Clinical Support Manual.

Duke T, Perna J: The ventricular assist device as a bridge to cardiac transplantation, *AACN Clin Issues* 10(2):217-228, 1999.

Lewandowski A: The bridge to cardiac transplantation: ventricular assist devices, *Dimens Crit Care Nurs* 14(1):17-24, 1995.

Maccioli GA, editor: *Intra-aortic balloon therapy,* Baltimore, 1997, Williams & Wilkins.

Quaal SJ: Caring for the intra-aortic balloon pump patient: most frequently asked nursing questions, *Crit Care Nurs Clin North Am* 8:471-476, 1996.

Quaal SJ: Maintaining competence and competency in the care of the intra-aortic balloon pump patient, *Crit Care Nurs Clin North Am* 8:441-450, 1996.

Stahl M et al: Ventricular assist devices: developing and maintaining a training and competency program, *J Cardiovasc Nurs* 2002 16(3):34-43, 2002.

Permanent Pacemakers

Margaret C. Herbst

1. What is the purpose of a permanent pacemaker?

Permanent pacemakers are implanted for the purpose of electrically stimulating the myocardium in the event that the patient's own heart rate is inadequate to meet the body's hemodynamic demands.

2. What are the most common indications for implantation of a permanent pacemaker?

Most commonly, pacemakers are implanted for treatment of symptomatic bradycardia caused by sinus node dysfunction or atrioventricular (AV) nodal block (heart block) that is believed to be nonreversible. Pacemaker therapy may also be indicated in the setting of chronotropic incompetence, which is the failure of the sinus rate to appropriately increase in response to the body's demand for increased cardiac output, such as with exercise. Patients with congestive heart failure (CHF) may meet the indication for implantation of a biventricular pacemaker if they have reduced left ventricular function and a widened QRS complex and are receiving optimal medical therapy.

3. What is symptomatic bradycardia?

Symptoms associated with bradycardia result from decreased perfusion of the central nervous system directly related to a reduced heart rate. They include syncope, presyncope, confusion, dizziness, or more vague symptoms such as fatigue, dyspnea, or exercise intolerance.

4. What are possible causes of symptomatic bradycardia?

Possible causes of bradycardia are many and include intrinsic and extrinsic etiologies.

Intrinsic causes include:
- Degenerative disease or damage to the cardiac conduction system, which occurs when fibrotic tissue replaces healthy nodal tissue or in the setting of infarction, ischemia, infiltrative disease (such as sarcoidosis or amyloidosis), collagen vascular disease, infectious disease, muscular dystrophy, or surgical trauma.

Extrinsic causes include:
- Drug therapy (beta adrenergic blockers, calcium channel blockers, clonidine hydrochloride, digoxin, or various antiarrhythmic therapies).
- Electrolyte, neurologic, or thyroid abnormalities.
- Neurally mediated effects such as carotid sinus hypersensitivity, neurocardiac syncope, and actions that would result in increased vagal tone, such as vomiting, coughing, or defecation.

The nurse should be aware of the following patient conditions or nursing actions, which may cause increased parasympathetic stimulation with resulting bradycardia:
- Increased intracranial pressure
- Sleep
- Intubation
- Suctioning

The treatment of bradycardia and the decision to implant a pacemaker is based on severity of the bradycardia, symptoms, and degree to which to the symptoms correlate with the arrhythmia.

5. What are the components of a permanent pacemaker?

The primary components of a pacemaker are the pulse generator and lead system. The pulse generator consists of circuitry and a lithium battery sealed in a titanium case, which is approximately 10 mL in volume (roughly the size of a silver dollar). The system also contains a reed switch, which responds to magnet application and can be used to inactivate the pacemaker's sensing function.

The pulse generator is connected to the pacemaker lead system, which is composed of an insulated lead wire that conducts impulses between the pulse generator and lead tip. The lead is most often positioned with fluoroscopy in the right ventricle or right atrium. (For additional details regarding device implantation procedure, see Chapter 25, Implantable Cardioverter Defibrillators.) The lead is attached to the myocardium with either active fixation, in which case a screw at the lead tip is attached to the endocardium, or passive fixation with "tines" or "fins" at the lead tip. The tines catch in the atrial appendage or right ventricular trabeculae (muscular connections inside the ventricular cavity) and thereby hold the lead in place.

6. How does the pacemaker function?

The pacemaker system constantly attempts to sense the patient's native (intrinsic) rhythm. The intrinsic atrial and ventricular activity is noted in millivolts. The pacemaker's ability to detect the intrinsic rhythm (sensitivity) can be programmed. For example, a 10-mV QRS complex is obviously larger than a 4-mV complex; however, if the sensitivity of the pacemaker is programmed to measure only QRS complexes greater than 5 mV, it does not "see" (sense) the 4-mV complex. For the smaller QRS complex to be sensed, the pacemaker must be made more sensitive by increasing the sensitivity to a level permitting the smaller complexes to be seen (sensed). In our example, decreasing the sensitivity setting to 2 mV (making the device more sensitive) would allow sensing of the 4-mV QRS complex. The sensitivity of the pacemaker (its ability to see the P wave or QRS complex) is increased by decreasing the millivolts for which it will detect (sensitivity setting). (See the following figure.)

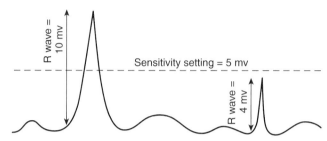

If the sensitivity setting of the pacemaker is programmed to 5 mV, it only sees (senses) R waves that are ≥ 5 mV and does not see (sense) the smaller 4-mV R wave. The pacemaker sensitivity setting must be made more sensitive by decreasing the setting to 2 mV so that 4-mV R wave is sensed.

If the pacemaker does not sense an intrinsic beat, it emits a stimulus (paces). If the stimulus is sufficient, depolarization of the chamber being paced results. This is known as capture and is dependent on adequate output of the pacemaker (known as amplitude and expressed in volts), delivered over a specified amount of time (known as pulse width and expressed in milliseconds). If the pacemaker output or the contact of the lead with the myocardium is not adequate, the stimulus may fail to depolarize, or capture, the chamber being paced. For example, a transvenous lead that is dislodged after implant and that no longer has good contact with the myocardium is not be capable of delivering an adequate pacing stimulus to activate the endocardium and therefore does not capture.

7. What other factors can affect the pacing threshold and capture?

The pacing threshold is the minimum amount of pacemaker output that results in capture. The nurse should be aware that a variety of factors can increase the pacing threshold, such as myocardial infarction, fibrosis, various drugs, and electrolyte imbalance. A malfunction of the lead may also result in lack of capture or an increase in pacing threshold.

8. What is the average longevity of the pacemaker components?

The average longevity of a permanent pacemaker pulse generator is approximately 6 to 8 years, depending on the percentage of time of pacing and the pacemaker settings that determine output (amplitude and pulse width).

Leads usually have a greater longevity than the pulse generator and are often retested and reused at the time of pulse generator replacement. Occasionally, leads malfunction and a new lead implant is required. Although leads generally last longer than the pacemaker pulse generator, the incidence rate of actual malfunction is higher for leads than for pulse generators.

9. How do the types of pacemakers vary?

Pacemaker leads can be inserted epicardially (directly on the outside surface of the heart) or endocardially via transvenous approach. The lead system can use one lead in the atrium or ventricle (a single-chamber pacemaker) or two leads, one each in the atrium and ventricle (a dual-chamber pacemaker). Less commonly, biventricular systems are also implanted for treatment of CHF (see Question 24). The pacemaker can operate at a fixed rate or can be programmed to a rate-responsive mode, which means that it paces at a gradually accelerated rate in the setting of increased patient activity.

10. What does the pacemaker code tell us about the function of the pacemaker?

A detailed explanation of the pacemaker code devised by the North American Society for Pacing and Electrophysiology and the British Pacing and Electro-physiology Group was published in 1987 and was summarized in 1991. The meaning and options for each of the various position codes are as follows. The options for the first two position categories are O (none), A (atrium), V (ventricle), or D (atrium and ventricle).
- The first letter indicates the chamber of the heart that is *paced*.
- The second letter indicates the chamber that is *sensed*.
- The third letter indicates the pacemaker's *response to sensing*. Options here are O (none), T (triggered, in which a response is triggered when a beat is sensed), I (inhibited, a response is inhibited when a beat is sensed), or D (dual, in which triggered and inhibited responses both occur).
- The fourth letter is used to describe *possible programming features*; the letter R is most commonly found in this position and indicates that the pacemaker is in the rate-responsive mode.
- Options for each position include:
  - A = Atrium
  - V = Ventricle
  - D = Atrium and ventricle (first and second position)
  - D = Triggered and inhibited (third position)
  - T = Triggered
  - I = Inhibited
  - R = Rate-responsive
  - O = None

For example, a DDDR pacemaker paces and senses both the atrium and ventricle. The third letter in this case, D, indicates that both a triggered and inhibited response will occur. This means that an intrinsic beat sensed in the atrium or ventricle will inhibit the paced beat in that chamber if it falls within a certain window of time. An atrial sensed or paced beat will be followed by a triggered ventricular paced beat at a preset interval (the programmed AV delay) if the atrial beat is not intrinsically conducted to the ventricle. The fourth letter, R, indicates that the pacemaker has an active rate-responsive sensor (see the following table).

Example of a pacemaker programmed to the DDDR mode

Chamber Paced	Chamber Sensed	Response to Sensing	Programmable Features
D	D	D	R
Atrium and ventricle are paced	Atrium and ventricle are sensed	A sensed beat can trigger or inhibit a response	The pacemaker has an active rate-responsive sensor

11. How does the pacemaker's rate-responsive sensor function?

Most pacemakers currently implanted are rate responsive and have a sensor component as part of the pulse generator circuitry. Ideally, a sensor should be able to mimic the function of the patient's sinus node. The circuitry in the pacemaker allows information about the patient's activity level obtained by the sensor to be converted to an increased pacing rate. Some sensors monitor vibration, which increases with the patient's movement, such as stair climbing or walking. This type of sensor can also result in an increase in heart rate with nonphysiological stimuli, such as tapping or pressure on the pulse generator. Another type of common sensor is an accelerometer that senses movement (acceleration or deceleration). A pacemaker with a "minute ventilation"–type sensor measures transthoracic impedance changes that result during respiration and that tend to correlate well with oxygen consumption. Some pacemakers provide rate responsiveness based on other types of sensors, or a single device may use more than one kind of sensor to optimize the pacemaker's ability to respond to physiological demands.

12. How is the decision made to implant a dual-chamber versus a single-chamber pacemaker?

In patients with sinus node function, a dual-chamber, rate-responsive pacemaker is usually recommended, unless the patient is bedridden, because this type of pacemaker has shown improved outcome and less long-term morbidity. The dual-chamber pacemaker can operate in four manners (A = atrial; V = ventricular):
- AV sequential pacing: both the atrium and ventricle are paced with a fixed AV delay, or

- A paced/V sensed: the atrium is paced, but intrinsic conduction is intact and the conducted QRS complex occurs before the programmed AV delay times out, or
- A sensed/V paced: the sinus node functions above the pacemaker lower rate, and the patient's intrinsic AV nodal conduction is longer than the programmed AV delay, resulting in ventricular pacing at the end of the AV delay interval, or
- A sensed/V sensed: sinus and AV nodal function are intact at a rate greater than the programmed lower rate, so atrial and ventricular pacing output is inhibited.

Patients with chronic atrial fibrillation have no need for an atrial lead and generally receive a VVIR pacemaker. Implantation of a pacemaker with a "mode switch" option is important for patients with paroxysmal atrial tachyarrhythmias to prevent tracking of the atrial arrhythmia resulting in ventricular pacing at the programmed upper rate limit.

13. How does the mode switch parameter of the pacemaker function?

If a pacemaker has the mode switch option activated, the device converts to a mode that does not sense the atrium if the atrial rate exceeds a preset limit. During the atrial tachyarrhythmia, atrial sensing and pacing are disabled and the pacemaker functions in a VVI mode. When the arrhythmia terminates (and the atrial rate is less than the preset limit), the pacemaker resumes pacing in the dual-chamber mode.

14. What are the important topics to be addressed during preoperative teaching for the patient with a pacemaker?

The patient should understand the indication for pacemaker implant and the general implant procedure. Most transvenous pacemaker implants are done with intravenous sedation rather than general anesthesia. The risks and benefits of the surgery, and the details of the implant procedure, should be explained to the patient and family by the physician before consent is obtained.

15. What complications can occur during or after pacemaker implantation?

The nurse should monitor the patient for signs and symptoms associated with the following possible complications: cardiac tamponade from perforation, lead dislodgement, arrhythmias, hematoma, venous thrombosis, erosion of the generator, and infection.

16. What is the role of the nurse in postoperative teaching of the patient with a pacemaker?

Postoperative care for the patient with a pacemaker is similar to that for patients who have had an implantable cardioverter defibrillator (ICD) implanted (see Chapter 25, Implantable Cardioverter Defibrillators). Patients are instructed to keep the incision site clean and dry for 7 to 10 days and to allow the Steri-Strips to fall off rather than removing them intentionally. They should report any sign of infection such as fever, chills, erythema (redness) or drainage at the pacemaker site promptly to their health care provider. Arm movement above shoulder height on the ipsilateral side (same side) is limited for a few weeks to prevent dislodgement. After a few days of recovery, there is usually no driving limitation, although if there is a question about the etiology of a patient's syncopal episode, the physician or nurse practitioner may limit driving. Patients are instructed to carry their pacemaker identification card, received at the time of surgical implantation, at all times and to inform their health care providers regarding the presence of the pacemaker.

A transtelephonic monitor is usually provided to the patient by the pacemaker staff before discharge, and use of this device is demonstrated. Transtelephonic follow-up on a regularly scheduled basis (usually every 3 months) is important to confirm battery and lead function. Patients are seen in the clinic for complete evaluation of the pacemaker every 6 to 12 months.

17. What is the effect of a magnet on a pacemaker?

Application of a magnet directly over the pacemaker results in asynchronous pacing (pacing without sensing) and may demonstrate the presence of capture. The magnet rate of the pacemaker also provides information about the battery status. Each pacemaker manufacturer has a preset rate that occurs with magnet placement, and the pacing rate during magnet application changes as the battery nears the "end of life" (EOL). Rhythm strips with and without magnet placement are routinely performed during transtelephonic follow-up checks, which allows regular evaluation of the battery function.

18. What is electromagnetic interference (EMI), and how does it affect pacemaker function?

As technology continues to advance, EMI has raised increased concerns for patients with permanent pacemakers and cardioverter defibrillators. In a worst-case scenario, EMI can result in a variety of pacemaker problems, including inappropriate inhibition or triggering of the device, asynchronous pacing, device reprogramming, or circuitry damage. Potential sources of EMI that can, in close proximity, interfere with pacemaker function are discussed subsequently. Patients are advised to discuss possible exposure to these sources with their nurse practitioner or physician. Cell phone use is permitted, although patients are asked to use the contralateral (opposite) ear and to refrain from carrying the phone in the shirt pocket over the pulse generator. Electronic surveillance systems, often found on either side of store entryways, are not an issue as long as the patient does not lean on or stand in close proximity to the device.

19. What sources of medical EMI can result in pacemaker malfunction?

Various medical equipment and procedures can result in alteration of pacemaker function and are listed in the following box. For this reason, it is important that the patient be instructed to inform all health care providers of the presence of the implanted pacemaker.

Sources of Potential Electromagnetic Interference (EMI)

Occupational or Situational EMI
- High-voltage power lines
- Transformers
- Degaussing coils
- Arc welding equipment
- Induction furnaces
- Running alternators

Medical Sources of EMI
- Magnetic resonance imaging (MRI)
- Electrosurgical instruments (electrocautery)
- Nerve stimulators
- External cardioversion of defibrillation
- Therapeutic diathermy
- Radiotherapy
- Lithotripsy
- Radiofrequency ablation

In the event of elective cardioversion, a pacemaker programmer should be available and a transcutaneous pacemaker should be applied before the procedure. The adhesive electrodes for cardioversion should ideally be positioned in the anterior-posterior direction as far from the pacemaker pulse generator and lead system as possible. If paddles on the anterior chest are to be used for cardioversion, positioning of the paddles as far away from the pacemaker system as possible (>5.0 cm) is important. After cardioversion, the patient should be monitored for appropriate pacemaker function and the device should be interrogated and evaluated.

Diagnostic radiology does not interfere with pacemaker function. However, in the event that radiation therapy is indicated in the region of the pacemaker, the device should be relocated to the opposite side. Shielding of the pulse generator should be maximized, and patients who are pacemaker dependent should have continuous electrocardiogram (ECG) monitoring during therapy sessions. The device should be interrogated and evaluated after the radiation therapy session. Patients undergoing radiofrequency ablation should have backup transcutaneous pacing available, and a temporary ventricular pacing wire should be inserted before application of radiofrequency energy.

In the event the patient with a pacemaker is to undergo a surgical procedure requiring electrocautery, bipolar cautery is preferred to unipolar and patients should have continuous ECG monitoring during the procedure. Preoperative device reprogramming may be warranted and should be discussed with the patient's cardiologist. After surgery, ECGs with and without magnet should be performed for evaluation of device function.

Magnetic resonance imaging in generally contraindicated for patients with pacemakers.

20. What possible pacemaker malfunctions can occur that would prompt nursing intervention?

The potential pacemaker problems of which the nurse should be aware are failure to capture and problems with sensing.

Failure to capture (as discussed earlier in Question 6) can be the result of pulse generator failure, lead dislodgement or fracture, or altered thresholds from a variety of causes. If a patient who is pacemaker dependent has failure to capture, the nurse should promptly notify the nurse practitioner or physician and prepare for placement of a transcutaneous or transvenous pacemaker.

Sensing problems can be the result of oversensing or undersensing. In the case of oversensing, the device sees artifact that it considers an intrinsic beat. This oversensing may be from electrical noise or inappropriate sensing of T waves or the sensing of pacing output in a different chamber of the heart. Oversensing results in "underpacing" because the pacemaker incorrectly interprets the artifact as the intrinsic depolarization. In patients without an underlying rhythm, oversensing can result in asystole because the pacemaker does not pace as needed. Undersensing results when the pacemaker does not sense the intrinsic rhythm and may be to the result of various causes including acute myocardial infarction, drugs, electrolyte disturbances, myocardial fibrosis, lead malfunction, or device programming (a sensitivity setting that is inadequate to see the intrinsic P wave or R wave). Undersensing results in "overpacing," meaning pacing stimuli are delivered when not needed. Pacing stimuli could occur inappropriately during the T wave and possibly result in malignant ventricular arrhythmias. Rarely, the pacemaker system may fail to generate an output because of circuitry failure or battery depletion.

21. How should the nurse assess for appropriate pacemaker function?

The nurse should elicit a history from the patient, including the reason for the initial pacemaker implantation, the type of pacemaker, the programmed pacemaker settings if possible, and any recent symptoms. The ECGs should be reviewed, and evidence of intrinsic activity and paced beats should be evaluated. Because the usual position for the ventricular lead is in the right ventricular apex of the heart, the paced ventricular rhythm resembles a left bundle branch block pattern with a wide QRS complex. Bipolar leads produce a small pacing artifact (vertical mark preceding the paced complex) that may not be obvious on the surface ECG; however, pacemaker artifact generated from a unipolar lead results in an obvious pacing spike initiating the paced beat. The relationship of the paced or sensed P waves to the paced or sensed QRS complexes should be evaluated as should the heart rate. This information helps the nurse determine whether or not the device is pacing, capturing, and sensing appropriately. Evidence that the device is not functioning properly should be brought to the nurse practitioner's or physician's attention. If obvious pacemaker malfunction is resulting in severe patient symptomatology, preparation for transcutaneous pacing and eventual placement of a transvenous pacemaker should be expedited.

22. What is hysteresis, and how does this affect pacemaker function?

A pacemaker programmed with hysteresis can easily fool many people. Hysteresis is a programmable feature that allows a longer escape interval to occur before pacing is activated at the basic lower rate. For example, if the patient's intrinsic rate is 80 bpm and the pacemaker is programmed in the VVI mode at a lower rate of 60 bpm with hysteresis programmed to 40 bpm, the patient's intrinsic rate needs to decrease to 40 bpm before the pacemaker is activated. It then paces at the lower rate of 60 bpm. This is normal functioning for this pacemaker and not an oversensing problem as one might initially suspect in evaluation of the ECG strip. This function is not commonly used but is occasionally utilized for patients with neurally mediated syncope.

23. What possible new indications for pacing have recently been introduced?

New indications for pacemaker implantation are rapidly evolving. The most recent applications of pacemaker therapy include prevention of paroxysmal atrial fibrillation, neurally mediated syncope, and treatment of hypertrophic obstructive cardiomyopathy (HOCM) and CHF.

Ongoing trials are evaluating the possibility that dual-site atrial pacing for patients with paroxysmal atrial fibrillation may improve the likelihood of maintaining sinus rhythm and increase arrhythmia-free intervals. Because atrial fibrillation is the most frequently occurring arrhythmia seen in clinical practice, an approved indication for pacing therapy intended to decrease episodes of paroxysmal atrial fibrillation would likely impact a substantial number of patients.

Neurally mediated syncope, also called vasovagal syncope or neurocardiogenic syncope, results from a disorder of autonomic cardiovascular regulation. A complex interaction between vasodilation (decreased preload), afferent neural stimuli, and an efferent reflex response may result in syncope associated with bradycardia and hypotension. Although some patients can undergo successful treatment with medication, dual-chamber pacemaker implantation may help prevent syncope when significant bradycardia or asystole is believed to be the major contributor to the patient's symptomatology.

Certain subsets of patients with HOCM may benefit from dual-chamber pacing, although this indication is controversial. Patients with HOCM have a dynamic obstruction of the left ventricular outflow tract (LVOT). Pacing in this patient group is intended to reduce the LVOT gradient by pacing the heart with an AV delay shorter than the intrinsic conduction interval. The patients with HOCM who may benefit from pacing therapy are those with refractory symptoms despite medical therapy in the presence of a significant LVOT gradient and those who have prominent hypertrophy of the basal portion of the interventricular septum and modest mitral regurgitation. Pacing in these patients improves LVOT obstruction by moving the septum away from the outflow tract. Because the septum is the major cause of obstruction in this disorder, cardiac output improves with pacing; however, studies have not shown consistent results with regard to symptomatic improvement.

24. What is biventricular pacing, and how does it benefit the patient with severe CHF?

Some patients with CHF have dyssynchronous (uncoordinated) contraction of the ventricles as evidenced by a left bundle branch block or intraventricular conduction delay on ECG. This lack of ventricular synchrony results in decreased left ventricular filling time and a decrease in left ventricular function. Biventricular pacing restores synchronous contraction by pacing the ventricles simultaneously through leads placed in the right ventricle and the coronary sinus and may result in increased stroke volume, improved New York Heart Association (NYHA) Functional Class, increased 6-minute walk duration, and improved quality of life. Present indications for use of biventricular pacing in CHF include patients with CHF at a NYHA Functional Class III or IV level who are already on optimal stable CHF medications and who have a left ventricular ejection fraction of 35% or less and a QRS duration of 130 ms or more. Ongoing trials continue to evaluate biventricular pacing therapy in this seriously ill and functionally limited group of patients.

 Key Points

- The pacing mode provides details regarding the function of the pacemaker. The first letter indicates the chamber paced, the second letter indicates the chamber sensed, and the third letter indicates the pacemaker's response to a sensed beat. If an R is the fourth letter, the device is rate responsive.

- A pacemaker with the rate-responsive mode turned on results in acceleration of the patient's lower pacing rate in response to increased activity or ventilation.

- Patients are usually restricted from lifting the arm on the same side as the new pacemaker implant above shoulder level for a few weeks after surgery to prevent lead dislodgement.

- Placement of a magnet over the pacemaker results in asynchronous pacing with the pacemaker not sensing intrinsic beats.

- Biventricular pacemakers can be implanted in patients with severe CHF and left ventricular dysfunction who have dyssynchrony of ventricular contraction on ECG. Many of these patients have an increased exercise tolerance, improved ventricular function, and decreased hospitalizations for CHF after implantation of this device.

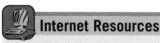

Internet Resources

NASPE Heart Rhythm Society:
www.naspe.org

American Heart Association:
www.americanheart.org

American Heart Association: Pacemakers:
http://www.americanheart.org/presenter.jhtml?identifier=24

American Heart Association: Cardiac Conduction System:
http://www.americanheart.org/presenter.jhtml?identifier=68

American Heart Association: Sinus Disturbances:
http://www.americanheart.org/presenter.jhtml?identifier=55

American Heart Association: What Are Arrhythmias?
http://www.americanheart.org/presenter.jhtml?identifier=560

American Heart Association: Heart Block:
http://www.americanheart.org/presenter.jhtml?identifier=42

Bibliography

Bernstein AD, Camm J, Fletcher RD et al: The NASPE/BPEG generic pacemaker code for antibradyarrhythmia and adaptive-rate pacing and antitachyarrhythmia devices, *Pacing Clin Electrophysiol* 10:794-799, 1987.

Glikson M, Hayes DL: Cardiac pacing: a review, *Med Clin North Am* 85(2):369-421, 2001.

Goldschlager N, Epstein A, Friedman P et al: Environmental and drug effects on patients with pacemakers and implantable cardioverter/defibrillators, *Arch Intern Med* 161:649-655, 2001.

Jacobson C, Gerity D: Pacemakers and implantable defibrillators. In Woods SL, Froelicher ESS, Motzer SV, editors: *Cardiac nursing*, ed 4, Philadelphia, 2000, Lippincott, pp 661-698.

Legge D, Leeper B: Management of heart failure: use of biventricular pacing, *J Cardiovasc Nurs* 16(3):72-81, 2002.

Linde C, Leclercq C, Rex S et al: Long-term benefits of biventricular pacing in congestive heart failure: results from the MUltisite STimulation In Cardiomyopathy (MUSTIC) study, *J Am Coll Cardiol* 40:111-118, 2002.

Mangrum JM, DiMarco JP: The evaluation and management of bradycardia, *N Engl J Med* 342(10):703-709, 2000.

Reynolds J, Apple S: A systematic approach to pacemaker assessment, *AACN Clin Issues* 12(1):114-126, 2001.

Teplitz L: Classification of cardiac pacemakers: the pacemaker code, *J Cardiovasc Nurs* 5(3):1-8, 1991.

Wolbrette DL, Naccarelli GV: Emerging indications for permanent pacing, *Curr Cardiol Rep* 2:353-360, 2000.

Implantable Cardioverter Defibrillators

Margaret C. Herbst

1. What is an implantable cardioverter defibrillator (ICD)?

An ICD is a device that detects and attempts to electrically convert ventricular tachyarrhythmia and ventricular fibrillation. It consists of a lead system (positioned inside the heart) that is connected to a battery pack (pulse generator).

2. How does an ICD function?

The lead implanted inside the right ventricle constantly monitors the heart rate, and if the heart rate exceeds a programmed value called the rate cut off, the device delivers therapy to convert the rhythm to normal. Therapies for conversion of tachyarrhythmias include:
- Synchronized cardioversion ("little shock").
- Unsynchronized defibrillation ("big" shock of approximately 30 J delivered internally, which is equivalent to approximately 360 J delivered externally).
- Antitachycardia pacing (fast pacing or "overdrive pacing").

In addition, the ICD can treat slow rhythms by functioning as a standard pacemaker.

3. Which patients need an ICD?

The current recommendations for ICD implantation include those patients with any of the following conditions:
- Cardiac arrest caused by ventricular fibrillation (VF) or ventricular tachycardia (VT) not from a transient or reversible cause.
- Spontaneous sustained VT.
- Syncope of undetermined origin and a positive electrophysiology (EP) study (clinically relevant, hemodynamically significant sustained VT or VF induced during the study).
- Nonsustained VT with coronary disease, prior myocardial infarction (MI), left ventricular (LV) dysfunction, and inducible VF or sustained VT at EP study that is not suppressible by a class I antiarrhythmic drug.

In addition, ICDs have proven beneficial for the following groups:
- Patients at high risk for life-threatening arrhythmias, such as those with a history of MI and decreased LV function (ejection fraction, <31%).

- Individuals at high risk because of conditions such as long QT syndrome, hypertrophic cardiomyopathy, Brugada syndrome, or arrhythmogenic right ventricular dysplasia.

4. How is the ICD implanted?

Early generation ICD implants used epicardial patches placed via a subxiphoid, thoracotomy or open chest (sternotomy) incision. These patch leads then were connected to a pulse generator implanted in the abdomen.

Present day ICD lead systems are almost always positioned endocardially (inside the heart) through a transvenous approach. After an incision is made slightly below the mid clavicle, the lead is inserted through the subclavian or cephalic vein and advanced into position in the right ventricle with fluoroscopic guidance. A second lead may be placed in the right atrium if a dual-chamber system is believed to be advantageous to the patient. The lead tips are secured to the endocardial surface with either a screw or a tine (like a fishhook) mechanism. The tined lead becomes firmly attached to the endocardial surface in a few weeks. The pulse generator then is attached to the lead and placed inside a subcutaneous or submuscular pocket formed by the physician (see the following figure). The system is tested by inducing VF to assure that the ICD can properly detect and convert the arrhythmia to a normal rhythm.

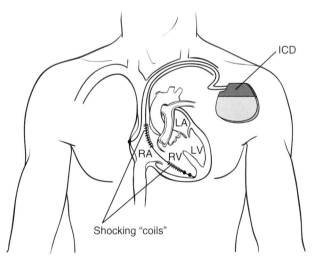

ICD system implanted via transvenous approach.

After successful testing, the incision is closed and a transparent dressing or sterilized strips are applied and covered with a pressure dressing.

5. **What is the typical length of hospital stay for these patients?**

Most patients who are already in the hospital can be discharged home on post-operative day 1 after the dressing is changed and a chest radiograph (with posteroanterior [PA] and lateral views) is performed to confirm proper lead position. In those patients for whom the ICD is implanted for a primary prevention indication, the surgery may be performed on a same-day basis or the patient may stay overnight in the hospital for observation.

6. **What are the essential components of preoperative teaching that should be discussed with a patient who is scheduled for ICD implantation?**

The patient and family must understand the indication for the surgery and the basic details of the implant procedure. Fears and concerns of the patient and family members should also be discussed.

7. **What postoperative nursing care is necessary for patients undergoing ICD implantation?**

- Frequent vital sign checks should be performed as ordered by the physician or nurse practitioner.
- Patients are usually kept on bed rest the evening after surgery and need assistance with activities of daily living such as voiding, eating, and dressing.
- Postoperative intravenous antibiotics are given as prescribed.
- Comfort measures such as positioning and administration of analgesic medication should be addressed.
- The patient should be on telemetry monitoring and be continuously observed for any occurrence of arrhythmia.
- The incision may be covered by a dressing until removal the next morning by the physician or nurse practitioner. The sterilized strips used to close the external layer of skin at the incision site are lightly covered with a 4 × 4 gauze and paper tape or transparent dressing. The dressing and incision site should be observed by the nurse for any signs of increased drainage, erythema, or hematoma that need to be reported to the physician or nurse practitioner.
- Before hospital discharge, the patient should have a standing PA and lateral chest radiograph. The nurse should remind the patient not to raise the arm on the side of the ICD implant above shoulder level.

8. **What postoperative issues should be discussed with the patient and family before discharge?**

The following issues should be addressed:

- **Wound care:** The wound should remain clean and dry for 10 days, after which the patient may wash gently over the incision. The sterilized strips should be allowed to fall off on their own, and patients should be instructed not to remove the sterilized strips prematurely.
- **Signs/symptoms of infection:** Any evidence of swelling, increased drainage, or erythema (redness) at the ICD pocket site or development of fever or chills

should be reported by the patient to the health care provider immediately. The patient should be provided with contact phone numbers in the event any sign or symptom of infection is seen.

- **Activity restrictions:** The arm on the same side as the ICD implant should be kept at or below shoulder level, and the patient should avoid all heavy lifting (greater than a few pounds) with the affected arm for a few weeks after surgery. This recommendation may vary based on the request of the implanting physician. Rough contact or forceful blows to the ICD site should always be avoided.
- **Driving:** Driving restrictions vary among patients based on the indication for ICD implant and physician preference. Patients who have had VT or VF associated with cardiac arrest or syncope are generally instructed not to drive for 3 to 6 months. Asymptomatic patients who have either documented sustained arrhythmias or who were found to be inducible at EP study may have an abbreviated driving restriction, although commercial driving is prohibited in both of these patient groups. Patients undergoing ICD implantation for primary prevention (no history of ventricular tachyarrhythmias) are usually not prohibited from driving after the first few days of recovery.
- **Return to work:** Resumption of regular work may be affected by many factors, including underlying cardiac disease and associated symptoms, the need to drive to or from work or driving as a condition of employment, and degree of physical activity associated with work. Patients who are employed predominantly with deskwork, such as computer work, can return to work within a week of surgery if they are not limited by concomitant health problems. Patients who perform physical labor as part of their job may need an extended absence or may need a written request for lighter work duty. The nurse should convey this need to the patient's doctor or nurse practitioner before discharge. Patients with ICDs who drive commercially (except those patients who undergo implantation for primary prevention purposes) are permanently disabled from their prior form of employment; this may present a significant form of financial and emotional hardship for the patient and family. The nurse should request the services of a social worker to assist with the patient's application for disability or possible employment retraining through vocational rehabilitation programs.
- **Need to carry identification (ID) card:** Patients are given an ID card that provides information about the implanted leads and pulse generator. They should be instructed to keep this with them at all times, especially when traveling away from home. In addition, patients are generally advised to wear ID jewelry, such as a necklace or bracelet, identifying that they have an ICD.

9. What effect does electromagnetic interference (EMI) have on an ICD, and what instructions should be given to the patient about EMI?

If a patient with an ICD comes into contact with a strong magnetic field, the device may be "blinded." This means that while the ICD is exposed to the magnetic field, the device will not detect any tachyarrhythmia, which could result in the ICD inappropriately withholding necessary therapy.

Household equipment and appliances such as microwaves, televisions, and electric blankets do not interfere with ICD function. Patients should avoid arc welding or close contact with a running alternator, large generators, or any strong magnetic field. Cellular phones should be used on the contralateral (opposite) side. Potential medical sources of EMI include magnetic resonance imaging (MRI) scanners (contraindicated in patients with ICDs), radiation therapy, and electrocautery. Patients should be advised to contact the physician who provides ICD care before any surgical procedure. Use of electrocautery in the patient may cause oversensing of the cautery output and result in inappropriate delivery of therapy to the patient despite the presence of a normal rhythm.

Some ICDs attempt to differentiate atrial from ventricular tachyarrhythmias (atrial fibrillation versus VF, for example). If the device is unable to make this distinction, a patient possibly may receive ICD therapy inappropriately if the rate of atrial fibrillation exceeds the ICD rate cut off. If a patient receives multiple inappropriate shocks for atrial fibrillation, the physician may ask the nurse to apply a magnet over the ICD to inhibit detection and prevent recurrence of the inappropriate shocks while plans for rate control or conversion of the atrial fibrillation are initiated.

10. What happens if the patient with an ICD walks through a metal detector or an electronic surveillance system?

Patients with an ICD can walk through a metal detector without harm to the device, but they may activate the alarm as a result. At that point, the patient should be instructed to present the device ID card to security personnel and request a hand search if necessary. Close exposure (usually up to 12 in) to hand-held wands containing magnets used for scanning the body should be avoided by patients with an ICD. Electronic surveillance devices (used for theft detection purposes at store doorways) are not likely to interfere with the ICD as long as prolonged close proximity is avoided, and patients are instructed to walk normally through such systems.

11. What does the patient feel when ICD therapy is delivered?

Activation of antitachycardia pacing therapy for conversion of a tachyarrhythmia is often not felt by the patient, although the arrhythmia itself may result in symptoms of palpitations and dizziness or syncope from rate-related hypotension. An electrical discharge of the ICD for cardioversion or defibrillation is generally felt as a strong jolt or shock to the anterior chest and has been described as a kick in the chest or like touching a cattle fence.

12. Will an individual who touches a patient with an ICD when the device discharges feel or be harmed by the shock?

Individuals in direct contact with a patient during an ICD discharge may feel a tingling sensation, but they are not harmed. Likewise, if a patient with an ICD is found to be without signs of life (not moving, breathing, or talking), cardiopulmonary resuscitation (CPR) should be performed as recommended by the Basic Life Support (BLS) protocol even if the ICD appears to be discharging because, on rare occasions, ICD shocks may fail to convert the potentially lethal ventricular arrhythmias.

13. What instructions are given to the patient regarding the occurrence of ICD discharges?

Patients are instructed to sit or lie down if they feel the onset of tachyarrhythmia symptoms or if the ICD discharges. In the event that the ICD discharges only once and the patient feels stable after the shock, they are instructed to call their ICD care provider. If the ICD discharges more than once in succession or the patient continues to feel chest pain, dyspnea, or presyncope, he or she should call 911 for transport to the closest emergency department for attention. In the event that the patient is rendered unresponsive and remains so after apparent ICD discharge, the family is instructed to dial 911 and begin CPR if the patient has no spontaneous respiration or signs of life.

14. Do patients with ICDs also require antiarrhythmic medications?

Approximately half of patients with ICDs also take an antiarrhythmic medication, which is intended to limit the number of ICD discharges.

15. How long does the pulse generator (battery) of an ICD last?

Although early models lasted only 2 to 3 years, present generation ICDs last approximately 5 to 6 years. The longevity of the pulse generator is affected by the percentage of time the pacemaker is in use and the number of defibrillation episodes.

16. How does the patient know when the ICD pulse generator needs to be changed, and how is this procedure performed?

Patients are seen for ICD interrogation approximately every 3 months and at each visit the battery and lead functions are evaluated. When the pulse generator reaches the estimated replacement index (ERI), the patient is scheduled for an elective pulse generator change. At that time, an incision is made over the site and the pulse generator is unhooked from the previously implanted lead system. The lead is tested, and if it is functioning properly, a new pulse generator is attached. The device then is tested, and the incision is closed. If any apparent malfunction of the lead system is found, new leads are implanted and attached to the pulse generator.

17. What information is stored in the ICD in the event that it is used to convert a tachyarrhythmia?

The ICD stores a recording of the tachyarrhythmia, the therapy used to convert the arrhythmia, and the postconversion rhythm, which can be printed out at a later time for review by the clinician.

18. **How do patients respond emotionally after ICD implant?**

Patients who have undergone ICD implant may have a variety of emotional, psychological, and social concerns in addition to the obvious physical issues. They may experience fear, anxiety, a sense of loss of control, depression, anger, difficulty sleeping, or alteration in body image or sexuality. Fear and anxiety may result from concerns regarding the pain associated with possible ICD shocks, potential for device malfunction or death, role changes, and financial or employment issues.

19. **How can the nurse help the patient and family address the many psychological and quality of life issues faced after ICD implant?**

The nurse should encourage patients and their families to discuss feelings and concerns in a supportive atmosphere and target feedback and education to these issues. It is important to assure the patient and family that their fears and concerns are normal and to provide accurate information in response to specific questions and referral to outside means of support, such as vocational rehabilitation for employment issues, social services for financial concerns, patient support groups for social support, or additional mental health services if needed. The nurse also can assist the patient and family by taking an active role in recovery. Providing encouragement and hope for the future is essential. Nurses should aid the patient and family in developing positive coping strategies and emphasizing resumption of everyday activities after discharge home.

Key Points

- An ICD detects and attempts to convert ventricular tachyarrhythmias.
- Modern day ICDs are capable of the following functions: synchronized cardioversion, unsynchronized defibrillation, antitachycardia pacing, bradycardia pacing, and biventricular pacing.
- If the ICD is exposed to a strong magnetic field, the device does not detect tachyarrhythmias.
- Patients should be instructed to keep their ICD identification card with them at all times.
- If a patient's ICD discharges while they are touching another person, that individual is not harmed.

Internet Resources

NASPE Heart Rhythm Society:
www.naspe.org

American Heart Association:
www.americanheart.org

Internet Resources   *continued*

American Heart Association: Pacemakers:
http://www.americanheart.org/presenter.jhtml?identifier=24

American Heart Association: Cardiac Conduction System:
http://www.americanheart.org/presenter.jhtml?identifier=68

American Heart Association: Sinus Disturbances:
http://www.americanheart.org/presenter.jhtml?identifier=55

American Heart Association: What Are Arrhythmias?
http://www.americanheart.org/presenter.jhtml?identifier=560

American Heart Association: Heart Block:
http://www.americanheart.org/presenter.jhtml?identifier=42

Bibliography

Ahmad M et al: Patients' attitudes toward implanted defibrillator shocks, *Pacing Clin Electrophysiol* 23:934-938, 2000.

Dougherty CM et al: Domains of nursing intervention after sudden cardiac arrest and automatic internal cardioverter defibrillator implantation, *Heart Lung* 29:79-86, 2000.

Eads AS et al: Supportive communication with implantable cardioverter defibrillator patients: seven principles to facilitate psychosocial adjustment, *J Cardiopulm Rehabil* 20:109-114, 2000.

Greene HL: The implantable cardioverter-defibrillator, *Clin Cardiol* 23:315-326, 2000.

Gregoratos G et al: ACC/AHA guidelines for implantation of cardiac pacemakers and antiarrhythmia devices, *J Am Coll Cardiol* 31(5):1175-1209, 1998.

Kohn CS et al: The effect of psychological intervention on patients' long-term adjustment to the ICD: a prospective study, *Pacing Clin Electrophysiol* 23(pt I):450-456, 2000.

Ocampo CM: Living with an implantable cardioverter defibrillator: impact on the patient, family, and society, *Nurs Clin North Am* 35(4):1019-1030, 2000.

Thomas SA et al: Living with an implantable cardioverter-defibrillator: a review of the current literature related to psychosocial factors, *AACN Clin Issues* 12(1):156-163, 2001.

White E: Patients with implantable cardioverter defibrillators: transition to home, *J Cardiovasc Nurs* 14(3):42-52, 2000.

Heart Transplantation

Scott Kowalczyk

1. How many transplants are performed annually in the United States?

The number of available donors has plateaued, and the demand for organs continues to greatly outnumber the supply. Data from the Organ Procurement and Transplantation Network (OPTN) website are presented in the following table.

Year	1999	2000	2001	2002	2003
Transplants	2188	2199	2202	2155	1897

2. What are the indications for heart transplant?

Survival without transplant after all appropriate conventional surgical and maximal medical therapies have been instituted is expected to be less than one year. Major diagnoses that lead to transplant are coronary artery disease and nonischemic cardiomyopathies. Common nonischemic cardiomyopathy etiologies are idiopathic, viral, familial, postpartum, sarcoid, lupus, valvular disease, myocarditis, and cardiotoxic agents like alcohol or doxorubicin (Adriamycin). Retransplantation for rejection, restrictive/constrictive disease, and transplant vasculopathy (chronic rejection) is a less frequent occurrence.

3. What are the absolute contraindications to transplant?

Although they vary among centers, common contraindications are:
- Patient does not want a transplant, despite what the family has to say in the matter. The medical regimen can be demanding, and to have a reasonable chance of a successful outcome, the patient must be fully committed.
- Active drug, tobacco product, or alcohol use. Some transplant centers require candidates to sign contracts and agree to random drug testing for a specified period of time before the patient is listed for transplant.
- No means of social support, no stable home, no one to call for assistance with acute events, or no transportation available for scheduled or nonscheduled returns to the hospital.
- Unresolved insurance issues. Medication costs alone during the first year after transplant can be thousands of dollars per month.

- Documentation of medical noncompliance (nonadherence to the medical plan). A contract may be made to monitor compliance in the heart failure clinic for a specified period of time, allowing for reevaluation of behavior. A transplant listing could then become a possibility.
- A history of active cancer or history of cancers likely to reoccur with immunosuppressive medications. Some cancers are confined and considered unlikely to reoccur after a specified period of time, and then transplant becomes an option.
- The presence of kidney, lung, liver, or other organ system disease that limits the life of the candidate separate from heart failure. However, some patients may be eligible for multiorgan transplants. Examples would be heart/kidney or heart/double-lung transplants. Double-organ transplants are becoming more common.
- Irreversible pulmonary hypertension. Although transplant centers' specific criteria vary, an example is a fixed pulmonary vascular resistance (PVR) greater than 5 Wood's units and inability for the pulmonary artery systolic pressure to be reduced to less than 50 mm Hg.

4. Are there age limits for a heart transplant?

Transplant surgeons and cardiologists have varied opinions regarding age-related inclusion/exclusion criteria. In the past, transplant programs excluded patients age 65 years and older from transplant. However, many programs now consider those patients. The patient's other organ systems must be without disease, increasing the likelihood of a successful outcome for the older candidate.

5. When should a patient be referred for transplant evaluation?

Whether the patient has adequate time to complete the work-up process should be considered. This time includes examination at a heart failure clinic, evaluation, listing, and waiting for an acceptable/compatible organ. A limited supply of organs exists for those patients who are truly running out of time. Premature listing of patients creates extensive waiting lists and causes more of a crisis than already exists. After the appropriate maximal medical and surgical therapy has been attempted, patients with the following conditions should be referred:

- Peak VO_2 <12 to 14 mg/kg/min and major physical limitation.
- Recurrent unstable cardiac ischemia that is not amenable to revascularization (percutaneous coronary intervention or bypass grafting).
- Difficulty maintaining fluid balance and renal function in the absence of fluid and dietary indiscretion or medication nonadherence.
- Symptomatic ventricular arrhythmias that fail to respond to conventional therapies.

Patients are recommended for referral to heart failure physicians for transplant evaluation when, despite the use of maximal conventional therapies, they continue to have heart failure symptoms that severely limit quality of life.

6. **What testing is involved when a patient is referred for a transplant evaluation?**

Variability is seen among transplant centers; however, typical testing includes the following:

- **Blood analysis:** A comprehensive bloodwork analysis is completed; this includes hemoglobin (Hgb) A1C, complete blood cell count (CBC) with differential, chemistry panels, coagulation studies, fasting lipid panel, liver function tests, and thyroid function testing. The infectious disease serological lab work analysis includes HIV, hepatitis, and cytomegalovirus (CMV) antibodies, among others. The ABO blood type is identified, and panel reactive antibody (PRA) testing is performed.
- **Other lab studies:** Urine is collected for analysis/culture, and 24-hour collection is performed for creatinine clearance and protein. A stool culture may be indicated.
- **Cardiac studies:** Echocardiography (Echo), radionuclide ventriculography, cardiopulmonary exercise stress testing with myocardial oxygen uptake measurements (VO_{2max}), right/left heart catheterization, and 12-lead electrocardiography (ECG) are included.
- **Other organ systems:** Right upper quadrant ultrasonography (for evaluation of the gallbladder, kidneys, and liver), pulmonary function testing (spirometry with volumes and room air arterial blood gas [ABG]), and chest radiography are ordered. Also a purified protein derivative (PPD) test with controls to rule out tuberculosis (TB) is done.
- **Other possible testing:** A colonoscopy should be performed if there is a history of polyps or a family history of colorectal cancer. A bone density scan may be performed to acquire a baseline before chronic steroid use after the transplant. Carotid Doppler or other vascular studies may be indicated. A nutritional and dental screening is performed. All patients undergo a social work evaluation and psychological examination.
  - In women who are older than 40 years, a Papanicolaou (PAP) smear, pelvic and breast exam, and mammogram are performed if these have not been done within the last 12 months.
  - For men, a prostate exam is performed. If the patient is greater than 50 years old, a prostate specific antigen (PSA) is drawn.

7. **How is pulmonary pressure measured during the transplant work-up, and what is considered high pulmonary pressure?**

Pulmonary pressure is measured directly with a pulmonary artery catheter. Pulmonary artery systolic, diastolic, mean, and capillary wedge pressures are measured, and the PVR is calculated. The unit of measure most commonly used is Woods units. The formula for calculation of the PVR is as follows: PVR = mean pulmonary artery pressure – pulmonary capillary wedge pressure ÷ cardiac output. The procedure is performed at the bedside in the intensive care unit (ICU) or in the cardiac catheterization laboratory. Systolic pressure greater than 50 mm Hg and PVR greater than 3 Woods units are considered high.

8. Why are high pulmonary pressures worrisome for patients undergoing heart transplantation?

One of the more common causes of acute graft failure after cardiac transplant is right-sided heart failure from high pulmonary pressure measured as PVR. The transplanted heart is taken from a donor with normal pulmonary pressure. If transplanted in a recipient with pulmonary hypertension, severe right heart failure could develop and cause graft failure and death.

9. Is pulmonary hypertension potentially reversible?

Pulmonary hypertension is potentially reversible with a "drug challenge." Typically the course of events consists of a pulmonary artery catheter inserted into the patient and identification of pulmonary hypertension. An intravenous vasodilator medication, such as nitroprusside, nitroglycerin, or milrinone, is used in an attempt to lower the pressure. If the pressures are not adequately reduced with the drug challenge, a heart/double-lung transplant or a heterotopic heart transplant (see Question 16) may be considered.

10. What does it mean when someone is "listed?"

The United Network of Organ Sharing (UNOS) holds a federal contract to maintain a scientific, equitable, and medically sound organ allocation system for the country. Policies and bylaws are in place to govern organ allocation. UNOS membership includes transplant centers, organ procurement organizations (OPOs), and tissue typing laboratories. The United States is divided into 11 regions, and organs are allocated within those regions. Listing refers to the entering of the patient's name and vital statistics into UNOS's waiting list database. The patient's name, blood type, height, weight, cardiac disease, pulmonary artery pressures, and other clinical and nonclinical information, such as education level and insurance coverage, are entered (listed) into electronic registration forms. Information gathering, as required by UNOS, is an ongoing responsibility of the different transplant centers. UNOS maintains a public website at www.unos.org. Transplant information is maintained for public use and review. Confidential patient information is password protected and accessible to transplant centers on a secure website.

11. What is the status system for the heart transplant waiting list?

Each solid organ has an individual status system for its respective lists. The heart transplant system uses four different statuses: 1A, 1B, 2, and 7. Each status indicates a medical urgency.

| 1A | Inpatient with one or combination of following: Right or left ventricular assist device for less than 30 days. 1A status is kept after 30 days if device-related medical complication exists. Total artificial heart. |

continued	
1A	Intraaortic balloon pump. Mechanical ventilation. Pulmonary artery catheter *and* high-dose intravenous inotrope. Life expectancy less than 7 days without any of previous criteria.
1B	Patient is not required to be located at listing center and has one of following: Continuous intravenous inotrope. Left or right ventricular assist device for more than 30 days.
2	Patient is actively listed without any of previous therapies.
7	Patient remains on waiting list, but status is inactive. Patient is not accruing waiting time.

For example, a typical waiting list would be as follows:
1A (<5% of the list)
1B (<10% of the list)
2 (>50% of the list)
7 (<30% of the list)

From the previous list, of those patients who underwent transplantation in a single year's time, 34% were 1A, 37% were 1B, and 26% were status 2. Of the total patients listed, with all diagnoses taken into account, during the past 5 years, 650 patients were removed from the waiting list each year because of death.

12. What factors are considered in the matching of organs with waiting patients?

- Blood type.
- Body size.
- Medical urgency.
- Accrued waiting time.
- Pulmonary pressures of the recipient: higher pressures require a bigger donor organ.
- Panel reactive antibody: a recipient with a high PRA needs a prospective crossmatch with the donor's blood.
- Geographic location of the donor hospital: the ischemic time (total time the heart remains outside a body without blood flow) must be limited to less than 6 hours.
- Viral hepatitis status: a hepatitis-positive donor organ is offered only to a similarly hepatitis-positive recipient.

13. How does blood type influence waiting time for a heart transplant?

According to the UNOS sharing annual report, the size of the heart waiting list has been fairly stable since 1998. There were 4096 registrants at the end of 2001.

The OPTN published data in the following table reflect the typical waiting time for a heart transplant according to blood type.

Blood Type	Waiting Time for Transplant (d)	Blood Groups as Compared with Total Transplants (2181)
0	363	(856) 39.2%
B	162	(269) 12.3%
A	158	(928) 42.5%
AB	60	(128) 5.9%

14. What are the survival rates for heart transplant?

Survival rates are reported at 1, 3, and 5 years. Recent rates were 85.5% at 1 year, 76.9% at 3 years, and 69.8% at 5 years. The longest survivor to date is a male who underwent transplant at 20 years of age and has survived more than 22 years.

15. What are the basic steps involved in the typical cardiac transplant?

The most common technique used in cardiac transplantation is the orthotopic biatrial technique (see Question 16). The patient undergoes intubation, and routine cardiac surgical intravenous drug/monitoring lines are inserted. The operation does not begin until the team at the recipient hospital receives a call from the retrieval surgeon that the donor heart looks acceptable. The donor heart has been cooled with a special cold saline (cardioplegia) solution, packed in double plastic bags, and placed on ice for transport in a picnic-type cooler. When the heart arrives, cardiopulmonary bypass is initiated and body temperature is cooled to 32° C. The recipient aorta is cross clamped, and the aorta is excised near the aortic valve. The pulmonary artery is circumferentially cut above the pulmonic valve. The right atrium is sculpted at the level of the atrioventricular groove, with the superior and inferior vena cava left intact. The left atrium is also excised, and the pulmonary veins are left undisturbed. The recipient's diseased heart then is removed. The donor heart is prepared with removal of the pulmonary veins for creation of a left atrial cuff. The left atrium then is sutured to the recipient left atrial cuff. The donor right atrium is opened from the inferior vena cava orifice to the right atrial appendage. This cuff is sutured to the recipient right atrial cuff. The great vessels are sized accordingly by the surgeon and are anastomosed. Air is vented from the aorta. Blood is allowed to fill the heart. The lungs are ventilated, and the cross clamp is removed. When blood begins surging through the heart, most hearts begin beating without the assistance of defibrillation. Holes created for venting are repaired. Temporary epicardial external pacing wires are sewn in place to the right atrium and right ventricle. Finally, the patient is weaned from cardiopulmonary bypass, the cannulas are removed, and the chest is closed in routine fashion. The patient then is transported to the ICU.

16. **Is the native (original) heart always removed when a patient undergoes cardiac transplantation surgery?**

The most common technique used in cardiac transplantation is the orthotopic biatrial technique, which is the removal of the native heart at the mid atrium. The atrial remnants of the native heart provide anchoring for sewing in the donor heart. Alternatively, a heterotopic technique is used in which the native heart remains and the donor heart is piggy-backed onto the native heart. This approach is rarely used.

17. **What are common postoperative problems and responsive care in the immediate postoperative period?**

Problem	Causes	Goal	Treatment	Note
Bradycardia	Intraoperative trauma, cardiac cellular edema, denervation of excised heart (lack of sympathetic and parasympathetic nerve supply), reperfusion cellular injury, sinus node ischemia.	Target heart rate, 90-120 bpm. Higher prescribed heart rates support higher cardiac outputs and assist in "retraining" heart as it wakes from cold ischemia.	External, temporary epicardial pacing wires. Intravenous isoproterenol drip. Oral theophylline (after several postoperative days). Permanent pacemaker (if prescribed rate does not return after 1-2 weeks).	Detection of two distinct atrial P waves is possible: one from preserved sinus node of native heart (cannot cross suture line) and second from donor atria (controls heart rate). Patients receiving amiodarone before surgery may have bradycardia until drug clears.
Delayed heart rate response to exercise	Denervation of transplanted heart.	Change in patient behavior.	Instruction to perform warm-up exercises before activity, which causes release of adrenaline, thereby increasing heart rate via bloodstream instead of direct sympathetic nervous system.	Patients in early postoperative period may have shortness of breath with activity. They should be encouraged to persist with activity because their heart rate increases and they can then breathe comfortably. Physical reconditioning can take some time.

Continued

continued

Problem	Causes	Goal	Treatment	Note
Atrial fibrillation/ tachycardia	Rejection, cardiac cell edema, pulmonary hypertension, cold ischemia, fluid overload.	Normal sinus rhythm.	Intravenous steroids to treat rejection. Otherwise, conventional antidysrhythmic medications/ electrical cardioversion.	When rejection is cause and is successfully treated, patient may have spontaneous conversion back to normal sinus rhythm.
Stiff ventricle and development of right ventricular failure	Cold ischemic injury, pulmonary hypertension.	Pulmonary vascular resistance <5 Wood's U. Pulmonary gradient < 10 mm Hg. Cardiac index >2.5 L/m^2.	Intravenous inotropic and vasodilatory drugs, such as: dobutamine, milrinone, prostaglandin, nitroprusside, and nitroglycerine. If drugs fail, intraaortic balloon pump or ventricular assist device.	Treatment is guided with use of pulmonary artery catheter.
Systemic hypertension	Increased cardiac output, steroids, postoperative fluid volume excess, immunosuppressive drugs (cyclosporine/ tacrolimus, steroids).	Systolic and diastolic blood pressure as prescribed.	Intravenous antihypertensives are used initially; later oral agents are used.	Integrity of cardiac suture lines must be protected. Occasionally patients have headache from unaccustomed higher systemic pressures.
Bleeding	Preoperative anticoagulation therapy, cardio- pulmonary bypass, large mediastinal space (from enlarged native heart), previous sternotomy.	Low cumulative chest tube outputs.	Close observation of chest tube outputs, cytomegalovirus- negative blood products, protamine sulfate, vitamin K.	
		Coagulation studies within normal limits.	Return to operating room for exploration.	

18. **What typical information is helpful in teaching patients and families about heart transplantation?**

It must be stressed that the wait could be long. The most difficult part of the wait is the inability to control disease progression and the helpless feeling that family members have about their loved one's future. Education can be comforting. The patient and family are taught about routine expectations after cardiac surgery. This education includes descriptions of ventilators, pulmonary artery catheters, temporary pacemakers, chest tubes, urinary drainage catheters, and continuous intravenous medications typically administered in the ICU. Escorting patients/family members to the thoracic or surgical ICU may be beneficial. Routine coughing, deep breathing, and early mobilization from bed to chair and the rationales related to those activities should be reviewed and reinforced. Pretransplant education includes a review of immunosuppressive and other drugs that are part of the institution's cardiac transplant protocol. Signs and symptoms of infection and rejection are taught, and the information is reinforced. Factual understanding of the waiting list, medical urgency statuses, and basic organ allocation procedures is helpful in preventing patient and family confusion and frustration. A frequent question from those waiting on a transplant list is exactly where they are on that list. Knowledge of where to refer patients for accurate transplant information is extremely useful. A program-based post–cardiac transplant care manual on hand with a unit's reference material is invaluable for patients, family, and staff.

19. **What are the essential components of patient and family teaching in the immediate period after transplant?**

Patients and their families can be taught a number of things that contribute to the best outcome after heart transplantation. A thorough understanding of the medications, the possible side effects, and the importance of taking medications as prescribed is necessary. A typical list of transplant medications can be reviewed (see Question 28). Patients and family members should be instructed that the transplant team members are to be notified of medication side effects. A medication plan can then be formulated to lessen or better tolerate those effects. Ongoing education provides expectations related to the physical and emotional changes that can occur with certain medications or dose changes. Signs and symptoms of rejection and infection are taught (see Question 25). Early identification of problems could significantly affect outcome. Frequent clinic appointments, including an endomyocardial biopsy, are part of routine posttransplant surveillance (see Question 21). Teaching aides, such as illustrations of the jugular vein, right ventricle, right ventricular septum, and bioptome in the right ventricle, are helpful.

20. **What is determined with an endomyocardial biopsy?**

Microscopic evaluation of the biopsy tissue is used to determine whether any cellular rejection exists. Biopsy specimens are fixed in solution, processed in wax, and shaved into layers. These individual layers are evaluated with the microscope. Rejection is spotty and does not involve the whole biopsy piece unless the rejection is quite severe. Rejection is a process in which lymphocytes recognize the transplanted heart as foreign and infiltrate the myocardium, surrounding individual cells. Various stages of lymphocytic infiltration and cell death (see Question 23) indicate rejection.

21. How often are biopsies performed?

Although variation may exist among centers, endomyocardial biopsies are performed weekly for a specified period and then every 2 weeks, monthly, bimonthly, trimonthly, and every 6 months or annually. Rejection and treatment alter the schedule.

22. How is the biopsy specimen obtained?

Access is gained through the right internal jugular vein, right/left femoral vein, or left subclavian vein. The most common approach is through the right internal jugular vein. The bioptome is inserted through a sheath and then guided with fluoroscopy courses into a vena cava, to the right atrium, through the tricuspid valve, and into the right ventricle. The bioptome's pinchers then are opened and rested against the right ventricular septum, and a small piece of endocardium is cut and withdrawn for analysis. Three to four specimens are obtained.

23. How are myocardial cells graded for rejection severity?

A standardized grading system constructed by the International Society of Heart and Lung Transplantation (ISHLT) is used (see the following table).

Grade	Histological Description
0	No evidence of rejection (NER)
1A	Focal infiltrate, no cellular necrosis
1B	Diffuse but sparse infiltrate, no necrosis
2	One focus of aggressive infiltrate or necrosis
3A	Multifocal aggressive infiltrates or necrosis
3B	Diffuse inflammatory process with necrosis
4	Diffuse aggressive infiltrates, edema, hemorrhage, vasculitis, with necrosis

24. How is rejection handled?

Rejection is treated per the institutional protocols in place. Biopsies are performed frequently in the first months after transplant because rejection could be present but asymptomatic. Therefore biopsy evaluation can be used to identify the presence of rejection before symptoms occur. A typical treatment protocol to address rejection is as follows:

- Biopsies are performed per protocol (as previously mentioned).
- Early asymptomatic rejection is identified with scheduled biopsies.
- If asymptomatic rejection is diagnosed, treatment is started per the institutional drug protocol for rejection.
- Patients undergo rebiopsy for evaluation of therapy effectiveness.
- If patients become symptomatic with rejection (i.e., arrhythmias, hypotension, syncope), then they are typically hospitalized.

25. What are the signs and symptoms of rejection?

Most patients remain asymptomatic during early rejection (see Question 24). The possible signs/symptoms of acute rejection are fatigue, shortness of breath, sudden edema or weight gain, change in vital signs, irregular heart rate, or flu-like aches, chills, dizziness, nausea, or vomiting. Patients are instructed to report any new symptom or change in condition. For clinicians, the identification of a new atrial or ventricular dysrhythmia must be assumed to be acute rejection until proven otherwise with an endomyocardial biopsy. Other signs or symptoms are enlargement of the cardiac silhouette on chest radiograph, S3 gallop, new murmur or change in murmur intensity, distended neck veins, and crackles on lung exam. Low cardiac output symptoms can mimic gastrointestinal illness, with symptoms of anorexia, nausea, vomiting, and diarrhea. If progressive, the rejection can lead to lethal dysrhythmia or circulatory collapse.

26. How is acute cellular rejection treated?

Biopsy Result	Therapy/Therapy Options
0	No changes/may consider steroid wean
1A, 1B	No changes/may consider adjustment in immunosuppressants
2	No change/rebiopsy sooner than next scheduled biopsy per protocol/maximize present immunosuppressive drugs/oral prednisone bump and taper
3A	Intravenous (IV) steroids for 3 d/oral prednisone bump and taper/optimize present immunosuppressants/rebiopsy in 2 wk
3B	IV steroids/oral prednisone bump and taper/optimize present immunosuppressants/ OKT3/antilymphocyte globulin (ALG)/antithymocyte globulin (ATG)/rebiopsy in 1-2 wk
4	IV steroids/OKT3/ALG/ATG/rebiopsy 1-2 wk/hemodynamic supportive therapy

27. What is the difference between acute and chronic rejection?

Two types of acute rejection exist. The more common type is cellular rejection with lymphocytic infiltration (see Question 23). Less common is humoral rejection, which is antibody mediated. Signs and symptoms of rejection are present without evidence of cellular infiltration on biopsy slides. Diagnosis can be obtained with immunofluorescence staining of the specimen. Plasmapheresis is the therapy of choice for humoral rejection. Chronic rejection is also referred to as cardiac allograft vasculopathy. The lumens of the major branches of the coronary arteries narrow, leading to myocardial infarction, or distal side branches occlude, often referred to as a "pruning effect." The disease is progressive and usually diffuse, typically not amenable to percutaneous coronary intervention. Aggressive treatment of acute rejection, viral infection, hyperlipidemia, or alteration of the immunosuppressive regimen, may lessen the likelihood of graft vasculopathy.

28. What maintenance immunosuppressive drugs are used?

The typical medical regimen includes the following triple immunosuppressive drug regimen:

- Corticosteroids (prednisone, intravenous methylprednisolone). Postoperative protocols include intravenous administration of 500 mg of methylprednisolone after the aortic cross clamp is removed and then 125 mg every 8 hours for a 24-hour period. An oral prednisone taper then is begun according to institutional protocol. After a maintenance prednisone dose is obtained, the prednisone wean is driven predominantly by biopsy result.
- Calcineurin inhibitors (cyclosporine: Sandimmune or Neoral; tacrolimus: Prograf). These T cell lymphocyte activity inhibitors are begun after stable postoperative renal function has been assured. Target trough blood drug levels guide drug dosing. The target troughs vary according to the length of time from the date of surgery, history of rejection, and renal function. Common side effects of these drugs are renal insufficiency and hypertension. Cyclosporine has relatively the same side effect profile as tacrolimus but can also include gingival hyperplasia and hirsutism.
- The third agents vary in drug action (azathioprine: Imuran; mycophenolate mofetil [MMF]: CellCept). Azathioprine is a purine metabolism antagonist that decreases white blood cell (WBC) counts. The most common side effect is bone marrow suppression. Doses are adjusted according to the WBC count, with a target count of 5000/mm³. MMF is a T and B lymphocyte inhibitor. It too can cause neutropenia. Common side effects are nausea and diarrhea. Administration of a proton pump inhibitor, such as omeprazole, can prevent or lessen this effect.
- Several medications can increase or decrease immunosuppressive drug levels when administered concomitantly. Frequent offenders that increase levels are certain antifungals (itraconazole, fluconazole), antibiotics (erythromycin, azithromycin), and the calcium channel blocker diltiazem hydrochloride. Drugs that decrease levels are antiseizure medications (carbamazepine, phenobarbital, phenytoin) and antituberculosis agent (rifampin).

29. What are some common posttransplant infections?

Posttransplant infections are caused by organisms, such as primary bacterial/viral infections, or reactivation of a latent virus. The following table outlines the usual sequence of infections after organ transplantation.

Timeline	Type of Infection
First month after transplant	Mostly conventional infections such as: • wound infections • catheter-related or intravenous-related infections • pneumonia
1 to 6 months after transplant	Mostly unconventional infections such as: Viral: Herpes simplex virus; onset of cytomegalovirus; Epstein-Barr virus; varicella zoster virus, such as shingles, influenza, respiratory syncytial virus, and adenovirus; hepatitis B and C Fungal: *Candida, Pneumocystis, Aspergillus, Cryptococcus* Bacterial: *Nocardia, Listeria,* tuberculosis Parasitic: *Leishmania, Strongyloides, Toxoplasma, Pneumocystis carinii*
More than 6 months after transplant	Mostly chronic infections, particularly viral infections, such as: • Chronic hepatitis • CMV gastritis, colitis, or pneumonia • Common community-acquired infections such as influenza, pneumococcal pneumonia, urinary tract infections • Geographically restricted endemic fungal infections • Posttransplantation lymphoproliferative disease

30. What medications are used to prevent the most common posttransplant infections?

Prophylactic antibiotics are used to prevent common infections. Ganciclovir is prescribed for a high risk of CMV infection, such as when a CMV-negative donor receives a CMV-positive organ. After a certain period of time, the risk of development of the infection lessens from weaning of the immunosuppressive drug doses. Acyclovir is given to prevent herpes simplex (HSV) infection. Trimethoprim sulfate is given to prevent *Pneumocystis carinii* pneumonia (PCP). Pyrimethamine is used for toxoplasmosis prophylaxis. Lastly, nystatin is used to prevent oral thrush or candidiasis.

31. What is on the horizon for outcome improvement with transplant or alternatives to transplant?

Scientists are pursuing the best devices to replace hearts and the most effective drugs to prevent rejection without harming the transplant recipient.
• In November 2002, left ventricular assist devices were approved by the US Food and Drug Administration (FDA) as destination therapy for patients who are not

candidates for heart transplantation on the basis of the REMATCH trial (Randomized Evaluation of Mechanical Assistance for the Treatment of Congestive Heart Failure).

- Ongoing human studies are evaluating implantable mechanical devices as an alternative to human heart transplant. These studies are enrolling patients who are not candidates for transplant because of advanced age, comorbidity, or other exclusion for transplant. The device used today, the AbioCor (Abiomed Corp), is a totally implantable, self-contained, electric artificial heart with the hope of success as a permanent end-stage heart failure therapy.
- Improvements in immunosuppressive drug therapy, particularly the development of more selective immunosuppressive drugs that prevent rejection without increasing the transplant recipient's tendency to acquire other infections, are in the research and development process.

Key Points

- Heart transplant is a consideration only after conventional medical and other indicated surgical therapies have failed.
- The best recipient outcomes are obtained with patient medication compliance, adequate social/financial support, and the lack of substance abuse and other comorbid conditions.
- Patients are referred to transplant centers to undergo an initial evaluation process. Numerous steps are involved in the process that leads to listing for a heart transplant.
- Irreversible pulmonary hypertension is a contraindication to heart transplant. A heart/double-lung transplant may be considered if pulmonary hypertension rules out a heart transplant alone.
- The UNOS maintains the nation's organ waiting lists and a continually updated transplant center–specific informational website.
- Tissue matching is not necessary in heart transplant. Major matching considerations are blood type, body size, and medical urgency.
- Endomyocardial biopsies are the gold standard for detection of rejection.
- Most rejection is symptom-free. This is a major indication for endomyocardial biopsies according to standard protocol.
- Acute rejection refers to the possibility of cellular damage whereas chronic rejection refers to the development of coronary artery disease.
- The use of immunosuppressant drugs and follow-up care at the transplant center are necessary for a lifetime.

Internet Resources

United Network for Organ Sharing:
www.unos.org

Organ Procurement and Transplantation Network (OPTN):
www.optn.org

International Society for Heart and Lung Transplantation:
www.ishlt.org

Transplant Patient Partnering Program (Roche Laboratories):
www.tppp.net/heart.html

Novartis Transplant (Novartis Pharmaceuticals Corporation):
www.novartis-transplant.com

International Transplant Nurses Society:
www.itns.org

American Society of Transplant Surgeons:
www.asts.org

Noncompliance in Heart Transplantation: A Role for the Advanced Practice Nurse:
http://www.ncbi.nlm.nih.gov/entrez/query.fcgi?cmd=Retrieve&db=PubMed&list_uids=128
93976&dopt=Abstract

Bibliography

Becker C, Petlin A: Heart transplantation: minimizing mortality with proper management, *Am J Nurs* 99(suppl):8-14, 1999.

Holmes E: The AbioCor totally implantable replacement heart, *J Cardiovasc Nurs* 18(1):23-29, 2003.

Mill M: Cardiac transplantation. In Tintinalli JE, Kelen GD, Stapczynski JS: *Emergency medicine: a comprehensive study guide,* ed 5, New York, 2001, McGraw-Hill, pp 422-428.

Rourk T et al: Heart transplantation: state of the art, *AACN Clin Issues* 10(2):185-201, 1999.

Stevenson LW: Medical management before cardiac transplantation. In *Handbook of cardiac transplantation,* Philadelphia, 1996, Hanley & Belfus, pp 1-9.

Section V

Cardiovascular Pharmacology

Thrombolytic Therapy

Deborah D. Smith and Leslie Davis

1. What is thrombolytic therapy?

Thrombolytic therapy drugs or "clot busters" dissolve red fibrin-rich clots that are responsible for the partial or total occlusion of coronary arteries that causes myocardial infarction (MI). Ideally the best thrombolytic is fibrin specific and thus acts directly at the site of the infarct clot instead of throughout the general circulation. Nonspecific lytics cause more bleeding. Fibrinolysis occurs when a plasminogen activator (human tissue-type plasminogen activator [t-PA] or a lytic agent) converts plasminogen to plasmin. Plasmin then degrades the fibrin in clots into soluble fibrin degradation products (FDPs) that promote clot lysis.

2. Which patients qualify for thrombolytic therapy?

To qualify for lytic therapy, patients must have ST elevation MI as evidenced by:
- Ischemic symptoms, with onset of less than 12 hours.
- Diagnostic 12-lead electrocardiogram (ECG) to include either ST elevation of 1 mm or more in at least two contiguous leads or a new left bundle branch block.

3. How soon should thrombolytic therapy be given after the symptoms of an acute MI (AMI) start?

Thrombolytic therapy is most effective when given early, preferably in the first 3 hours but no longer than 12 hours after the onset of acute symptoms. Target "door-to-drug" time should be within 30 minutes of patient arrival to the hospital.

4. Which patients should *not* receive thrombolytic therapy?

There are absolute and relative contraindications for use.
Absolute contraindications include:
- Active internal bleeding.
- History of cerebrovascular accident.
- Recent intracranial bleed or known intracranial neoplasm.
- Suspected aortic dissection.

A relative contraindication means that potential risk is involved for the patient with the thrombolytic therapy. In this situation, the physician makes the judgment whether the patient's potential risk of side effects outweighs the potential benefits of the therapy. Minimal bleeding is worth major myocardial salvage.

Relative contraindications include:
- Severe uncontrolled hypertension at presentation (blood pressure [BP] >180/110 mm Hg).
- Known bleeding disorders (thrombocytopenia, von Willebrand's syndrome).
- Current use of therapeutic doses of anticoagulants (warfarin).
- Noncompressible vascular puncture.
- Active peptic ulcer.
- Pregnancy.
- Recent trauma within the past 2 to 4 weeks, including head trauma.
- Traumatic or prolonged cardiopulmonary resuscitation (>10 minutes).
- Recent internal bleeding (2 to 4 weeks).

The previous list was adapted from the American College of Cardiology/American Heart Association (ACC/AHA) guidelines 1999.

5. Why is obtaining a portable chest radiograph before administration of thrombolytic therapy important?

Patients with a dissecting aortic or leaking aneurysm could bleed to death with thrombolytic therapy.

6. What are the most common current agents available, and how are they administered?

	Dose	Administration Infusion Time	Weight Adjusted (Y/N)	Half-life (min)	Antigenicity (Y/N)	Metabolism
Streptokinase*	1.5 × 1.6 IU	Infusion: 1.5 million IU infused × 1 hr.	N	23	Y	Hepatic
Tissue plasminogen activator (Alteplase [Activase])	100 mg max	Bolus + infusion. Bolus: 15 mg intravenously (IV). Then 0.75 mg/kg next 30 min (no >50 mg). Then 0.50 mg/kg for 60 min (no >35 mg). Infusion: 90 min.	Y	5	N	Hepatic

continued

	Dose	Administration Infusion Time	Weight Adjusted (Y/N)	Half-life (min)	Antigenicity (Y/N)	Metabolism
Recombinant plasminogen activator (r-PA) (Reteplase [Retavase])	20 U	Double bolus. First 10 U IV bolus for 2 min. Then 30 min later, second bolus 10 U. Normal saline solution flush before and after each.	N	18	N	Renal
TNKase (Tenecteplase)	50 mg max	Single bolus: 30-50 mg.	Y	20	N	Hepatic
Anisoylated plasminogen-streptokinase activator complex (APSAC) (Anistreplase)	30 mg	Single bolus: 30 mg for 5 min.	N	95	Y	Renal

7. A patient has just received a diagnosis of ST elevation MI, and thrombolytic therapy has been ordered. What are the immediate nursing actions?

- Continuous ECG monitoring to catch changes in rhythm.
- The resuscitation equipment should be near.
- Assurance that a chest radiograph has been obtained and interpreted.
- Initiation of at least two to three IV lines. All invasive lines should be inserted before therapy because of bleeding risks.
- Insertion of a Foley catheter if the need for one is anticipated.
- Baseline labs—coagulation labs (prothrombin time [PT], partial thromboplastin time [PTT]), hematocrit (Hct) and hemoglobin (Hgb), and platelets—should be drawn.
- Assessment of baseline neurological status and charting of assessment for potential intracranial bleeding.
- Additional staff should be secured during the initiation of thrombolytic therapy.
- Assessment of the patient for continued signs of ischemia or ECG and hemodynamic changes.

8. **What other medications are given as adjunct therapy with thrombolytic agents?**
   - Aspirin: on arrival to hospital and daily to prevent further thrombosis of the coronary artery.
   - Heparin: either unfractionated intravenous (IV) heparin (UFH) or low–molecular-weight heparin (LMWH).

9. **What is the most common complication of thrombolytic therapy?**

   Bleeding is the leading complication of thrombolytic therapy, with intracranial bleeding the most devastating. Contraindications to therapy are targeted to exclude patients in high-risk bleeding categories. The nurse can be instrumental in history taking and screening for these red flags, such as history of stroke or uncontrolled hypertension. The patients at the highest risk for bleeding are those who are elderly, have a lower weight, and are female.

10. **What nursing interventions can prevent/minimize bleeding in patients who have received thrombolytic therapy?**

    To avoid bleeding, the nurse should:
    - Avoid intramuscular (IM) injections and invasive lines.
    - Inspect/test all body fluids for occult blood (i.e., guaiac emesis and stools).
    - Minimize traumatic procedures.
    - Monitor vital signs (especially increased heart rate) and labs (PT, PTT, Hct, platelet count).
    - Assess any known potential bleeding sites (lines, old wounds, and catheter sites).
    - Assess neurological status regularly, and remember that any changes could represent intracranial bleeding.
    - Monitor adjunctive therapies (for example, if IV heparin therapy is given, monitor PTTs every 6 hours and make adjustments in the drip rate based on the PTT).
    - Be especially cautious and assess frequently for signs of bleeding with other anticoagulants/antithrombin/antiplatelet agents (warfarin, dipyridamole, or clopidogrel bisulfate) because of the higher risk of bleeding.
    - Be alert for possible retroperitoneal bleed (bleeding in the retroperitoneal area), which is manifested by bruising, bleeding at the groin site, a drop in Hgb or Hct, or tachycardia, with post–thrombolytic therapy and an interventional procedure (percutaneous coronary intervention [PCI]) within the same 12 to 24 hours.

11. **What nursing actions are done if a patient has bleeding after thrombolytic therapy?**
    - Frequent assessment of vital signs for hemodynamic compromise (including oxygen saturation, heart rate, and BP).
    - Reporting of findings to the physician.
    - Checking of lab results (such as Hgb, Hct, PT, PTT).

- Discontinuation of the thrombolytic agent and any heparin (if used) if major bleeding is suspected.
- Application of pressure to the bleeding sites.
- Consideration of transfusion therapy with packed red blood cells, platelets, or fresh frozen plasma for severe bleeding that causes hemodynamic compromise.
- Administration of saline ice rinses for gingival bleeding.

Note that minor bleeding, such as oozing from venous or arterial puncture sites or the gums, should not require stopping the thrombolytic therapy. However, the nurse should alert the health team to have a higher suspicion for major bleeding.

12. What percentage of patients have successful reperfusion from thrombolytic therapy?

Thrombolytic therapy is successful in 50% to 60% of patients. A patient may have partial or complete reperfusion. However, some patients may not have successful reperfusion or may in some cases have opening of the infarct-related artery and then reocclusion. Nursing assessment is critical for signs of reperfusion, failed perfusion, and reocclusion (which usually occurs within the first 24 hours after thrombolytic therapy).

This assessment includes watching the ECG for ST changes, vital sign changes, symptoms of chest discomfort, shortness of breath, or decreased oxygen saturation, and arrhythmias that may indicate ongoing ischemia.

13. How does the nurse know whether thrombolytic therapy has worked?

Evidence of clinical reperfusion includes:
- Relief of the patient's ischemic symptoms (chest pain or anginal equivalent).
- Resolution of ST segment changes on the 12-lead ECG; serial ECGs need to be done every 2 to 4 hours for evaluation of whether ST segments are returning to normal.
- Reperfusion dysrhythmias (see Question 14).
- Earlier, rapid peak in creatine kinase isoenzyme MD (CK-MB) may be seen as enzymes are flushed into circulation by reperfused arteries and overall lower levels.

The nurse should ensure that the patient is monitored in the lead that displays the most significant ST segment changes to capture ischemia during continuous monitoring.

14. What alternative therapy is initiated if evidence of reperfusion after thrombolytic therapy is not seen?

Patients may have all or none of the previous signs of reperfusion. However, for clinical decompensation or for continuing signs of ischemia on ECG and symptoms of chest pain, nausea, and diaphoresis after lytic therapy, alternative reperfusion therapies, such as PCI or emergent coronary artery bypass surgery (CABG), should be instituted.

15. What is a reperfusion dysrhythmia, and what should the nurse expect?

Reperfusion dysrhythmias are common after thrombolytic therapy and occur when a closed coronary artery is suddenly opened with successful reperfusion treatment. Ventricular tachycardia (V tach) is the most likely dysrhythmia to occur 7 to 9 hours after thrombolysis. Less serious dysrhythmias, such as sinus bradycardia, heart block, idioventricular rhythm, and nonsustained V tach, may also occur. Reperfusion dysrhythmias are usually self-limiting and do not require therapy. However, the nurse should be prepared for a cardiac arrest situation, with all code equipment nearby, including antiarrhythmic medications.

16. What education should the nurse provide for those patients who undergo thrombolytic therapy?

The nurse should explain that the patient is having a heart attack, which is caused by a blood clot blocking one of the coronary arteries that supplies the heart with blood. The symptoms of a heart attack are the result of the lack of oxygen reaching the heart muscle. Patients should know that they are being given a clot buster drug that may dissolve the clot and open the artery so that more blood with oxygen gets to the heart. Because a clot buster usually busts other blood clots in the body, it may cause bleeding. The patient should be reassured that the nurse will be at the bedside to assist them, observe for side effects, and administer medication for pain. The patient may sometimes have reperfusion arrhythmias when circulation is restored. Therefore the patient should be informed that irregular heartbeats may be felt. The nurse needs to emphasize to the patient that improvement or worsening or symptoms may indicate effectiveness of therapy. Encouraging patients to report any symptom changes is imperative. Patient education is key to the patient notifying the nurse of the potential return of ischemic symptoms.

17. What nursing actions should be taken if a patient who has presumably had successful reperfusion has a return of ischemic symptoms?

- An immediate 12-lead ECG should be obtained.
- The physician should be notified.
- Oxygen should be administered.
- Nitroglycerine or morphine should be administered.
- Changes in vital signs should be assessed.
- The patient should be prepared for potential emergent intervention.

18. What is the nurse's role for patients with failed reperfusion with thrombolytic therapy who then go to the cardiac catheterization lab for alternative treatment?

Early anticipation of failed reperfusion and the need for alternative treatment and nursing intervention is important. All patients with failed reperfusion with thrombolytic therapy should have a minimum of two to three IV lines in place. The nurse should be prepared to report all interventions, medications, and other assessment data to the catheterization lab team. The patient is at higher risk for bleeding complications because of the thrombolytic therapy; therefore the prethrombolytic lab work (especially the Hgb, Hct, platelet count, PT, and PTT) should be reported to the team. A current type and screen for blood type should be done in the event blood products are necessary for the patient.

19. What lab values are affected by thrombolytic therapy?

The following lab results may be affected and should be measured at baseline and monitored by the team during the course of therapy:
- Hematocrit: should remain in the normal range, unless bleeding occurs; important to know baseline for future assessments of bleeding.
- Coagulation parameters, such as platelet count, PT, and PTT, may be affected by IV heparin therapy used in conjunction with lytics.

20. What can an institution do to improve time to treatment with thrombolytic therapy?

The GUSTO (Global Utilization of Streptokinase and Tissue Plasminogen Activator for Occluded Arteries) Time to Treatment nursing study showed that those hospitals that collected time to treatment data, reported the data to a multidisciplinary team, implemented strategies to decrease delays, and continued to give monthly feedback, were able to decrease time to treatment significantly. Strategies that have been successful in reducing thrombolytic treatment times include:
- A multidisciplinary team approach.
- Monthly quality improvement time data review with feedback.
- Tools, care maps, and algorithms that expedite treatment like routine orders, "clot boxes."
- Assessment tools for indications/contraindications of therapy.
- Prehospital ECGs.
- Collaborative review of triage procedures, treatment times, and patient transfer issues between emergency medical services, emergency department staff, cardiologists, and emergency department physicians.

21. What is combination therapy for AMI?

Combination therapy is the combined use of lowered doses of approved thrombolytic agents with antithrombin agents and glycoprotein IIb/IIIa receptor blocker agents as the strategy of choice for reperfusion therapy. The use of all three classes of agents helps facilitate degradation of the red fibrin-rich clot (lytic agents), block thrombin action (heparin), and block formation of the white platelet-rich portion of the clots (IIb/IIIa inhibitors) to synergistically improve the chances of opening the infarct-related artery and maintain an open vessel after therapy. Clinical trials are underway that examine the best "cocktail" or combination of these three classes of medications. The challenge for nursing is to be alert to potential increased bleeding risk of combinations of these potent therapies.

22. What areas are under current investigation in regard to the future of thrombolytic therapy for patients with AMI?

- Combination therapies with lower doses of thrombolytics and glycoprotein IIb/IIIa inhibitors with the goal to achieve an additive or synergistic effect with one agent targeting fibrin and one targeting platelets (see Question 21).
- Thrombolytics followed by immediate PCI are being studied, also known as "facilitated PCI."
- Determination of which is the better antithrombin agent to use with thrombolytic agents (i.e., IV UFH versus LMWH versus direct thrombin inhibitors).
- Complement activation in AMI is an important mediator of inflammatory damage and is associated with worse outcomes (larger MI). Complement inhibitor trials are ongoing to determine efficacy for improved outcomes.
- Patient-specific thrombolytic regimens that consider patient personal risk profile. For example, elderly patients with an AMI have a higher risk of intracranial bleed if given thrombolytic therapy; therefore the risks of thrombolytic therapy may far outweigh the benefit. Thus primary PCI may be the choice of reperfusion therapy.
- Prehospital thrombolysis. Nurses may soon receive patients after the patient has received the thrombolytic agent in the field.
- Newer thrombolytic agents like Saruplase (prourokinase) are being studied.
- National quality improvement (QI) initiatives to improve rapid identification and treatment of patients through streamlined guidelines, comparison with other institutions, and Joint Commission quality measures to ensure accountability for high standards of practice nationally.
- Public campaigns to encourage patients to arrive at the hospital earlier.
- Institution-specific guidelines and algorithms to target decreased treatment times.
- Wireless transmission of ECG data from EMS to help triage potential AMI patients and prevent treatment delays.

23. Are there any current controversies in the field of thrombolytic therapy?

One area of controversy is whether primary PCI is superior to thrombolytic therapy in the treatment of AMI. The latest review of multiple clinical trials indicates that primary PCI (angioplasty or stent to the infarct-related artery) has a mortality advantage (fewer deaths), less complications, and greater long-term survival benefits as compared with thrombolytic therapy after AMI. Feasibility of patient transfer to angioplasty sites and availability of facilities to perform urgent PCI remain issues of concern/controversy. (Please see Chapter 10, Myocardial Infarction, for further discussion of this issue.)

Key Points

- A detailed nursing history can target the risk factors for bleeding. One should watch out for the red flags of increased bleeding risks: history of stroke/transient ischemic attacks, uncontrolled hypertension (180/110 mm Hg), age >75 years, low body weight, and treatment with other antithrombin/platelet agents like clopidogrel bisulfate, warfarin, or LMWH. A high level of suspicion for bleeding should be maintained.

- After thrombolytic therapy has finished, the nurse should continue to assess for signs of ischemia by watching for chest pain or the patient's anginal equivalent, ongoing or new ST elevation or depression, hemodynamic changes, or shortness of breath. If any of these symptoms arise, a repeat ECG is needed immediately.

- Baseline labs (Hct, platelets, PT, and PTT) should be obtained. These lab results should be rechecked if bleeding after therapy is suspected, especially in the setting of new or worsened tachycardia.

- One should focus on time to treatment delays in the facility and participate in QI efforts to grease the system and decrease delays. The AHA has resources to help the team "Get with the Guidelines."

Internet Resources

Journal Article: Primary Angioplasty for Acute Myocardial Infarction—Is it Worth the Wait?
http://content.nejm.org/cgi/content/short/349/8/798

ACC/AHA Guidelines for the Management of Patients With Acute Myocardial Infarction
www.acc.org/clinical/guidelines/nov96/1999/jac1716ftl.htm

Journal Article: Combination Therapy for Acute Myocardial Infarction: Glycoprotein IIb/IIIa Inhibitors Plus Thrombolysis
http://www.ncbi.nlm.nih.gov/entrez/query.fcgi?cmd=Retrieve&db=PubMed&list_uids=10492852&dopt=Abstract

MDBrowse.com Specialty Spotlight: Thrombolytic Therapy
http://www.mdbrowse.com/Speciality/Cardiology/ThrombolyticTherapy.htm

CME Cardiology Series: Duke Cardiology Series 2002
http://cme.cybersessions.org/

Genentech, Inc: TNKase Patient Profiles
www.gene.com/gene/products/profiles/tnkase.jsp

American Heart Association
www.americanheart.org

American Heart Association Journals
http://www.ahajournals.org

American Heart Association Emergency Cardiovascular Care
www.cpr-ecc.org

MedLine Plus Health Information Medical Encyclopedia: Thrombolytic Therapy (Tissue Plasminogen Activator—tPA)
http://www.nlm.nih.gov/medlineplus/ency/article/007089.htm

Cardiosource: A Collaboration of American College of Cardiology Foundation and Elsevier:
http://cardiosource.com

Bibliography

ASSENT-2 Investigators: Single-bolus tenecteplase compared with front-loaded alteplase in acute myocardial infarction: the ASSENT-2 double-blind randomized trial, *Lancet* 354:716-722, 1999.

ASSENT-3 Investigators: Efficacy and safety of tenecteplase in combination with enoxaparin, abciximab, or unfractionated heparin: the ASSENT-3 randomized trial in acute myocardial infarction: the Assessment of the Safety and Efficacy of a New Thrombolytic Regimen, *Lancet* 358:605-613, 2001.

Braunwald E: *Essential atlas of heart diseases,* ed 2, Philadelphia, 2001, McGraw-Hill, p 58.

Glys K, Gold M: Acute coronary syndromes: new developments in pharmacological treatment strategies, *Crit Care Nurse* 20:1-15, 2000.

Keeley E, Boura J, Grines C: Primary angioplasty verses intravenous thrombolytic therapy for acute myocardial infarction: a quantitative review of 23 randomized trials, *Lancet* 361:13-20, 2003.

Kline E, Martin J, Smith D: New era of reperfusion in acute myocardial infarction, *Crit Care Nurse* 19:21-31, 1999.

Ohman M, Harrington R, Cannon C et al: Intravenous thrombolysis in acute myocardial infarction, *Chest* 119(1 suppl):253S, 2001.

Pifarre R, Scanlon P: *Evidence-based management of the acute coronary syndrome,* Philadelphia, 2001, Hanley & Belfus, pp 147-163.

Roettig M, Tanabe P: Emergency management of acute coronary syndromes, *J Emerg Nurs* 26(suppl):S1-42, 2000.

Ryan TJ, Antman EM, Brooks NH et al: 1999 update: ACC/AHA guidelines for the management of patients with acute myocardial infarction: executive summary and recommendations: a report of the American College of Cardiology/American Heart Association Task Force on Practice Guidelines (Committee on Management of Acute Myocardial Infarction), *Circulation* 110:1016-1030, 1999.

Topol E, editor: *Acute coronary syndromes,* New York, 2001, Marcel Dekker.

Van de Werf F, Baim D: Clinical update: reperfusion for ST segment elevation myocardial infarction: an overview of current treatment options, *Circulation* 105:2813-2816, 2002.

Antiplatelet and Antithrombotic Agents

Deborah D. Smith and Leslie Davis

1. What are the most common medications that alter the clotting cascade?

A thrombus contains platelets, fibrin, clotting factors, and other cellular elements of the blood. For this reason, several classes of medications affect formulation or extension of a thrombus. These medications are as follows:

- Anticoagulants. This class includes antithrombin agents such as unfractionated heparin (UFH; intravenous [IV] heparin) or low–molecular-weight heparin (LMWH; enoxaparin, dalteparin sodium, and others). Also included are oral agents like warfarin (see Chapter 29, Chronic Anticoagulation).
- Antiplatelet agents. This class includes oral agents, such as aspirin (ASA), clopidogrel bisulfate (Plavix), ticlopidine hydrochloride (Ticlid), or dipyridamole (Persantine), or IV agents, such as glycoprotein IIb/IIIa (GP IIb/IIIa) inhibitors (abciximab, eptifibatide, or tirofiban).
- Thrombolytic (fibrinolytic) agents. This class includes agents such as alteplase, anistreplase, reteplase, streptokinase, and tenecteplase (see Chapter 27, Thrombolytic Therapy).

2. What is the goal of treatment for the use of antithrombin and antiplatelet agents in patients with cardiovascular (CV) disease?

The primary goal of this class of agents is prevention of platelet aggregation, which leads to thrombosis. The pathogenesis of acute coronary syndrome (ACS) involves rupture of plaque and exposure of subendothelial collagen and the lipid-rich plaque core. Platelet activation and aggregation follow vessel injury, which leads to platelet-rich thrombus formation. Several current therapies target prevention of platelet aggregation and subsequent clot formation. Platelet-rich thrombi, associated with unstable angina (USA) and non-ST elevation myocardial infarction (MI; NSTEMI), are composed primarily of white clot and are more resistant to thrombolysis than the erythrocyte-rich thrombi seen in acute ST elevation MI (STEMI), which are composed primarily of red clot. Currently many research endeavors are working to develop strategies to target both the white clot and the red clot in the ACS patient population.

3. Why is ASA so important in the treatment of ACS?

Aspirin inhibits platelet cyclooxygenase irreversibly for the life of a platelet (5 to 10 days). Combined studies in more than 100,000 patients have shown a 29% reduction in MI incidence rate in patients treated early with ASA. The American

Heart Association (AHA) guidelines recommend ASA 81 to 325 mg per day for all patients with ACS. ASA should be the initial pharmacological intervention in the ACS setting.

4. What are the most common oral platelet inhibitors used today?

See the following table.

Drug	Action	Dose	Indications	Side Effects	Precautions	Peak Onset of Action
Aspirin (ASA)	Irreversibly inhibits production of thromboxane A2	81-325 mg/d	First line therapy for all patients with acute coronary syndrome (ACS): early	Gastrointestinal (GI) upset, bleeding	Watch for allergies; bleeding precautions	Minutes to hours
Clopidogrel bisulfate (Plavix)	Adenosine diphosphate (ADP)-induced platelet aggregation	75 mg/d; 300 mg loading dose is sometimes given after percutaneous coronary intervention (PCI)	In unstable angina and non-ST elevation myocardial infarction; in addition to ASA if patient not likely to have emergent coronary artery bypass grafting (CABG); after PCI including stenting, usually given in catheterization lab	Neutropenia, thrombotic thrombocyto-penic purpura (TTP), GI upset, diarrhea	Caution if invasive surgery such as CABG (should be stopped 5-7 d before); caution with impaired liver function	Antiplatelet effect within 1 hr (with loading dose) lasting up to 5 d for platelet inhibition
Ticlopidine hydro-chloride (Ticlid)	Inhibits and antagonizes ADP receptor and may inhibit interactions of glycoprotein IIb/IIIa receptor with fibrinogen	250 mg twice daily	Allergy to ASA; second line treatment to clopidogrel bisulfate; primary and secondary prevention of ACS; after PCI	Neutropenia (1%-3% of patients), TTP (0.03%), GI upset, diarrhea	Monitor complete blood cell count; platelet effects irreversible (up to 1 week)	3-5 d

5. In what settings are combination antiplatelet agents used?

Combination therapies with clopidogrel bisulfate and ASA have shown a significant decrease in death and nonfatal acute MI in patients at high risk for ischemia. Current AHA guideline changes recommend clopidogrel bisulfate with ASA initially in patients with ACS when invasive therapies are not expected. Dipyridamole (Persantine) has not been shown to provide greater benefit than ASA alone in these patients.

6. What are GP IIb/IIIa inhibitors?

The GP IIb/IIIa receptor is the primary receptor that binds fibrinogen. Fibrinogen forms a bridge between adjacent platelets, resulting in platelet aggregation. GP IIb/IIIa inhibitors block the receptors from binding fibrinogen and thus prevent this process.

7. What are indications for GP IIb/IIIa inhibitor use?

Glycoprotein IIb/IIIa inhibitors are indicated for patients at high risk of ACS (with USA or NSTEMI) or for patients undergoing percutaneous coronary intervention (PCI; including balloon angioplasty or stent placement). Clinical trials have shown that use of GP IIb/IIIa inhibitors decreases the incidence of death, MI, and other complications, such as acute stent closure and reinfarction. Patients with ACS who are most likely to benefit from GP IIb/IIIa therapy have chest pain at rest for at least 10 minutes in duration within 24 hours and any of the following:
- ST segment depression of more than 0.5 mm on electrocardiogram (ECG)
- T-wave inversion of more than 1 mm on ECG
- Cardiac enzyme elevations greater than the upper limit of normal

8. Which patients should not undergo GP IIb/IIIa therapy?

Absolute contraindications to GP IIb/IIIa therapy are similar to the contraindications for thrombolytic therapy and include:
- A history of bleeding diathesis (disorders).
- Evidence of active abnormal bleeding within the last 30 days.
- Severe uncontrolled hypertension (systolic blood pressure [BP] > 200 mm Hg or diastolic BP > 110 mm Hg not controlled with antihypertensive therapy).
- Platelet count of less than 100,000/mm^3.
- Serum creatinine level of 4.0 mg/dL or more or renal dialysis dependence.
- History of stroke within 30 days or any history of hemorrhagic stroke.
- Major surgery within preceding 6 weeks.
- Known hypersensitivity to any component of the product.
- Current or planned administration of another IV GP IIb/IIIa inhibitor.

Relative contraindications to GP IIB/IIIA inhibitor use include:
- Anticipation of a central line (some central vessels are considered noncompressible and therefore not responsive to manual pressure if bleeding occurs).
- Pregnancy; no studies have examined the side effects.

- Patient weight and age; the bleeding incidence rate is higher in the elderly and patients with lower weights.
- Use of medications that may affect hemostasis—such as thrombolytics, oral anticoagulants, nonsteroidal antiinflammatory drugs (NSAIDs; like ibuprofen), dipyridamole, ticlopidine hydrochloride, and clopidogrel bisulfate—all could potentially increase bleeding risk.

9. How are GP IIb/IIIa inhibitors used?

Generic Name (Brand Name)	Approved Indications	Half-Life	Dose and Administration	Average Duration of Therapy
Abciximab (ReoPro)	In conjunction with planned percutaneous coronary intervention (PCI)	12-24 hr affects platelet function	Intravenous (IV) bolus 0.25 mg/kg for 10-60 min, then 0.125 mg/kg continuous IV infusion	6 hr, maximum 10 mcg/min for 12 hr
Eptifibatide (Integrilin)	Unstable angina/non–Q–wave myocardial infarction (NQWMI), acute coronary syndrome (ACS) managed medically or with PCI	4 hr	IV bolus 180 mcg/kg for 2 min, then continuous IV infusion of 2 mcg/kg/min	Up to 72 hr
Tirofiban (Aggrastat)	ACS, managed medically or with PCI	4 hr	IV bolus of 0.4 mcg/kg/min for 30 min; plus continuous IV infusion of 0.1 mcg/kg/min	12-24 hr

Adapted with permission from Roettig M, Tanabe P: Emergency management of acute coronary syndromes, *J Emerg Nurs* 26:6, Dec 2000.

10. Is dosing of GP IIb/IIIa inhibitors different in lower weight or elderly individuals?

All GP IIb/IIIa inhibitors must be weight adjusted. Packet inserts and charts are available at most institutions for bolus dosing and titration instructions. Lower weight and elderly patients are at a higher risk of bleeding, so all dosing must be adjusted downward to prevent bleeding. Other important considerations for these therapies include:
- Administration on controlled infusion pump is necessary.

- Lower dose adjustments are necessary for patients with renal impairment (tirofiban and eptifibatide).
- Duration of therapy varies based on the individual patient, procedures initiated, and anticoagulants already being administered.
- GP IIb/IIIa inhibitors are usually given in conjunction with UFH or low–molecular-weight heparin.

11. What laboratory values may be affected by GP IIb/IIIa therapy?

- Glycoprotein IIb/IIIa therapy may increase the activated clotting time (ACT) level or partial thromboplastin time (PTT) synergistically if given with anticoagulants (such as heparin).
- Bleeding times may be prolonged.
- Platelet count may decrease; therefore caution should be used if it decreases to less than 100,000 mm^3 (or if it drops by more than 50% from the baseline).
- With eptifibatide or tirofiban, the platelet count returns to baseline within 4 hours; with abciximab, within 12 to 24 hours.

12. What important nursing actions should be considered before, during, and after GP IIb/IIIa inhibitor therapy administration for patients with USA?

BEFORE INFUSION:
- Assessment for the presence of any contraindications to therapy.
- Assessment of hemodynamic parameters, such as vital signs.
- Assessment of baseline neurological status.
- Assessment of potential bleeding sites.
- Initiation of two peripheral IV lines before start of therapy.
- Confirmation of adjunctive heparin therapy choice: UFH versus LMWH.
- Minimization of vascular and other trauma: placement of IV lines and Foley catheters before initiation of therapy, and caution with the placement of nasotracheal intubation and gastric tubes.
- Assessment of baseline lab results: hematocrit (Hct), hemoglobin, platelet count, serum creatinine level, and prothrombin time (PT) and activated PTT (aPTT).
- Measurement of a baseline ACT, if PCI is to be performed.

DURING INFUSION:
- Assessment for neurological status changes.
- Maintenance of bleeding precautions; Hct repeated daily.
- Assessment for signs of ischemia—chest pain, ECG changes (repeat of ECG for recurrent or new symptoms), and serial enzymes/ECGs.
- Minimization of venipunctures as well as arterial punctures
- Monitoring of aPTT every 6 hours with UFH or institutional specific standing orders for heparin to prevent excessive heparin dosing, which may increase the risk of bleeding.
- Discontinuation if platelet count decreases to less than 100,000/mm^3.

- Monitoring of renal status daily (may require lower dosing adjustments).
- Watching for any hemodynamic changes that may be early signs of bleeding.

FOLLOWING INFUSION:
- Continuation of monitoring for signs of recurrent ischemia.
- Careful assessment of bleeding, especially at femoral access sites, with increased physical activity after sheath removal.
- Assurance that oral antiplatelet medications such as clopidogrel bisulfate or ASA are given.

13. What nursing actions are needed for a patient on GP IIb/IIIa inhibitor therapy who develops tachycardia and bleeding from the gums?

Although this patient may certainly have more serious bleeding, from the information given, bleeding from the oral cavity (or oozing from venipuncture sites) is not serious and does not warrant discontinuation of infusion. However, tachycardia that is new for the patient should raise the level of suspicion for bleeding and should be assessed thoroughly. Actions include assessment for any bleeding and monitoring of the complete blood cell (CBC) count, specifically the platelet count and hematocrit. The platelet count should not be less than 3% from the initial count or less than 100,000 cells overall. If this decrease occurs, then there is significant thrombocytopenia.

14. What should the nurse do with a significant drop in the platelet count (or if thrombocytopenia occurs) after initiation of GP IIb/IIIa therapy?

- Notify the physician or nurse practitioner.
- Check coagulation lab results (PT/PTT) and hemoglobin and Hct.
- If bleeding is serious, discontinue the infusion and consider platelet or blood transfusions.
- Maintain a level of suspicion for a retroperitoneal bleed if patient has had a recent groin stick (cardiac catheterization or PCI).

15. What actions should be taken if a patient on GP IIb/IIIa inhibitor therapy has to have emergent coronary artery bypass grafting (CABG) surgery?

The risk for bleeding in patients receiving GP IIb/IIIa therapy is a significant concern. The IV infusion of GP IIb/IIIa should be discontinued at least 2 to 4 hours before surgery. In the case of the small molecule agents (such as eptifibatide or tirofiban) with short half-lives (4 hours), platelets should normalize within 4 to 6 hours. With abciximab, which actually coats and deactivates the platelet for the half-life of the platelet (10 days), a higher risk of bleeding may exist with early surgical interventions. These patients may need a platelet transfusion during or before CABG. Patients should have a platelet count and Hct performed before surgery and a current type and screen.

For patients with multivessel coronary artery disease (CAD) and a high risk of CABG, the use of the smaller molecule agents is recommended upfront for shorter half-lives in the event surgery becomes necessary.

16. **What should occur before discontinuation of a femoral sheath in a patient on GP IIb/IIIa therapy?**

- Discontinuation of IV heparin 3 to 4 hours before removal of the sheath.
- Coagulation status check and assurance that the aPTT is less than 45 seconds or the ACT is less than 150 seconds before removal.
- Assessment of vascular access site for bleeding.
- Application of manual or mechanical pressure for 10 to 30 minutes according to institutional protocol.

ONCE SHEATHS ARE PULLED:
- The patient should ambulate early.
- Reassessment should be performed for bleeding and circulation with a check of pulses below the femoral access site.

17. **When are heparin therapies used in patients with CV and why?**

Heparin is indicated for patients with suspected or confirmed ACS before, during, and after coronary intervention. Heparin works by activating anti-thrombin, which in turn inhibits thrombin and activated factor X (Xa). Because thrombin plays a pivotal role in platelet aggregation, inhibition of thrombin prevents further development of the fibrin-rich clots responsible for ACS.

18. **What is the difference between UFH and LMWH?**

Both types of heparin can inactivate factor Xa, but only UFH inactivates factor IIa (thrombin) because it requires a larger molecule. LMWHs are chemically processed heparins with significantly smaller molecules, somewhere between 4000 and 6000 d. UFH molecular weight ranges between 12,000 and 15,000 d. LMWHs are given subcutaneously and have a more predictable anticoagulant effect (see Question 19). See the following table for more information about the similarities and differences of UFH and LMWHs.

Heparin Agent	Unfractionated Heparin (UFH) Given Intravenously*	Low–Molecular-Weight Heparin (LMWH); Prototype: Enoxaparin
Action	Inhibits platelet function Binds endothelial cells, macrophages, and plasma proteins to prevent thrombus at site of injury Inactivates factor Xa and IIa (thrombin)	Inhibits platelet function (but to lesser extend than UFH) Inactivates factor Xa
Dosing	Initial bolus of 60 U/kg not to exceed 4000 U Maintenance infusion: 12 U/kg/hr, adjusted to maintain activated partial thromboplastin time (aPTT) of 50-70 s; maximum infusion rate is 1000 U/hr For patients >70 kg: bolus maximum is still 4000 U; infusion maximum is 1000 U/hr	1 mg/kg subcutaneously every 12 hr for several days dependant on disease and intervention

Continued

continued		
Heparin Agent	**Unfractionated Heparin (UFH) Given Intravenously***	**Low–Molecular-Weight Heparin (LMWH); Prototype: Enoxaparin**
Duration of therapy	Usually 24-72 hr	Usually 48-72 hr
Onset of action and half-life	Onset of action: immediate Half-life: dose-dependent; <4 hr	Long plasma half-life
Monitoring	PTT every 6 hr Nomogram used to adjust doses based on target therapeutic aPTT of 2.5-3 times control Measure activated clotting time before percutaneous coronary intervention and before sheath removal	No routine monitoring of lab results If lab tests needed: serum anti-Xa factor activity may be measured
Side effects	Bleeding Thrombocytopenia Use cautiously in patients with bleeding diathesis, renal insufficiency, or gastrointestinal ulceration	Bleeding Thrombocytopenia
Antidote	Protamine sulfate	Protamine sulfate

*UFH may be given intravenously or subcutaneously. However, for patients with ACS, it is given intravenously.

19. What advantages does LMWH have over UFH?

- Lower weight molecule
- Longer half-life
- Subcutaneous twice daily dosing
- Improved bioavailability; dose-dependant clearance
- More predictable anticoagulant response because of low protein binding ratio; therefore less individual variability (so no need for lab monitoring)
- No rebound effect like that seen with UFH when it is discontinued; this rebound causes a paradoxical effect of procoagulation
- Can be self-administered safely if needed after discharge

20. What are other examples of LMWH?

See the table on the facing page for review of LMWH agents on the market.

Generic Name of LMWH (Trade Name)	Dose	Peak Effect
Ardeparin (Normiflo)	50 antifactor Xa U/kg subcutaneously (SC) every 12 hr*	2-4 hr
Dalteparin sodium (Fragmin)	25,000–50,000 IU SC daily*	4 hr
Enoxaparin (Lovenox)	30 mg SC every 12 hr	3-5 hr
Tinzaparin (Innohep)	175 anti-Xa IU/kg SC daily*	3-5 hr

*Dosing for deep venous thrombosis prophylaxis indication.

21. Which type of heparin is the agent of choice for patients with ACS?

Some controversy remains as to which agent is the best for patients with ACS. Previous studies have shown that patients have a lower rate of death, MI, and coronary revascularization with LMWH versus UFH. Other studies have shown that the use of LMWH is associated with a lower mortality rate and a lower rate of serious cardiac ischemic events compared with IV UFH and is preferable in patients with USA/NSTEMI in conjunction with GP IIb/IIIa inhibitors in the absence of renal failure and surgical intervention within 24 hours. The current standard of care for patients undergoing PCI or CABG is to use IV UFH for more readily reversible anticoagulant effects. However, ongoing clinical trials are studying the comparison between UFH and LMWH in the ACS patient population with planned PCI (the SYNERGY study). Some of the questions currently being addressed in ongoing clinical trials are the use of LMWH with combination therapies, including GP IIb/IIIa inhibitors and thrombolytics.

22. What is heparin-induced thrombocytopenia (HIT)?

Heparin-induced thrombocytopenia is an antibody-mediated adverse reaction to heparin that can result in venous and arterial thrombosis. The clinical/serological features are:
- Unexplained fall in platelet count of 50% or more usually 5 to 15 days after initiation of heparin therapy
- Skin lesions at heparin injection sites

Hematology should be consulted to make the diagnosis, which requires special activation and antigen assays that may need to be sent to specialized facilities for analysis.

23. How is HIT treated?

Treatment is to discontinue heparin and initiate another type of antithrombin agent, typically argatroban (Acova), which binds to the active thrombin sites to inhibit any platelet aggregation, formation of fibrin, or activation of other coagulation factors. Another agent used may be hirudin (Lepirudin), a direct thrombin inhibitor. For rapid therapeutic anticoagulation, a loading dose of 0.4 mg/kg IV bolus is followed by a maintenance dose of 0.15 mg/kg/h, with adjustments made to maintain aPTT 1.5 to 2.5 times median normal range. Direct thrombin inhibitors, such as lepirudin, are a good alternative to heparin when HIT is confirmed or suspected.

24. What is bivalirudin (Angiomax), and when is it used?

Bivalirudin is a reversible direct thrombin inhibitor indicated for use in patients with USA undergoing PCI. It has a renal excretion, and the dose can be adjusted for patients with renal impairment. Bivalirudin prolongs the ACT, PT, and aPTT. Coagulation times return to baseline within 1 hour of discontinuation of the drug. Bivalirudin is given IV bolus 1.0 mg/kg followed by a 4-hour infusion at a rate of 2.5 mcg/kg/h. After the first 4 hours, an additional infusion may be initiated of 0.2 mg/kg/h for up to 20 hours. Ongoing clinical trials are assessing its use in patients with HIT. This drug is still in early phases of use, with its safety and efficacy in conjunction with platelet inhibitors other than ASA, such as the GP IIb/IIIa inhibitors, not yet established. It is one of the promising new agents that may have advantages over heparin when more data are available.

25. What are the ongoing controversies with thrombin and platelet inhibitor therapies?

- The best GP IIb/IIIa inhibitor agent.
- Early invasive versus early conservative strategies: access to catheterization labs and plans for transfer of patients and drug therapy based on availability of aggressive therapies.
- Unfractionated heparin versus LMWH, especially in patients undergoing acute coronary interventions. Interventional cardiologists prefer to measure ongoing levels of heparin with frequent change and nature of lesions. Trials exploring best combination with GP IIb/IIIa therapy are ongoing.
- Costs of drugs and availability (cost versus benefit); the newer agents are expensive.
- Risk stratification for aggressive strategies with multiple and combination of thrombin and platelet inhibitors.
- The best combination treatment cocktail to open arteries and keep them open long term with the least bleeding complications; modifications of dosing based on combinations are being tested.
- How much bleeding is worth the risks of the newer agents?

Key Points

- Current antithrombin and antiplatelet therapies for patients with CV target the platelet aggregation process that occurs in thrombosis.
- Current AHA guideline changes recommend clopidogrel bisulfate with ASA initially in patients with ACS when invasive therapies are not expected.
- Glycoprotein IIb/IIIa inhibitors should be considered early in treatment of patients with high-risk ACS with any of the following:
- ST segment depression more than 0.5 mm on ECG.
- T-wave inversion more than 1 mm on ECG.
- Cardiac enzyme elevations greater than the upper limit of normal.
- The following nursing actions are required when administering GP IIb/IIIa therapies:
  - Awareness of contraindications to therapy.
  - Attention to changes in hemodynamics and vital signs.
  - Scrutiny of neurological status and changes.
  - Knowledge of lab parameters like Hct, hemoglobin, platelet count, serum creatinine, PT, and aPTT.
  - Recognition and continued assessment of potential bleeding sites.
  - Attention to adjunctive therapies that may increase bleeding (heparin, clopidogrel bisulfate).
  - Ensuring continued multivenous access.
  - Monitoring continuously for signs of new ischemia, like chest pain, ECG changes, and cardiac enzyme levels.
- The following lab values may be affected by the use of GP IIb/IIIa therapy:
  - ACT level.
  - aPTT.
  - Platelet count.
- Weight adjustment is crucial for all IV antithrombin and antiplatelet agents. Dosing calculations should be double checked with another colleague.
- Most weight charts for antiplatelet or antithrombin therapy are available in the drug insert. Lower weight and elderly patients are at a higher risk of bleeding, so all dosing must be adjusted downward to prevent bleeding.
- Glycoprotein IIb/IIIa agents should be discontinued at least 2 to 4 hours before surgery. With eptifibatide or tirofiban, platelets should normalize within 4 to 6 hours. With abciximab, the half-life of the platelet is much longer; therefore use of this agent may pose a higher risk of bleeding with early surgical interventions.

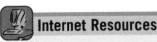

Internet Resources

Scottish Intercollegiate Guidelines Network: Antithrombotic Therapy Guideline:
http://www.sign.ac.uk/guidelines/fulltext/36/index.html

CME course: Treating the Post MI Patient: Preventing Future Atherosclerotic Events (sponsored by George Washington University)
www.antiplatelet.net

Journal Article: Thrombolytic, Antithrombin, and Antiplatelet Treatment of Acute Coronary Syndromes:
http://www.aoa-net.org/publications/jaoa/supplements/1100puma.pdf

American College of Chest Physicians:
www.chestnet.org/guidelines

Bibliography

Bates S, Weitz J: The mechanism of action of thrombin inhibitors, *J Invasive Cardiol* 12(suppl F):27-31F, 2000.

Braunwald E, Altman E, Theroux P, for the Committee on the management of Patients with Unstable Angina on ACC/AHA Practice Guidelines: ACC/AHA 2002 update for the management of patients with non-ST-segment elevation myocardial infarction—summary article: a report of American College of Cardiology, *J Am Coll Cardiol* 40(7), 1366-1374, 2002.

Bryan R: Plavix (clopidogrel bisulfate): effective against atherosclerotic events, *Adv Nurs* 5:37, 2001.

Futterman L, Lemburg L: Low-molecular-weight heparin: an antithrombin agent whose time has come, *Am J Crit Care* 8(1):520-523, 1999.

Glys K, Gold M: Acute coronary syndromes: new developments in pharmacological treatment strategies, *Crit Care Nurse* 20(2):1-15, 2000.

Goodman S, Cohen M et al: Unfractionated heparin for unstable coronary artery disease one year results of the Essence study, *Am Coll Cardiol* 36(3):693-698, 2000.

Hirsch J, Annund S: Guide to anticoagulant therapy: heparin: a statement for healthcare professionals from the American Heart Association, *Circulation* 103:2994, 2001.

Lui H: Dosage, pharmacological effects and clinical outcomes for bivalirudin in percutaneous coronary intervention, *J Invasive Cardiol* 12(supp F):41-52F, 2000.

Ross A, Molhoek P et al: Randomized comparison of low-molecular weight heparin: with unfractionated heparin adjunctive to recombinant tissue plasminogen activator thrombolysis and aspirin: Second Trial of Heparin and Aspirin Reperfusion Therapy (HART II), *Circulation* 104:608, 2001.

The Clopidogrel in Unstable Angina to Prevent Recurrent Events (CURE) Trial Investigators: Effects of clopidogrel in addition to aspirin in patients with acute coronary syndromes without ST-segment elevation, *N Engl J Med* 345(7):494-502, 2001.

Turpie A, Antman E: Low-molecular-weight heparins in the treatment of acute coronary syndromes, *Arch Intern Med* 161:1484-1490, 2001.

Vogt A, Neuhaus KL: Antithrombin therapy in acute coronary syndromes. In Topol E, editor: *Acute coronary syndromes,* ed 2, New York, 2001, Marcel Dekker, pp 515-540.

White H, HERO-2 Investigators: Thrombin-specific anticoagulation with bivalirudin verses heparin in patients receiving fibrinolytic therapy for acute myocardial infarction: the HERO-2 randomized trial, *Lancet* 358:1855-1863, 2001.

Chapter 29

Chronic Anticoagulation

Mary Jo Goolsby

1. What are the most common indications for chronic anticoagulation therapy?

Chronic anticoagulation therapy is usually prescribed to treat venous thrombosis and prevent recurrence, to treat pulmonary emboli (PE), and to prevent the formation of systemic emboli in patients who have tissue or mechanical heart valves, who have had a myocardial infarction (MI), or who have atrial fibrillation. In some cases, anticoagulation therapy is used to prevent recurrent MIs.

2. What types of chronic anticoagulation therapy are most often used?

Most commonly, ambulatory patients who need chronic anticoagulation therapy are prescribed an oral form—warfarin (Coumadin). For women who are pregnant or individuals with other contraindications to warfarin therapy, one of the low–molecular-weight heparins (LMWHs) may be used for chronic anticoagulation therapy. Otherwise, the use of alternatives, such as LMWH, greatly increases the cost and complexity of self-treatment because the patient or a family member must inject the medication (see Chapter 28, Antiplatelet and Antithrombotic Agents).

3. How is warfarin used?

Warfarin is taken orally and should be taken daily at approximately the same time. The typical regimen calls for late afternoon/early evening dosing, around the time of dinner. With treatment for actual venous thrombosis or with a need to induce an anticoagulation state more rapidly than can be achieved with warfarin alone, warfarin is usually started while the patient receives either an unfractionated heparin or a LMWH. Regardless, treatment is usually started at 5 mg and the dose is then adjusted to achieve a therapeutic value. Once the therapeutic dose of warfarin is achieved, the heparin or LMWH is discontinued.

4. Is the starting dose ever greater or less than 5 mg?

With an urgent need to establish an anticoagulant state but without the necessity for parenteral anticoagulation, 7.5 to 10 mg of warfarin a day may be used initially. However, because a start with the anticipated actual dose has been found to be best, the higher doses are not routinely used. In contrast, a lower initial dose may be necessary for patients who have liver disease, are malnourished, are at high risk for bleeding, or are elderly. The dose is selected that allows anticoagulation while avoiding the complication of bleeding.

5. How does one know whether the dose is therapeutic? How is the effect of warfarin monitored?

The effect of warfarin on coagulation can be measured with two tests: the pro-thrombin time (PT) and the international normalized ratio (INR). The PT has long been used to monitor warfarin therapy and is reported in seconds. This test relies on thromboplastin reagents that may differ from institution to institution, resulting in the potential for significant variation in results. Compared with the PT, the INR provides a more reliable method, reporting a value reflecting the ratio of the patient's PT over the mean, local, and normal PT. The INR is the preferred determinant of whether the dose is within a therapeutic range because it relies on a standardized thromboplastin reagent, without institutional variation.

6. How often is the PT or the INR measured to assess the warfarin dose?

When treatment is first started, the INR should be measured daily until the desired range is achieved and maintained for 2 days. Once the therapeutic range appears stable, monitoring is decreased to two or three times a week for the next 2 weeks to ensure that the INR remains stable. At that point, monitoring is further decreased but should be performed at least every 4 weeks.

7. What is the usual time for a therapeutic level to be achieved?

A therapeutic range is usually achieved in about 5 days.

8. Once a therapeutic dose is achieved, is the INR monitoring maintained indefinitely every 4 weeks?

The INR is generally monitored every 4 weeks for the duration of therapy. However, each patient's provider determines the frequency with which the INR should be monitored, and if the patient is at higher than normal risk for development of bleeding or another complication of warfarin therapy, a shorter interval between INRs may be chosen. Yet any time the warfarin dose is changed, a nontherapeutic range is suspected, or the patient has a condition or treatment that could alter the effectiveness of the warfarin or alter the INR, the INR should be repeated. When the warfarin dose must be altered or the INR is not within a therapeutic range, monitoring should be performed more frequently until the therapeutic range is once more established and stable.

9. What INR levels suggest a therapeutic level and dose of warfarin?

The level that is therapeutic differs, according to the reason for warfarin therapy. Generally, an INR of 2.5 (2.0 to 3.0) is desirable for most patients. A slightly higher INR of 3.0 (2.5 to 3.5) is suggested for patients who are prescribed warfarin to prevent recurrence of an acute MI and for those with most mechanical heart valves. See the following table.

Indication	Therapeutic International Normalized Ratio (INR)
Prophylaxis of venous thrombosis	2.0-3.0
Treatment of venous thrombosis	2.0-3.0
Treatment of pulmonary emboli	2.0-3.0
Prevention of systemic embolism (tissue heart valves, acute myocardial infarction [AMI], valvular heart disease, atrial fibrillation)	2.0-3.0
Mechanical prosthetic valves	2.5-3.0
Bileaflet mechanical valve in aortic position	2.0-3.0
Prevention of AMI (note that dosage used to prevent AMI is higher than that used to prevent systemic emboli in patients with AMI)	2.5-3.5

10. What actions are generally taken if the INR is subtherapeutic?

A decision regarding whether to increase the dosage is based on how low the INR is and whether any condition or situation might explain why it is decreased (for instance, the patient recently forgot one or more doses of warfarin). If the INR is only slightly decreased, the previous dose may be maintained and the INR checked again in 2 to 3 days. Otherwise, the dosage is increased and the INR is monitored again in 2 to 3 days. The warfarin dosage is usually increased only 10% to 20% at any given time. Any time the dosage is changed, it is crucial that the patient understand the new dosing schedule and when to expect to follow-up for another INR.

11. What actions are typically taken for patients with an INR that is too high?

The response to an elevated INR also depends on the degree to which it is elevated. This situation is more complicated because the response depends on how much risk is indicated by the elevation and the patient's status. The general recommendations are summarized in the following table. Knowledge and careful following of the orders specific to each individual patient are important in response to an elevated INR.

International Normalized Ratio (INR)	Patient Characteristics	General Response*
INR > therapeutic, but <5.0	No significant bleeding	Dose may be continued and INR rechecked Or One dose may be held and lower dose resumed.
INR >5.0 but <9.0	No significant bleeding	1-2 doses held, INR frequently monitored, lower dose when resumed Or Dose may be held and vitamin K administered orally (1-2 mg); lower dose once resumed.
INR >9.0	No significant bleeding	Doses held, oral vitamin K administered at higher dose than above (3-5 mg); lower dose once resumed.
INR >20	Serious bleeding	Doses held, vitamin K administered intravenously (10 mg) and repeated every 12 h as needed; fresh frozen plasma or prothrombin complex concentrate may also be infused if urgent need; admittance for treatment and monitoring.

*For all responses, patient is expected to be monitored as described in responses to Questions 6 and 8, unless otherwise indicated or ordered.

12. What medications affect INR values?

A myriad of other medications (prescribed and over-the-counter, herbal and traditional) are associated with warfarin interactions and either increase or decrease the INR. The Coumadin package insert has a comprehensive list of medications that are known to interact with warfarin. The following box summarizes some of the major classifications of drugs that may interact with warfarin:

Drugs that increase PT/INR

- Antacids
- Antiarrhythmics
- Antipsychotic agents
- Anticonvulsants
- Diuretics
- Enteral nutritional supplements
- Gastric acid/peptic ulcer agents
- Hypolipidemics
- Estrogen-containing oral contraceptives
- Vitamins

Drugs that decrease PT/INR

- Analgesics
- Antiarrhythmics
- Antibiotics
- Anticonvulsants
- Antidepressants
- Beta-adrenergic blockers
- Diabetes agents
- Diuretics
- Gastrointestinal agents
- Gout treatments
- Hypolipidemics
- Nonsteroidal antiinflammatory agents
- Steroids

This list is not exhaustive. Because so many medications interact with warfarin, identification of all medications, herbs, and vitamins taken by patients who need chronic anticoagulation therapy is important. Specifically important is inquiry about herbal/botanical agents, some of which alter the effects of warfarin, including: garlic, St. John's wort, ginkgo biloba, and coenzyme Q10. More frequent monitoring of the INR any time a new medication is added or stopped is important to determine whether an interaction has occurred. Sometimes, avoiding the use of a medication that is known to interact with warfarin is not possible, and more frequent monitoring allows for the warfarin dosage to be appropriately adjusted, avoiding complications.

13. What foods affect INR values?

Vitamin K is the antidote to warfarin; therefore foods that are high in vitamin K decrease the effectiveness of oral anticoagulation therapy. The amount of vitamin K is highest in green leafy vegetables. Patients who are taking warfarin must eat a consistent diet, with no major fluctuations in the amount of green leafy vegetables, so that the intake of vitamin K is more or less constant. They should not, for instance, go on a weight reduction diet consisting primarily of vegetables or start a multivitamin regimen with vitamin K because either of these situations is likely to result in a decreased INR and increased blood coagulability. Conversely, patients who have traditionally eaten diets high in vitamin K and who suddenly decrease the vegetable content of their diet are likely to have an increased INR and be at higher risk for bleeding.

14. Are there any other situations/conditions, other than specific medications or foods, that can affect the INR?

Other conditions that are associated with alteration of the INR include liver diseases, malnutrition, and hypermetabolic states (fevers or hyperthyroidism). Alcohol intake is also associated with increased INR, particularly with a history of liver damage.

15. Are there patients in whom warfarin therapy is contraindicated?

Warfarin is absolutely contraindicated during pregnancy. It has been associated with abnormalities of the central nervous system, fetal bleeding, and increased rate of fetal death. Pregnant women who need chronic anticoagulation therapy are treated with heparin or LMWH. The one potential exception to this contra-indication involves pregnant women with mechanical heart valves who are at increased risk of clot formation.

Other conditions exist for which chronic anticoagulation therapy has relative contraindications, and the potential risks must be carefully considered before initiation of warfarin. These conditions include alcoholism, drug abuse, dementia, and psychosis and instances in which persons are at higher than average risk for hemorrhage. Examples of patients who are considered to be at higher risk for hemorrhage and thus have a relative contraindication to chronic anticoagulation therapy include persons who have had a recent (within 2 months) stroke or intracranial hemorrhage, have uncontrolled severe hypertension, have had recent major trauma, or have hemorrhagic retinopathy.

16. What side effects are associated with chronic oral anticoagulation therapy?

The most frequent and serious side effect or adverse effect of oral anticoagulation therapy is hemorrhage. Warfarin-associated hemorrhage can involve the skin and mucous membranes, the lungs, the central nervous system, the urinary system, and the gastrointestinal tract. The other major potential adverse reaction is skin necrosis. This complication of therapy usually appears 3 to 8 days after the medication is started and involves thrombosis of venules and capillaries located within the subcutaneous fat. Patients in whom this reaction develops are usually thereafter treated with long-term heparin or LMWH therapy instead of with warfarin.

17. What key nursing assessments should be performed to detect potential adverse effects of chronic anticoagulation therapy?

Before a patient starts warfarin therapy, the history of adverse medication reactions should be reviewed, with assurance that there is no history of previous warfarin-related skin necrosis. During the first few days of therapy, completion of a skin examination and asking the patient about the development of any new skin lesions is important because as skin necrosis is most likely to become evident within the first week of treatment.

For the period that the patient needs warfarin, nursing assessment should include history and physical assessment directed towards identification of any bleeding. The signs of bleeding include hematuria, epistaxis, easy bruising, bleeding gums, melena, abdominal pain, and dizziness. Monitoring the vital signs of patients receiving warfarin or other chronic anticoagulation therapy and being attentive for hypotension or tachycardia, which may suggest bleeding, are important. The INR or PT should be monitored. Depending on the setting and the availability of equipment, point-of-care (POC) testing may be performed to determine the PT or INR as part of the assessment.

18. What is POC testing?

Point-of-care testing for INR uses a monitor that measures a thromboplastin-mediated clotting time and then converts it to either a PT or INR. The specimen can be obtained through a finger stick. The POC monitors are available for clinic settings and for home use. POC monitoring minimizes the need for the patient (or specimen) to be sent to the lab and the wait for results. When considering the potential for POC testing in a clinic or home setting, determination of the accuracy and limitations of all available monitors is extremely important. When POC testing is considered for home use by a patient, other considerations must include the patient's ability to perform, interpret, and appropriately respond to the test. Some studies have shown good outcomes associated with home POC testing and self-management by patients.

19. **What information must a patient undergoing chronic anticoagulation therapy with warfarin receive?**

The education of patients who need chronic anticoagulation therapy is a vital nursing role. The educational plan should include the following:
- The reason an anticoagulant is prescribed.
- The anticipated duration of treatment.
- The frequency, timing, and dose prescribed.
- The symptoms that should be reported (signs of skin reaction or bleeding).
- The purpose of PT/INR monitoring.
- The frequency and routine expected for the monitoring.
- Procedures if a dose is missed.

20. **Is warfarin the same substance commonly found in rat poison?**

Yes. It is helpful to inform the patient that this drug is the same agent used in many rat poisons but that the dose is small and they are carefully monitored. The number of people in the community who know this isolated fact about warfarin and the concern that occurs when patients are suddenly made aware that they have been taking "rat poison" is amazing. Regardless, it is important to provide the patient an opportunity to ask questions and express any concerns and to satisfactorily address these questions and concerns.

21. **What should a patient do if a dose of warfarin is missed?**

The procedure for a missed dose should be determined by the provider who prescribes the medication.

However, often the patient is instructed to take the missed dose if the lapse is realized by a certain time of day (perhaps by bedtime on the day it was to have been taken). But because patients often do not notice the missed dose until later the next day, they are usually told to omit the missed dose and to resume the normal schedule with the next dose. If two doses are missed in a short period of time, the nurse should work with the patient to identify strategies that help with adherence to the schedule in the future.

22. **Does the brand of warfarin a patient uses matter?**

Normally the answer to whether or not a specific brand is better than a generic form is debatable, and this is no exception. Coumadin (the major brand of warfarin) has been used for years, is inexpensive, and is used by most providers. In addition to the low cost of this brand, the pill colors are standardized for each dosage. When patients are instructed for any necessary dosage change, the knowledge that they only have Coumadin is comforting so that the appropriate tablet that they should be taking can be described. However, generic forms of warfarin are available and the bioavailability is supposedly equal to the brand form. The cost of generic warfarin is even lower than the brand Coumadin. Probably more important than a determination regarding whether a patient should be prescribed a generic or brand form, however, is the need for any given patient to receive one consistent form of warfarin—whether brand or generic.

Any time a patient changes from one form to another, the INR should be monitored to establish whether a dosage requirement must be made. Patients should be instructed to question any change in the appearance (by color, shape, or size) of their warfarin tablets and to report any changes to the pharmacist or provider before using the new supply.

23. How long must a patient take anticoagulation treatment?

The duration of treatment depends largely on the indication for which it is prescribed.

After venous thrombosis, warfarin is usually prescribed for 3 to 6 months. The longer period of time is associated with a lower incidence rate of recurrence. Treatment is typically indicated at least 6 months after PE. When patients have had more than one episode of idiopathic vein thrombosis, idiopathic PE, thrombosis associated with a malignant disease, homozygous factor V Leiden genotype, or antiphospholipid antibody syndrome, the treatment is indefinite. Similarly, anticoagulation therapy is indefinite for atrial fibrillation and prosthetic heart valves.

24. What happens when patients who are on chronic anticoagulation therapy also need surgery or another invasive procedure, with regard to risk of bleeding or hemorrhage?

All patients receiving chronic anticoagulation therapy must know the importance of all providers being aware of the treatment. Before any procedure, the patient should confirm that the person who performs the procedure is aware of the warfarin regimen.

Patients who take warfarin are instructed on when/how to withhold the warfarin dose before a procedure. The degree of risk for formation of thrombosis and risk of bleeding determines the actual order for preprocedure and postprocedure anticoagulation therapy. For instance, when the patient is deemed at low risk for thromboembolism (e.g., a patient who is more than 3 months after deep venous thrombosis [DVT] or who has atrial fibrillation but no history of cardiovascular accident [CVA]), the warfarin is held as much as 4 days before the procedure. Low-dose heparin can be administered, if ordered, once the procedure is completed. For patients who are at higher risk for development of thrombosis, the warfarin is held up to 4 days before the procedure, but low-dose heparin may be administered 2 days before and initially after the procedure.

25. Are there any new treatments for patients who need chronic anticoagulation therapy?

A variety of medications are currently on the market and prevent platelet adhesion; these are used for some patients in lieu of warfarin to prevent strokes and MIs. Examples include aspirin, dipyridamole, ticlopidine hydrochloride, and clopidogrel bisulfate. However, these are not purely anticoagulants. As the cost of the LMWH decreases, these may be used more frequently for chronic anticoagulation therapy. They have advantages over the unfractionated heparin in that they have greater bioavailability, require less (usually no) lab monitoring, can be administered once daily, and are associated with a lower risk of bleeding. (See chapter 28, Antiplatelet and Antithrombotic Agents.)

Key Points

- Compared with the PT, the INR more reliably reflects the patient's anticoagulation status.
- For most patients treated with warfarin, the INR should be maintained between 2.0 and 3.0.
- Because vitamin K is a warfarin antidote, patients on this drug should eat a diet that is consistent in the amounts of daily green leafy vegetables.
- The INR should be monitored each time a patient on warfarin therapy has some change in other medications (prescribed and over-the-counter).
- Warfarin is absolutely contraindicated in pregnancy.
- For all patients on warfarin and other chronic anticoagulation therapy, the nursing assessment should include vital signs and assessment for hematuria, epistaxis, easy bruising, bleeding gums, melena, abdominal pain, and dizziness.

Internet Resources

Family Practice Notebook: Hormonally Active Chemotherapy
www.fpnotebook.com/HEM163.htm

American Academy of Family Physicians:
www.afp.org

East Carolina University Department of Internal Medicine: Anticoagulation Resources:
www.ecu.edu/anticoagulation/

Bibliography

Ansell J, Hirsh J, Dalen J et al: Managing oral anticoagulant therapy, *Chest* 119(suppl):22S-38S, 2001.

Goolsby MJ: Clinical practice guideline: managing oral anticoagulant therapy, *J Am Acad Nurse Pract* 14:16-18, 2002.

Gorski LA: A clinical pathway for deep vein thrombosis, *Home Healthcare Nurs* 18:451-461, 2000.

Hirsch J, Dalen JE, Anderson DR et al: Oral anticoagulants: mechanism of action, clinical effectiveness, and optimal therapeutic range, *Chest* 119(suppl):8S-21S, 2001.

Lassiter TF: Medications used to prevent adhesion and clotting, *Prim Care Pract* 4:619-632, 2000.

Yacovella T, Alter M: Anticoagulation for venous thromboembolism: what are the current options? *Postgrad Med* 108:43-54, 2000.

Chapter 30

Diuretics and Nitrates

Margaret T. Bowers

1. How do diuretics work?

Diuretics promote water and sodium excretion at various sites of the nephron in the kidney. They reduce both intravascular (blood) and extravascular (edema) fluid.

2. Where do diuretics work, and what are the usual dosing parameters?

Diuretic Type	Action	Example	Oral Dose (Minimal/Maximal)	Intravenous (IV) Dose
Loop	Loop of Henle	Furosemide	20-80 mg/d single dose; maximal daily dose, 600 mg	IV dose usually $1/2$ oral dose; infusion: 40 mg loading dose (LD) then adjust to creatinine clearance (CrCl) 10-40 mg/hr
		Bumetanide	0.5-2 mg/d; maximal, 10 mg/d	IV 0.5-10 mg/d maximal dose; infusion: 1 mg LD then adjust to CrCl 0.5-2 mg/hr
		Torsemide	5 mg/d up to 100 mg/d	IV: oral dose; infusion: 20 mg LD then 5-20 mg/hr
Thiazide	Proximal distal renal tubule	Hydrochlorothiazide	25 mg/d as single dose up to 200 mg/d	Not applicable
		Metolazone	0.5 mg/d up to 20 mg/d	
Carbonic anhydrase inhibitors	Proximal renal tubule	Acetazolamide	250 mg/d with maximal 1000 mg/d	Not applicable
		Methazolamide	50-100 mg twice to three times a day	

Continued

continued				
Diuretic Type	**Action**	**Example**	**Oral Dose (Minimal/Maximal)**	**Intravenous (IV) Dose**
Potassium-sparing	Distal renal tubule and collecting duct	Spironolactone Amiloride hydrochloride	25 mg/d up to 400 mg/d in divided doses 5 mg/d up to 20 mg/d	Not applicable

3. What are the most common adverse effects of diuretics?

Ototoxicity may be seen with loop diuretics and is usually associated with high doses. Early recognition and diuretic dose adjustment can minimize prolonged ototoxicity. Skin reactions and interstitial nephritis are associated with both thiazide and loop diuretics. Spironolactone may cause gynecomastia in about 10% of patients for whom it is prescribed, but it usually resolves when the medication is discontinued.

4. How is it known if the patient is tolerant to a diuretic?

- Before determination of tolerance to a diuretic, placement on a sodium and fluid restriction may be necessary.
- If the patient does not respond to adequate doses of a particular diuretic, then combination therapy may be indicated. Because each category has a different site of action, a synergistic effect is seen with combination therapy.
- Some diuretics, such as furosemide, have a variable absorption rate. Different doses must be attempted before it is deemed ineffective.
- Torsemide and bumetanide are well absorbed, so their effectiveness is readily apparent.
- For the patient with renal insufficiency, escalating doses of diuretics are frequently necessary.

5. How often does a patient receive an oral diuretic?

Thiazide and potassium-sparing diuretics have long half-lives and may be dosed once daily. Loop diuretics have a short half-life (1 to 3 hours), so they may be dosed more frequently, usually twice daily. In addition, the effectiveness of the diuresis dissipates before the next dose being administered.

6. What are indications for administration of a diuretic?

- Hypertension
- Heart failure

- Pulmonary edema
- Hepatic cirrhosis
- Idiopathic edema
- Hypercalcemia
- Nephrolithiasis
- Nephrotic syndrome

7. What are important aspects of patient and family education that a nurse should include for patients receiving diuretics?

- Sleep disruption is minimized if the diuretic is taken in the morning.
- The patient and family should be instructed about dietary sources of potassium unless the patient is on a potassium-sparing diuretic.
- If patients have renal insufficiency or a high normal potassium level, then they may not be on a potassium supplement.
- Limiting dietary sodium intake may reduce the amount of diuretic needed.
- Patients with diabetes should be informed that glucose levels might increase when diuretic therapy is initiated and the diabetic regimen may need to be adjusted because of insulin suppression.
- Use of sunscreen and avoidance of prolonged sunlight exposure is necessary to prevent photosensitivity reactions.
- Concurrent use of nonsteroidal antiinflammatory drugs (NSAIDs) may reduce the effectiveness of the diuretic.
- Gout flares may occur as a result of decreased excretion of uric acid by the kidneys.
- Sudden position changes should be avoided to minimize orthostatic hypotension.

8. How is orthostatic hypotension managed in a patient receiving diuretics?

Orthostatic hypotension may result from overdiuresis or from a combination of medical therapy that affects the vascular system. If a patient develops orthostatic hypotension, a reduction in the dose of diuretic or a discontinuation for a period of time may be necessary. Cautious hydration with oral fluids may reduce the symptoms of weakness and lightheadedness. Orthostatic hypotension can be minimized by avoiding sudden position changes and with resting in a sitting position before standing to ambulate. In addition, the entire medication regimen should be reviewed and the dosing schedule should be adjusted to minimize hypotension throughout the day.

9. What lab or dietary implications exist for a patient receiving diuretics?

Diuretics cause shifts in electrolytes; therefore monitoring of potassium and magnesium levels is important. These electrolytes are found in many foods. Often supplementation can be achieved through dietary changes, but magnesium oxide or potassium chloride may be necessary to correct the imbalance. The following table lists foods that are rich in potassium.

Food	Amount	Calories	Potassium (mg)
Banana	1 medium	105	452
Cantaloupe	1 cup pieces	56	494
Honeydew melon	1 cup pieces	60	461
Kidney beans	1 cup boiled	113	357
Lentils	1 cup boiled	115	366
Milk (nonfat)	8 oz	86	406
Orange juice	8 oz (frozen)	112	473
Papaya	½ medium	60	391
Potato	Baked with skin, 4 oz	124	476
Spinach	1 cup boiled	21	419
Sweet potato	Baked with skin, 4 oz	117	397

10. What should be done if a patient becomes hyperkalemic?

- The patient should be asked if he/she is currently taking a potassium supplement tablet or potassium-sparing diuretic, which may be temporarily or permanently discontinued.
- Potassium-rich dietary sources to avoid, which are listed in the previous table, should be discussed.
- One should ask about the use of salt substitute, which usually contains potassium instead of sodium.
- Electrocardiographic (ECG) changes should be monitored. Peaked T waves are most common.
- The health care provider should be contacted regarding possible treatment with sodium polystyrene sulfonate (Kayexalate).

11. What other types of adverse reactions should be anticipated for a patient undergoing diuretic therapy?

- Orthostatic hypotension
- Dizziness
- Hearing impairment/tinnitus
- Nausea/vomiting
- Interstitial nephritis
- Anemia
- Urticaria
- Pruritus
- Hyperuricemia
- Hyperglycemia/glycosuria
- Weakness

- Muscle spasm
- Dysrhythmias
- Lipid abnormalities
- Metabolic alkalosis

12. When are nitrates used?

- Coronary artery disease, including stable and unstable angina
- Acute myocardial infarction
- Hypertension
- Heart failure

13. How do nitrates work?

Nitrates are in a class of drugs known as venodilators because they act by redistributing blood volume from the venous side of the heart into the systemic circulation, resulting in a reduction in preload. They are often used in combination with arteriolar dilators, such as hydralazine, to provide afterload reduction.

14. What are the routes of administration for nitrates, and what are the usual doses?

Route	Dose	Frequency
Sublingual	0.4 mg	One every 5 min up to maximum of three in 15 min
Spray	0.4 mg per metered dose	Maximum of three sprays in 15 min
Oral	5-60 mg 60-120 mg	Short acting every 4-6 hr Long acting once a day
Transdermal	0.2 mg/hr-0.8 mg/hr	Application for 12-14 hr then remove
Ointment	1/2 in-2 in	Application once every 6-8 hr with 10-hr nitrate-free interval
Intravenous	5 mcg-600 mcg/min	Continuous infusion

15. What are the main side effects of nitrates?

- Hypotension
- Nausea
- Tachycardia
- Vomiting
- Syncope
- Cutaneous vasodilation

- Headache
- Urinary frequency
- Dizziness
- Blurred vision
- Dyspnea
- Methemoglobinemia

16. What is meant by the term "nitrate holiday?"

A nitrate holiday is the interval when the patient is free of topical nitrates. This interval reduces the risk of development of a tolerance to nitrates. Transdermal nitrate patches should be applied for a 12-hour to 14-hour period and then removed for 10 to 12 hours before the next patch is applied.

Oral nitrates should be dosed either once, twice, or three times daily rather than every 4, 6, or 8 hours.

17. What type of patient education should be provided?

- Sublingual nitroglycerin is meant to be dissolved under the tongue and not swallowed.
- The patient should always sit or lie down before using rapid acting nitrates, such as sublingual or spray forms of nitroglycerin.
- Nitroglycerin spray is dispensed as 0.4 mg per metered spray, and usage should not exceed three sprays in 15 minutes.
- Medication should be stored at room temperature, and sublingual tablets should be discarded 6 months after the bottle is opened.
- Sudden position changes should be avoided to prevent orthostatic hypotension.
- Alcohol intake should be avoided because it may exacerbate orthostasis.
- The health care provider should know if the patient is taking Viagra. Nitroglycerin should never be used with Viagra because intractable hypotension can develop.

18. When are nitrates contraindicated?

- Anemia
- Glaucoma (use caution)
- Uncorrected hypovolemia
- Intracranial hemorrhage
- Constrictive pericarditis
- Cardiac tamponade
- Pericardial effusion
- Hyperthyroidism
- Hepatic disease (use caution)
- Pregnancy (category C)
- Breastfeeding
- With Viagra

19. Where should the topical nitroglycerin, either transdermal patch or nitropaste, be applied?

- Topical nitroglycerin should be applied to a hairless site without abrasions or calluses.
- Application over the distal extremities should be avoided.
- The site of application should be changed daily.
- The patch needs to be applied with firm pressure and replaced with another patch if it falls off.
- Patches may be worn during bathing or swimming because they are waterproof.
- Switching brands should be avoided because of dosage equivalency.
- To avoid burns, the patch should be removed before cardioversion or defibrillation.

 Key Points

- A nitrate holiday is the interval when the patient is free of topical nitrates to reduce the risk of development of a tolerance to nitrates. Transdermal nitrate patches should be applied for a 12-hour to 14-hour period and then removed for 10 to 12 hours before the next patch is applied.
- Patients should never use nitroglycerin with Viagra because intractable hypotension can develop.
- If a patient on diuretics develops orthostatic hypotension, a reduction in the dose of diuretic or discontinuation may be necessary for a period of time.
- Orthostatic hypotension may be treated as follows: cautious hydration with oral fluids, the client avoiding sudden position changes, and careful review of the entire medication regimen to potentially adjust the dosing schedule to minimize hypotension throughout the day.

 Internet Resources

Heart Center Online for Patients: Vasodilators
http://www.heartcenteronline.com/myheartdr/common/articles.cfm?ARTID=439

Heart Center Online for Patients: The Diuretics Center
http://www.heartcenteronline.com/myheartdr/home/splash1.cfm?sp_id=204&T_Id=463&searchterm=diuretic#

Valencia Community College: Mrs. Ludy's Nursing Notes: Pharmacology:
http://faculty.valencia.cc.fl.us/mludy/pharm1.htm

University of Utah School of Pharmacology: Diuretics:
http://lysine.pharm.utah.edu/netpharm/netpharm_00/notes/diuretics.html

Bibliography

Appendix 2: drugs influencing renal function. In Levine R: *Pharmacology: drugs actions and reactions,* ed 6, New York, 2000, Parthenon, pp 485-490.

Brater C: Drug therapy: diuretic therapy, *N Engl J Med* 339:387-395, 1998.

Carter B et al: Essential hypertension. In Young L, Koda-Kimble M, editors: *Applied therapeutics: the clinical use of drugs,* ed 6, Vancouver, 2001, pp 10-1–10-33.

Davies M, Gibbs C, Lip G: Management: diuretics, ACE inhibitors, and nitrates, *Br Med J* 320:428-431, 2000.

Ives H: Diuretic agents. In Katzung B: *Basic and clinical pharmacology,* New York, 2001, Lange Medical Books/McGraw-Hill, pp 242-260.

Johnson J et al: Heart failure. In Dipiro J et al, editors: *Pharmacotherapy: a pathophysiologic approach,* ed 5, New York, 2002, McGraw-Hill, pp 185-215.

Parker J, Tommaso G: Tolerance to the organic nitrates: new ideas, new mechanisms, continued mystery, *Circulation* 104:2263-2265, 2001.

Raehl C, Nolan P: Ischemic heart disease: anginal syndromes. In Young L, Koda-Kimble M, editors: *Applied therapeutics: the clinical use of drugs,* ed 6, Vancouver, 2001, Applied Therapeutics, pp 13-1–13-25.

Sowinski K: Ischemic heart disease. In Herfindal E, Gourley D, editors: *Textbook of therapeutics: drug and disease management,* ed 7, Philadelphia, 2000, Lippincott Williams & Wilkins, pp 917-936.

Talbert R: Ischemic heart disease. In Dipiro J et al, editors: *Pharmacotherapy: a pathophysiologic approach,* ed 5, New York, 2002, McGraw-Hill, pp 219-250.

Young J: Chronic heart failure management. In Topol E: *Textbook of cardiovascular medicine,* Philadelphia, 1998, Lippincott-Raven, pp 2273-2307.

Beta-Blockers and Calcium Channel Blockers

Sara Paul

BETA-BLOCKERS

1. How do beta-blockers work?

Beta-1 receptors are found primarily in the heart muscle and, when stimulated, increase heart rate, contractility, and atrioventricular conduction. Beta-2 receptors are present in smooth muscle, particularly bronchial and vascular smooth muscle. When these receptors are activated, vasodilation and bronchodilation occur. Beta-blocking drugs (also known as beta-antagonists) inhibit catecholamines, such as norepinephrine, at the beta-adrenoreceptor sites in cells and block the stimulating effects, resulting in decreased heart rate, decreased contractility, slowed atrioventricular conduction, and blunting of bronchodilatation. In addition, beta-blockers inhibit the adverse effects of the sympathetic nervous system in patients with heart failure (HF). In more than 20 published placebo-controlled trials, beta-blockers were found to lessen the symptoms of HF, improve the clinical status of patients, and reduce the risk of death and the combined risk of death or hospitalization.

2. What are some examples of beta-blockers?

Examples of commonly used beta-blocking drugs are: acebutolol, atenolol, bisoprolol fumarate, carteolol hydrochloride, carvedilol, esmolol hydrochloride, labetalol, metoprolol, nadolol, pindolol, propranolol, sotalol hydrochloride, and timolol maleate. See the following table for dosages.

Beta-blockers

Generic Name	Trade Name	Beginning Dose/Frequency	Maximum Dose
Acebutolol	Sectral	400 mg once a day	*1200 mg/d
Atenolol	Tenormin	50 mg once a day	100 mg once a day
Betaxolol hydrochloride	Kerlone	10 mg once a day	20 mg/d
Bisoprolol fumarate	Zebeta	5 mg once a day	40 mg once a day
	Ziac (bisoprolol/ HCTZ)	2.5 mg/6.25 mg once a day	10 mg/6.25 mg– 2 tabs once a day

Continued

Beta-blockers *continued*

Generic Name	Trade Name	Beginning Dose/Frequency	Maximum Dose
Carvedilol	Coreg	3.125 mg twice a day	25 mg twice a day
Esmolol hydrochloride	Brevibloc (intravenous only)	Supraventricular tachycardia: Start at 500 mcg/kg/min × 1 min, then 50 mcg/kg/min × 4 min, repeat if necessary (increase by 50 mcg each dose) Postoperative hypertension: 1 mg/kg × 30 s, then infuse at 150 mcg/kg/min	300 mcg/kg/min intravenous infusion
Labetalol	Normodyne Trandate	100 mg twice a day 100 mg twice a day	2.4 g/d 2.4 g/d
Metoprolol	Lopressor Toprol XL	*100 mg/d 12.5 mg once a day	*450 mg/d 200 mg/d
Nadolol	Corgard	40 mg once a day	320 mg/d
Penbutolol sulfate	Levatol	20 mg once a day	20 mg once a day
Pindolol	Visken	5 mg twice a day	*60 mg/d
Propranolol	Inderal	40 mg twice a day	*640 mg/d
Sotalol hydrochloride	Betapace	80 mg twice a day	*320 mg/d
Timolol maleate	Blocadren	10 mg twice a day	10 mg twice a day

*May be given in divided daily doses.

3. What is the difference between selective and nonselective beta-blockers?

Some beta-blockers selectively block only the beta-1 receptors, and other beta-blockers block both the beta-1 and beta-2 receptors equally and are known as nonselective beta-blockers. At higher doses, the selective beta-blockers also block the beta-2 receptors.

4. What are the indications for use of beta-blockers?

Beta-blockers are used in the treatment of stable and unstable angina pectoris, hypertension, acute myocardial infarction, congestive HF from systolic or diastolic dysfunction, and the therapy and prevention of some arrhythmias. Beta-blockers are also used to treat certain types of migraine headaches.

5. What are some contraindications to the use of beta-blockers?

Because beta-blockers can slow heart rate, they are contraindicated in patients with sick sinus syndrome or impaired atrioventricular conduction (heart block) unless an artificial pacemaker is implanted. Patients with severe bronchospastic disease such as asthma should not be placed on beta-blocker therapy because these agents prevent bronchodilation and may induce increased airway resistance. Beta-blockers should be used cautiously in patients with chronic obstructive pulmonary disease (COPD) for the same reasons. Beta-blockers should not be used in patients with asthma who are dependent on inhalers or in patients with COPD who need supplemental oxygen. Beta-blockers should be used with caution in patients with diabetes because they can mask the symptoms of hypoglycemia, such as sweating and tachycardia.

6. What are the side effects associated with beta-blocker therapy?

Cardiac side effects of beta-blocker therapy include worsening of congestive HF, hypotension, and significant bradycardia. Patients with mild bronchospastic disease who are on beta-blocker therapy may have increased wheezing and should have careful and frequent evaluation. In patients with severe peripheral vascular disease who are on beta-blocker therapy, extremities may feel cold and peripheral pulses may be absent. Patients with intermittent claudication may have worsening symptoms. Patients with diabetes may have hypoglycemia, and the early warning signs, such as sweating and anxiety, may be diminished or absent in the presence of beta-blockers. Other side effects may include dreams, hallucinations, insomnia, male impotence, depression, and fatigue.

7. What essential nursing assessments should be included in care for a patient who is started on beta-blocker therapy?

The patient's heart rate should be carefully monitored for 1 full minute and recorded, with assessment for changes and the presence of bradycardia. Breath sounds should be auscultated in each lung field every shift and more frequently in patients with bronchopulmonary disease. Peripheral pulses should be palpated and documented each shift for patients with peripheral vascular disease. Patients with HF who are started on beta-blockers should be monitored for signs and symptoms of worsening HF and fluid retention, such as edema, elevated jugular venous pulsations, pulmonary crackles, increased shortness of breath, orthopnea, and paroxysmal nocturnal dyspnea.

8. Are there drug interactions to be concerned about in a patient who is prescribed a beta-blocking drug?

Drugs that depress myocardial function or slow the heart rate, such as calcium channel blockers, digitalis, phenytoin (Dilantin), and amiodarone, are of particular concern when used with beta-blocker therapy. Beta-blockers may also increase lidocaine levels with the potential for toxicity.

9. What patient teaching is needed when starting a beta-blocker for the first time?

Patients must be informed that they should never abruptly discontinue beta-blocker therapy without consulting their health care provider and should be sure to have an adequate amount of medication on hand when traveling.

Patients and family members should be taught to look for symptoms of bradycardia, such as dizziness, fatigue, or syncope, and should be instructed in the technique to count the patient's pulse. Patients with HF should be educated to look for the symptoms of worsening HF, such as swelling, weight gain, orthopnea, increased shortness of breath, or fatigue. If these symptoms occur, patients should call their health care provider immediately. Extended-release beta-blockers should be taken with food to potentiate consistent breakdown of the pill in the gastrointestinal system. Ideally, beta-blockers should be taken 1 hour apart from other antihypertensive agents to avoid possible hypotension and dizziness. Beta-blockers should never be abruptly discontinued because acute withdrawal could cause serious side effects, including increased angina, myocardial infarction, or sudden death in patients with coronary artery disease. The beta-blocker dose should be slowly tapered before discontinuation.

10. Are there any controversies concerning beta-blocker therapy?

Although beta-blockers are clearly indicated for the treatment of systolic HF, their role in diastolic HF is unknown at this time. Many HF experts, however, recommend the use of beta-blockers for the treatment of diastolic HF.

The uptitration of angiotensin-converting enzyme (ACE) inhibitors concomitantly with beta-blockers in patients with HF has been a controversial issue. Some practitioners believe that the ACE inhibitor dose should be maximized before initiation of beta-blocker therapy; however, patients need not be taking high doses of ACE inhibitors before consideration for treatment with a beta-blocker. In patients taking a low dose of an ACE inhibitor, the addition of a beta-blocker produces a greater improvement in symptoms and reduction in the risk of death than an increase in the dose of the ACE inhibitor, even to the target doses used in clinical trials.

Several issues regarding beta-blocker use in the treatment of HF remain open for debate, including the role of beta-blockers in asymptomatic patients or patients who have severe (New York Heart Association [NYHA] class IV) HF. The COPERNICUS trial suggested that patients with severe HF can receive beta-blocker therapy, but no hard and fast rules exist for beta-blocker use in asymptomatic or severely symptomatic HF patients at this time. Consensus guidelines call for beta-blocker therapy in patients with HF who are mildly symptomatic to reduce the risk of disease progression. Conversely, patients with severe HF whose conditions are clinically unstable (intensive care unit stay, fluid volume overloaded or depleted, or recently in need of a positive inotropic agent) should not receive beta-blocker therapy until they are clinically stable.

CALCIUM CHANNEL BLOCKERS

1. How do calcium channel blockers work?

Calcium channel blockers (or calcium channel antagonists) block the initial calcium influx into cardiac cells and vascular smooth muscle cells. In the management of arrhythmias, verapamil hydrochloride and diltiazem hydrochloride affect the sinoatrial and atrioventricular nodes to slow depolarization and conduction, thus slowing or terminating supraventricular arrhythmias. Dihydropyridine calcium channel blockers cause significant vasodilation and a decrease in blood pressure that diminishes myocardial workload, consequently relieving angina pectoris. In addition, they vasodilate coronary arteries, reduce coronary resistance, increase coronary blood flow, and may enhance the formation of coronary collateral circulation. Dihydropyridine calcium channel blockers have little or no affect on the sinoatrial and atrioventricular nodes.

2. What are some examples of calcium channel blockers?

Examples of calcium channel blockers include: verapamil hydrochloride, diltiazem hydrochloride, and the dihydropyridines nifedipine, felodipine, amlodipine besylate, nicardipine hydrochloride, nisoldipine, and isradipine. See the following table for dosages.

Calcium Channel Blockers

Generic Name	Trade Name	Beginning Dose/ Frequency	Maximal Dose
Verapamil hydrochloride	Calan	80 mg three times a day	*480 mg/d
	Calan SR	180 mg once a day	*480 mg/d
	Covera-HS	180 mg at bedtime	480 mg at bedtime
	Isoptin SR	120-180 mg in AM	240 mg every 12 hr
	Verelan PM	200 mg at bedtime	400 mg at bedtime
Diltiazem hydrochloride	Cardizem CD	180-240 mg once a day	480 mg once a day
	Cardizem SR	60-120 mg twice a day	*360 mg/d
	Dilacor-XR	180-240 mg once a day	540 mg/d
	Tiazac	120-180 mg once a day	540 mg/d
Dihydropyridines			
Amlodipine besylate	Norvasc	5 mg once a day	10 mg once a day
Felodipine	Plendil	5 mg once a day	10 mg once a day
Isradipine	DynaCirc	2.5 mg twice a day	*20 mg/d
	DynaCirc CR	5 mg once a day	20 mg/d
Nicardipine hydrochloride	Cardene	20 mg three times a day	*120 mg/d
	Cardene SR	30 mg twice a day	60 mg twice a day
Nifedipine	Adalat CC	30 mg once a day	90 mg once a day
	Procardia	10 mg three times a day	30 mg/dose, 180 mg/d
	Procardia XL	30-60 mg once a day	90 mg once a day
Nisoldipine	Sular	20 mg once a day	60 mg once a day

*May be given in divided daily doses.

3. **What is the difference between dihydropyridine calcium channel blockers and other calcium channel blockers?**

Calcium channel blockers can be divided into two categories: dihydropyridines, which block the L-type calcium channels, and nondihydropyridines (verapamil hydrochloride and diltiazem hydrochloride). The dihydropyridines are potent vasodilators that have little or no negative effect on cardiac contractility or conduction. Verapamil hydrochloride and diltiazem hydrochloride decrease cardiac contractility, slow conduction, and are less potent vasodilators.

4. **What are the indications for use of calcium channel blockers?**

Calcium channel blockers are widely used in the treatment of hypertension, stable angina pectoris, vasospastic angina, and supraventricular arrhythmias. Because of their effect on sinus and atrioventricular tissue, verapamil hydrochloride and diltiazem hydrochloride are often used for management of supraventricular tachycardias and to slow the heart rate in atrial fibrillation and atrial flutter. Verapamil hydrochloride has also been used in the prophylactic treatment of cluster headaches.

5. **What are some contraindications to the use of calcium channel blockers?**

Because nondihydropyridines (verapamil hydrochloride and diltiazem hydrochloride) can depress cardiac contractility and slow conduction through the heart, they are relatively contraindicated in patients taking beta-blockers, patients who have left ventricular systolic dysfunction, and patients with existing conduction defects such as sick sinus syndrome or atrioventricular block. Speculation exists that large doses of short-acting calcium channel blockers, such as nifedipine, may increase mortality in patients immediately after myocardial infarction and thus should be avoided in these patients.

6. **What are the side effects associated with calcium channel blocker therapy?**

Side effects of the different calcium channel blockers vary from agent to agent. Those that are potent vasodilators can cause headache, dizziness or lightheadedness, flushing, and peripheral edema. The major side effect of verapamil hydrochloride is constipation.

7. **Are there any particular nursing assessment issues in care for a patient who is started on calcium channel blocker therapy?**

The patient's heart rate should be carefully monitored and recorded, with assessment for changes and the presence of bradycardia. The electrocardiogram should be continuously monitored if patients are being treated for supraventricular arrhythmias, with evaluation of the effectiveness of the calcium channel blocker in terminating or controlling the arrhythmia. Patients should also undergo assessment for the presence of new peripheral edema.

8. **Are there drug interactions to be concerned about in a patient who is prescribed a calcium channel blocking drug?**

   Drugs that depress myocardial function or slow the heart rate—such as beta-blockers, digitalis, phenytoin (Dilantin), and amiodarone—are of particular concern when used in the presence of calcium channel blocker therapy. Anticonvulsant drugs, such as phenytoin and phenobarbital, can decrease bioavailability of felodipine and nifedipine, requiring higher doses. Conversely, drinking grapefruit juice or eating unprocessed grapefruit can increase the plasma concentration of felodipine considerably. Propranolol, and presumably other beta-blockers, decreases hepatic blood flow and slows nisoldipine elimination.

9. **What patient teaching is needed when starting a calcium channel blocker for the first time?**

   Patients and family members should be taught to look for symptoms of bradycardia, such as dizziness, fatigue, or syncope, and should be instructed in the technique to count the patient's pulse. Patients should be taught to assess for peripheral edema and should contact their health care provider if edema occurs. They should be instructed to avoid drinking grapefruit juice or eating fresh grapefruit.

10. **Are there any controversies concerning calcium channel blocker therapy?**

    Calcium channel blockers have not been shown to be beneficial in the immediate postmyocardial infarction period and, in fact, may be harmful. Large doses of short-acting nifedipine may increase mortality in these patients from profound hypotension and sympathetic activation.

    Although the dihydropyridine calcium channel blockers may be used to treat hypertension or angina in patients with congestive HF, the negative inotropic effects of verapamil hydrochloride and diltiazem hydrochloride may increase mortality in these patients. Some short-acting calcium channel blockers (verapamil hydrochloride, diltiazem hydrochloride, and nifedipine) have been shown in some studies to increase mortality in patients with hypertension by increasing the risk for myocardial infarction. The findings in these studies were inconclusive and may have been caused by confounding variables, such as patient selection. Other studies suggested that short-acting nifedipine may increase mortality in elderly patients, short-acting verapamil hydrochloride or diltiazem hydrochloride may increase the risk of gastrointestinal hemorrhage, and short-acting verapamil hydrochloride or nifedipine may increase the incidence of various cancers. These results are controversial, and many of the studies have been criticized by experts. Furthermore, other studies have been published that show no increased risk from the longer acting calcium channel blockers. Consequently, current recommendations suggest that the use of short-acting calcium channel blockers should be curtailed but that the long-acting agents are safe when used appropriately. Experts suggest, however, that calcium channel blockers should not be used as a first-line drug in the treatment of most patients with hypertension because they lack the cardiovascular benefits of some other agents, such as ACE inhibitors and beta-blockers.

Key Points

- Beta-blocking drugs inhibit catecholamines, such as norepinephrine, at the beta-adrenoreceptor sites in cells and block the stimulating effects, resulting in decreased heart rate, decreased contractility, slowed atrioventricular conduction, and blunting of bronchodilatation.
- Beta-blockers are used in the treatment of stable and unstable angina pectoris, hypertension, acute myocardial infarction, congestive HF from systolic or diastolic dysfunction, and the therapy and prevention of some arrhythmias.
- Calcium channel blockers are widely used in the treatment of hypertension, stable angina pectoris, vasospastic angina, and supraventricular arrhythmias.
- Calcium channel blockers can be divided into two categories: dihydropyridines, which block the L-type calcium channels, and nondihydropyridines (verapamil hydrochloride and diltiazem hydrochloride).
- Because nondihydropyridines can depress cardiac contractility and slow conduction through the heart, they are relatively contraindicated in patients taking beta-blockers, patients who have left ventricular systolic dysfunction, and patients with existing conduction defects.

Internet Resources

Texas Heart Institute: Medicines for Cardiovascular Disease:
http://www.tmc.edu/thi/cardmeds.html

What You Need to Know About Heart Disease/Cardiology:
http://heartdisease.about.com/cs/cardiacdrugs/

Bibliography

Abernethy DR, Schwartz JB: Calcium-antagonist drugs, *N Engl J Med* 341(19):1447-1457, 1999.

Bailey DG, Arnold MO, Munoz C, Spence JD: Grapefruit juice—felodipine interaction: mechanism, predictability, and effect of naringin, *Clin Pharmacol Ther* 53(6):637-642, 1993.

Dangerfield L, Paul S: Calcium channel blockers: current and future trends, *Am J Nurs* 5(suppl):14-20, 1997.

Dargie HJ: Effect of carvedilol on outcome after myocardial infarction in patients with left ventricular dysfunction: the CAPRICORN randomised trial, *Lancet* 357(9266):1385-1390, 2001.

de Vries RJ, van Veldhuisen DJ, Dunselman PH: Efficacy and safety of calcium channel blockers in heart failure: focus on recent trials with second-generation dihydropyridines, *Am Heart J* 139(2 part 1):185-194, 2000.

Furberg CD, Psaty BM, Meyer JV: Nifedipine: dose-related increase in mortality in patients with coronary heart disease, *Circulation* 92(5):1326-1331, 1995.

Gottlieb S, McCarter R, Vogel R: Effect of beta blockade on mortality among high risk and low risk patients after myocardial infarction, *N Engl J Med* 343(6):1196, 2000.

Hall R, Chong C: A double-blind, parallel-group study of amlodipine versus long-acting nitrate in the management of elderly patients with stable angina, *Cardiology* 96(2):72-77, 2001.

Hjalmarson A, Goldstein S, Fagerberg B et al: Effects of controlled-release metoprolol on total mortality, hospitalizations, and well-being in patients with heart failure: the Metoprolol CR/XL Randomized Intervention Trial in Congestive Heart Failure (MERIT-HF), *JAMA* 283(10):1295-1302, 2000.

Julius S, Majahalme S, Palatini P: Antihypertensive treatment of patients with diabetes and hypertension, *Am J Hypertens* 14(11 pt 2):310S-316S, 2001.

Kennedy H: Current utilization trends for beta blockers in cardiovascular disease, *Am J Med* 110(5A):2S-6S, 2001.

Leone M, D'Amico D, Frediani F et al: Verapamil in the prophylaxis of episodic cluster headache: a double-blind study versus placebo, *Neurology* 54:1382-1385, 2000.

Opie LH: Calcium channel blockers in hypertension: reappraisal after new trials and major meta-analyses, *Am J Hypertens* 14(10):1074-1081, 2001.

Opie LH, Schall R: Evidence-based evaluation of calcium channel blockers for hypertension: equality of mortality and cardiovascular risk relative to conventional therapy, *J Am Coll Cardiol* 39(2):315-322, 2002.

Packer M: Current role of beta-adrenergic blockers in the management of chronic heart failure, *Am J Med* 110(7A):81S-94S, 2001.

Packer M, Bristow MR, Cohn JN et al, for the US Carvedilol Heart Failure Study Group: The effect of carvedilol on morbidity and mortality in patients with chronic heart failure, *N Engl J Med* 334(21):1349-1355, 1996.

Ryan TJ, Antman EM, Brooks NH et al: 1999 update: ACC/AHA guidelines for the management of patients with acute myocardial infarction: executive summary and recommendations, a report of the American College of Cardiology/American Heart Association Task Force on Practice Guidelines (Committee on Management of Acute Myocardial Infarction), *Circulation* 100:1016-1030, 1999.

Angiotensin-Converting Enzyme Inhibitors and Angiotensin-Receptor Blockers

Sara Paul

ANGIOTENSIN-CONVERTING ENZYME INHIBITORS

1. How do angiotensin-converting enzyme (ACE) inhibitors work?

Angiotensin II is a neurohormone that plays a role in regulation of intravascular fluid volume by promoting sodium and water retention. It increases vascular resistance by causing arteriolar vasoconstriction and elevates blood pressure. Angiotensin II contributes to the remodeling process of the left ventricle, leading to hypertrophy and heart failure, stimulates sympathetic system stimulation, and promotes the development of atherosclerosis, particularly in patients with hyperlipidemia. ACE inhibitors block the formation of angiotensin II by blocking the enzyme that combines with angiotensin I to form angiotensin II.

2. What are some examples of ACE inhibitors?

Examples of ACE inhibitors include alacepril, benazepril hydrochloride, captopril, cilazapril, delapril, enalapril, fosinopril sodium, imidapril, lisinopril, moexipril hydrochloride, omapatrilat, perindopril, quinapril hydrochloride, ramipril, spirapril, trandolapril, and zofenopril (see the following table).

Angiotensin-Converting Enzyme Inhibitors

Generic Name	Trade Name	Starting Dose/ Frequency	Maximum Dose
Benazepril hydrochloride	Lotensin	10-20 mg once a day	20 mg twice a day
Captopril	Capoten	6.25 mg three times a day	50 mg three times a day
Enalapril	Vasotec	2.5 mg twice a day	10-20 mg twice a day
Fosinopril sodium	Monopril	5-10 mg once a day	40 mg once a day
Lisinopril	Prinivil	2.5-5 mg once a day	20-40 mg once a day
Moexipril hydrochloride	Univasc	3.75 mg once a day	*60 mg once a day
Perindopril	Aceon	4 mg once a day	8 mg once a day
Quinapril hydrochloride	Accupril	10 mg twice a day	40 mg twice a day
Ramipril	Altace	1.25-2.5 mg once a day	10 mg once a day
Trandolapril	Mavik	1 mg once a day	8 mg once a day

*May be given in two divided doses.

3. What are the indications for use of ACE inhibitors?

Angiotensin-converting enzyme inhibitors are used in the management of patients with hypertension, congestive heart failure, and postmyocardial infarction and to protect renal function in diabetic and nondiabetic nephropathy.

4. What are some contraindications to the use of ACE inhibitors?

Patients with angioedema (swelling of the lips or tongue) should never use ACE inhibitors again, regardless of the dose or brand of drug. Soft tissue swelling of angioedema can proceed to the point of obstructing the airway, creating a life-threatening situation. Pregnancy is a contraindication to the use of ACE inhibitors, and they should be used cautiously in patients with aortic stenosis, hepatic dysfunction, hyperkalemia, hypotension, neutropenia, proteinuria, renal insufficiency, and renal artery stenosis. They should be avoided if possible during breastfeeding

5. What are the side effects associated with ACE inhibitor therapy?

The major side effects associated with ACE inhibitors include hypotension, acute renal failure, hyperkalemia, chronic cough, angioedema, and anaphylactic-type reactions. Impotence has been reported during therapy with various ACE inhibitors, and occasional gastrointestinal side effects, such as loss of taste, may occur.

6. Are there any particular nursing assessment issues in care for a patient who is started on ACE inhibitor therapy?

Patients should have a baseline electrolyte panel drawn before starting therapy with an ACE inhibitor, and electrolytes should be checked regularly, particularly if the patient is undergoing diuresis or is on a potassium supplement. If the patient's renal function is stable, electrolytes should be reevaluated when clinically indicated, such as with a change of condition. If the patient has renal insufficiency or if an electrolyte imbalance is suspected, electrolytes should be checked monthly. Patients should be checked for volume depletion, and blood pressure should be monitored at least each shift during a hospital stay. Blood pressures should be checked supine, sitting, and standing if the patient has any symptoms of orthostatic dizziness. Patients with symptoms of cough should be carefully evaluated to determine the cause. If the patient has any signs or symptoms of angioedema (mouth or lip swelling), the ACE inhibitor must be discontinued immediately and the physician or nurse practitioner notified.

7. Are there drug interactions to be concerned about in a patient who is prescribed an ACE inhibitor?

Some data suggest that higher doses of aspirin decrease the effectiveness of ACE inhibitors by blocking prostaglandin synthesis. The use of ACE inhibitors in patients receiving azathioprine has been reported to result in anemia or leukopenia. Concomitant use of ACE inhibitors and cyclosporine may decrease renal function. In a number of case reports, the concomitant use of lithium and ACE inhibitors has been reported to increase lithium levels by as much as threefold. Severe postural hypotension has been reported when ACE inhibitors are added to loop diuretic therapy, but this response is usually transient. Nonsteroidal antiinflammatory drugs may decrease the antihypertensive and sodium excreting effect of ACE inhibitors. ACE inhibitor therapy can result in potassium retention, causing severe hyperkalemia and arrhythmias when combined with potassium supplements or potassium-sparing diuretics.

8. What patient teaching is needed when starting an ACE inhibitor for the first time?

Patients should avoid alcohol when taking ACE inhibitors and should not use potassium-based salt substitutes in their diet. They need to notify their health care provider if they have any of the following symptoms: extreme weakness, hoarseness, lip or tongue swelling, trouble breathing or swallowing, dizziness, skin rash or hives, and yellowing of skin or eyes. Patients should monitor their blood pressure at home, especially when first starting an ACE inhibitor or when the dose is increased. ACE inhibitors should not be used during pregnancy.

9. Are there any particular concerns about ACE inhibitors in the presence of other comorbid conditions?

Angiotensin-converting enzyme inhibitors should be used with extreme caution in the presence of renal insufficiency.

10. Are there any controversies concerning ACE inhibitor therapy?

The question of aspirin/ACE inhibitor interaction is controversial. Many experts recommend using lower doses of aspirin in the presence of ACE inhibitors, but clinicians must weigh the benefits against the risks of aspirin therapy in these patients.

ANGIOTENSIN-RECEPTOR BLOCKERS

1. How do angiotensin-receptor blockers (ARBs) work?

Rather than blocking the formation of angiotensin II, ARBs block angiotensin II at the receptor site of the cells to prevent it from having an effect on the cell.

2. What are some examples of ARBs?

Examples of ARBs include: candesartan cilexetil, eprosartan, irbesartan, losartan potassium, tasosartan, telmisartan, and valsartan (see the following table).

Angiotensin-Receptor Blockers

Generic Name	Trade Name	Starting Dose/Frequency	Maximum Dose
Candesartan cilexetil	Atacand	8 mg once a day	*32 mg once a day
Eprosartan	Teveten	*400 mg once a day	*800 mg once a day
Irbesartan	Avapro	150 mg once a day	300 mg once a day
Losartan potassium	Cozaar	25 mg once to twice a day	100 mg once to twice a day
Telmisartan	Micardis	20 mg once a day	80 mg once a day
Valsartan	Diovan	80 mg once a day	320 mg once a day

*May be given in two divided doses.

3. What are the indications for the use of ARBs?

Angiotensin-receptor blockers are approved by the US Food and Drug Administration for use in hypertension but are sometimes used in patients with heart failure in whom an intolerance to ACE inhibitors develops. Extreme caution must be used in patients with angioedema from an ACE inhibitor because ARBs may also cause angioedema, although it is more uncommon. Currently, ARBs are being evaluated for first-line agents in heart failure, myocardial infarction, and diabetes with hypertension in place of ACE inhibitors.

4. What are some contraindications to the use of ARBs?

Angiotensin-receptor blockers are contraindicated in pregnancy and should be avoided if possible during breastfeeding. Reduced doses should be used in the presence of renal or hepatic impairment, although some ARBs are contraindicated in patients with severe hepatic impairment, cirrhosis, or biliary obstruction.

5. What are the side effects associated with the use of ARBs?

As with ACE inhibitors, the side effects of ARBs are usually mild and transient and include headache, dizziness, and orthostatic hypotension, particularly in patients with volume depletion. Hyperkalemia and myalgia have been reported, and more rarely, rash, angioedema, and elevated liver enzymes. Rare episodes of angioedema have been reported with ARB use. Anemia and neutropenia have also been reported.

6. Are there any particular nursing assessment issues with care for a patient who is started on an ARB?

The nursing assessment issues are the same for ARBs as they are for ACE inhibitors.

7. Are there drug interactions to be concerned about in a patient who is prescribed an ARB?

Co-administration of ARBs and potassium supplements or potassium-sparing diuretics may result in elevated serum potassium levels. Patients on an ARB and lithium may be at risk for lithium toxicity.

8. What patient teaching is needed when starting an ARB for the first time?

Patient teaching issues are the same for ARBs as they are for ACE inhibitors.

9. Are there any particular concerns about use of an ARB in the presence of other comorbid conditions?

Angiotensin-receptor blockers should be used with extreme caution in the presence of aortic or mitral valve stenosis, biliary cirrhosis or obstruction, hepatic dysfunction, hypotension, or renal artery stenosis.

10. Are there any controversies concerning ARB therapy?

- It remains to be proven that angiotensin II receptor antagonists have the same clinical benefits as ACE inhibitors aside from blood pressure reduction. Studies are currently ongoing to compare ACE inhibitors with ARBs and to combine the two drugs in the treatment of heart failure.
- In addition, ongoing clinical trials are evaluating the use of combination ACE inhibitor and ARB use in the treatment of heart failure. The Val-HeFT trial concluded that an ACE inhibitor and an ARB should be used concomitantly in patients with heart failure who cannot tolerate a beta-blocker. The use of all three drugs (ACE inhibitor, ARB, and beta-blocker) is not recommended.
- The LIFE study (more than 9000 patients aged 55 to 80 years) recently showed a clinical advantage of ARB and diuretic over beta-blocker and diuretic in the treatment of patients with hypertension with left ventricular hypertrophy. Although blood pressure reduction was similar in both groups, a greater reduction in cardiovascular death, fatal and nonfatal stroke, and new onset diabetes in the ARB-treated group was seen. Nonfatal and fatal MI was slightly less in the beta-blocker group.

 Key Points

- Angiotensin II is a neurohormone that contributes to the remodeling process of the left ventricle, leading to hypertrophy and heart failure, that stimulates sympathetic system stimulation, and that promotes the development of atherosclerosis, particularly in patients with hyperlipidemia.
- Angiotensin-converting enzyme inhibitors block the formation of angiotensin II by blocking the enzyme that combines with angiotensin I to form angiotensin II.

Continued

Key Points *continued*

- Angiotensin-converting enzyme inhibitors are used in the management of patients with hypertension, congestive heart failure, and postmyocardial infarction and to protect renal function in diabetic and nondiabetic nephropathy.
- Rather than blocking the formation of angiotensin II, ARBs block angiotensin II at the receptor site of the cells to prevent it from having an effect on the cell.
- Angiotensin-receptor blockers are approved for use in hypertension but are sometimes used in patients with heart failure who are intolerant to ACE inhibitors.

Internet Resources

Health A to Z: Angiotensin Converting Enzyme Inhibitors:
http://www.healthatoz.com/healthatoz/Atoz/ency/angiotensin-converting_enzyme_inhibitors.html

Personal Health Zone: ACE Inhibitors: Interactions and Warnings:
http://www.personalhealthzone.com/drug_interactions/ace_inhibitors.html

The Thomson Corporation: Angiotensin Converting Enzyme Inhibitors
http://www.ehendrick.org/healthy/000079.htm

Therapeutics Letter: Angiotensin II Receptor Blockers:
www.ti.ubc.ca/PDF/28.PDF

CoreyNahman.com (Internet Drug News): Angiotensin Receptor Blockers:
http://www.coreynahman.com/Angiotensinreceptorblockers_ARBs.html

Bibliography

Adams KF Jr, Baughman KL, Dec WG et al: HFSA guidelines for management of patients with heart failure caused by left ventricular systolic dysfunction: pharmacologic approaches, *Pharmacotherapy* 20(5):495-522, 2000.

Baruch L, Anand I, Cohen IS et al: Augmented short- and long-term hemodynamic and hormonal effects of an angiotensin receptor blocker added to angiotensin converting enzyme inhibitor therapy in patients with heart failure, *Circulation* 99:2658-2664, 1999.

Carson PE: Rationale for the use of combination angiotensin-converting enzyme inhibitor/angiotensin II receptor blocker therapy in heart failure, *Am Heart J* 140:361-366, 2000.

Cundy T: Diabetic nephropathy in indigenous populations: prevention and management of diabetic nephropathy, *Nephrology* 4:S76-S80, 1998.

Giles TD, Sander GE: Angiotensin II receptor (AT1) antagonists in heart failure after Val-HeFT—Quo Vadis? *Am J Geriatr Cardiol* 10(1):60-63, 2001.

Jorde UP, Ennezat PV, Lisker J et al: Maximally recommended doses of angiotensin-converting enzyme (ACE) inhibitors do not completely prevent ACE-mediated formation of angiotensin II in chronic heart failure, *Circulation* 101(8):844-846, 2000.

Krumholz H, Chen Y, Wang Y et al: Aspirin and angiotensin-converting enzyme inhibitors among elderly survivors of hospitalization for an acute myocardial infarction, *Arch Intern Med* 161:538-544, 2001.

Lindholm LH, Ibsen H, Dahlof B et al: The LIFE Study Group: cardiovascular morbidity and mortality in patients with diabetes in the Losartan Intervention For Endpoint reduction in hypertension study (LIFE): a randomised trial against atenolol, *Lancet* 359(9311):1004-1010, 2002.

Maschio G, Alberti D, Locatelli F et al: Angiotensin-converting enzyme inhibitors and kidney protection: the AIPRI trial, *J Cardiovasc Pharmacol* 33(suppl 1):S16-S20, 1999.

Pitt B, Poole-Wilson PA, Segal R et al: Effect of losartan compared with captopril on mortality in patients with symptomatic heart failure: randomised trial—the Losartan Heart Failure Survival Study ELITE II, *Lancet* 355:1582-1587, 2000.

Plum J, Bunten B, Nemeth R et al: Effects of the angiotensin II antagonist valsartan on blood pressure, proteinuria, and renal hemodynamics in patients with chronic renal failure and hypertension, *J Am Soc Nephrol* 9:2223-2234, 1998.

Ray KK, Dorman S, Watson RDS: Severe hyperkalaemia due to the concomitant use of salt substitutes and ACE inhibitors in hypertension: a potentially life threatening interaction, *J Hum Hypertens* 13:717-720, 1999.

Song JC, White CM: Pharmacologic, pharmacokinetic, and therapeutic differences among angiotensin II receptor antagonists, *Pharmacotherapy* 20(2):130-139, 2000.

Struthers AD: Angiotensin II receptor antagonists for heart failure, *Heart* 80:5-6, 1998.

Swedberg K, Held P, Kjekshus J et al: The CONSENSUS Trial Study Group: effects of enalapril on mortality in severe congestive heart failure, *N Engl J Med* 316:1429-1435, 1987.

The sixth report of the Joint National Committee on Prevention, Detection, Evaluation, and Treatment of High Blood Pressure, *Arch Intern Med* 157:2413-2446, 1997.

Warner KK, Visconti JA, Tschampel MM: Angiotensin II receptor blockers in patients with ACE inhibitor-induced angioedema, *Ann Pharmacother* 34(4):526-528, 2000.

Wright JM: Choosing a first-line drug in the management of elevated blood pressure: what is the evidence? 3: angiotensin-converting enzyme inhibitors, *Can Med Assoc* 163(3):293-296, 2000.

Digoxin and Other Positive Inotropic Agents

Jana M. Glotzer

1. What is an inotropic agent or inotrope?

Ino- is a Greek prefix defined as pertaining to a muscle or fiber, and the suffix *–tropic* is defined as affecting or changing. Therefore *inotrope* refers to a substance that alters the muscle fiber's contraction. A positive inotrope increases the myocardial fibers speed or force of contraction (FOC), and a negative inotrope adversely affects myocardial contraction. For the purposes of this chapter, inotrope always refers to a positive inotrope. The main physiologic objective in the treatment of chronic heart failure (HF) is not simply to make the heart pump harder but to enhance tissue perfusion. An inotrope enhances tissue perfusion by increasing the myocardial FOC, which raises the left ventricular ejection fraction (LVEF), thereby augmenting the cardiac output (CO) and the cardiac index (CI).

2. What are the most common inotropic agents used?

Inotrope	Agent	Trade Name	Strength	Indications
Digitalis glycoside	Digoxin	Lanoxin Digitek	↑	Chronic heart failure (HF) New York Heart Association class II-IV
Catecholamine	Dopamine	Intropin	↑↑↑↑	Symptomatic hypotension. To improve renal perfusion (at low doses). Rarely used in HF syndromes.
Synthetic catecholamine	Dobutamine	Dobutrex	↑↑↑	Acute decompensated HF (ADHF) with hypoperfusion syndrome.
Phosphodiesterase inhibitors	Milrinone	Primacor	↑↑	ADHF with hypoperfusion syndrome.

3. How many oral inotropes are on the US market?

Just one, the digitalis glycoside, digoxin.

4. Is digoxin still advocated in the treatment of chronic HF?

Yes. In the early 1990s, use of digoxin in the treatment of HF fell out of favor because it was determined to be a weak inotrope. However, since then, several rigorous clinical research studies strongly support the use of digoxin in HF. Both the 1999 HF guidelines established by the Heart Failure Society of America (HFSA) and the 2001 American College of Cardiology (ACC)/American Heart Association (AHA) advocate the use of digoxin in HF.

5. Why is digoxin still standard therapy in HF if it is such a weak inotrope?

For years, the benefit of digoxin in systolic HF was attributed solely to its inotropic action, which occurs by attenuating neurohormonal mechanisms in the cardiac muscle. More recent findings have found that the neurohormonal inhibition in other areas, such as the vagus nerve and kidneys, is more likely responsible for the improvement of clinical outcomes in patients with HF treated with digoxin. Autonomic dysfunction in HF is dampened by modulating enzyme production in the vagus nerve, which helps maintain the heart rate (HR) at a slower, more steady state. The action of digoxin in the atrioventricular (AV) node also helps achieve a slower steady rate. The kidneys respond to the enzyme inhibition properties of digoxin by producing natriuresis (sodium excretion), which modulates renin secretion.

Well-designed, placebo-controlled clinical trials have shown that digoxin reduces the need for hospitalization and the need for additional medical interventions, increases exercise tolerance, provides symptomatic improvement, and yields improved quality-of-life scores. In addition, retrospective analyses of these studies found that the withdrawal of digoxin in patients with only mild symptoms of HF significantly increases the risk of worsening HF and the need for hospitalization.

6. What is the normal serum digoxin concentration (SDC)?

The most widely used SDC level is 0.8 to 2 ng/mL. However, current analyses (March 2002) have shown that an SDC between 1 and 2 ng/mL provides no additional neurohormonal inhibition or symptomatic improvement than do those levels at the lowest range (0.5 to 0.9 ng/mL). The goal of ascertaining any therapeutic range is to maximize efficacy while minimizing the risks of toxicity.

Digoxin toxicity is a serious adverse event and can be life threatening. Because medications frequently prescribed in HF, such as beta-blockers, amiodarone, captopril, loop diuretics, spironolactone, and warfarin, can elevate the SDC, maintenance of a lower SDC may help minimize the risk of toxicity. Therefore a target SDC level of 0.5 to 0.9 ng/mL is advocated because additional efficacy is not attained with higher SDCs and the side effects and risk of toxicity are dose related.

7. Besides keeping the SDC level to less than 1 ng/mL, what strategies minimize the risks of digoxin?

- Monitoring electrolytes and organ function is important because hypokalemia, hyperkalemia, hypomagnesemia, hypercalcemia, and worsening renal, liver, and thyroid function can lead to digoxin toxicity. Loop diuretics promote kaluresis; therefore a brisk diuresis obviates increased frequency of electrolyte monitoring. Timing blood draws to ensure electrolyte disturbances are identified and treated before the daily digoxin administration is important. Monitoring of the blood urea nitrogen (BUN) and creatinine daily is advocated in hospitalized patients with HF because they are at a greater risk of renal insufficiency or failure for a variety of reasons (intravenous [IV] diuretics, low output syndrome).

- In initiation of digoxin therapy, the individual's creatinine clearance (refer to Chapter 4, Selected Laboratory Procedures) should be calculated to ensure proper dose selection. Remember the elderly and debilitated should be started on half the usual dose and have periodic evaluations of creatinine clearance.

8. Is routine monitoring of SDCs a suggested approach to minimize the risks of digoxin therapy?

No. Routine SDC levels are problematic for a number of reasons. Studies have found that 16% to 38% of SDCs that were considered toxic (>2 ng/mL) were drawn too soon after the last digoxin dose. An additional 22% were not appropriately marked as to the time drawn in relation to dosing, yielding them invalid. At a cost range of an average of $50 per test, this could represent a significant annual cost for uninterpretable SDCs. Furthermore, erroneously high SDCs can subject the patient to additional inconvenient, expensive, and often invasive tests to rule out digoxin toxicity.

9. Under what circumstances is monitoring of a patient's SDC appropriate?

- After a patient has achieved a stable state (usually 2 to 3 weeks) after initiation or titration of digoxin or the addition of a concomitant medication that affects SDC.
- If signs or symptoms of toxicity exist.
- If a significant decline in renal function is seen.
- After a steady state is achieved after initiation in the elderly.

10. How soon after a patient begins a dose should a digoxin level be drawn?

The gold standard, and the way all major clinical trials evaluate SDCs, is drawing a trough sample, which is just before the next dosing. However, it is not always possible or prudent to wait until the next dosage is due (24 to 48 hours), particularly in the outpatient setting or when the patient is seen at the hospital with acute signs or symptoms of digoxin toxicity. Consequently, a minimum of 6 hours after dosing is acceptable. If drawn any sooner, the level is completely inaccurate and no clinical decisions should be made based on the result. Good clinical practice dictates that documentation of the time the last dose was taken accompany every SDC drawn. Also, morning phlebotomy draws should be scheduled closest to the dosing, and the lab's window for acceptable draw times and the nursing unit's window for acceptable medication administration should be taken into account. Finally, if an inpatient's level is to be drawn on the next shift, communication in the report of the need to check that the level has been drawn before administering the next dose is helpful.

11. Which concomitant medications can affect the digoxin level?

It is advised to review a more comprehensive list before initiating any new medication. Some medications may cause a mild increase in SDCs, and others markedly boost SDCs by a mean of 115% (erythromycin). The following list includes those medications that are often prescribed in the patient with chronic HF that may affect SDC:

- Alprazolam
- Antacids
- Antiarrhythmics (amiodarone, dofetilide, propafenone hydrochloride, quinidine)
- Antibiotics (clarithromycin, doxycycline, erythromycin, indomethacin, metronidazole, neomycin, rifampin, trimethoprim, tetracycline)
- Barbiturates
- Beta-blockers
- Calcium channel blockers (except amlodipine)
- Captopril
- Corticosteroids
- Cyclosporine
- Diazepam
- Diuretics
- Herbal products (flaxseed, ginger, ginseng, hawthorn, St. John's wort)
- Lipid-lowering agents (cholestyramine, colestipol hydrochloride, high-dose atorvastatin calcium, fluvastatin, simvastatin)
- Spironolactone
- Warfarin

12. If the HR is less than 60 bpm, should the digoxin dose be withheld?

Sinus bradycardia is not a reason in itself to hold the digoxin dose. Patients with HF on beta-blocker therapy are considered to have therapeutic conditions when the rate is around 60 bpm, if asymptomatic. Therefore an individualized low HR limit from the prescriber is important. However, if the HR is less than 50 bpm, the current dose should not be given and the prescriber should be notified to determine whether a SDC should be drawn or the dose held or lowered. Bradycardia in the presence of sick sinus syndrome or AV blocks is worrisome and requires particular caution. Any new cardiac rhythm disturbances should be reported to the prescriber as soon as possible.

13. What are some of the signs and symptoms of digoxin toxicity?

See the following table.

System	Signs & Symptoms
Gastrointestinal	Nausea, vomiting, anorexia, abdominal pain, diarrhea, and constipation.
Visual	Change in color of vision (more yellow color), photophobia, blurred vision, light flashes, or halos around lights.

continued	
System	**Signs & Symptoms**
Neurological	Headache, dizziness, drowsiness, fatigue, symptoms of itching, tingling in hands or feet, confusion, personality changes, or acute psychosis.
Rhythm disturbances	Any cardiac arrhythmias, but in particular heart block, ventricular tachycardia, junctional tachycardia, junctional escape beats, atrial fibrillation with slow ventricular response, sinus bradycardia (<50 bpm), and sinus arrest.

14. Is it okay for patients to take generic digoxin?

In therapy initiation, generic digoxin is fine. However, once a therapeutic level is achieved on a stable dose, brand switching is discouraged because different brands can affect each patient uniquely. With hospitalization, brands are often changed for formulary restrictions; therefore monitoring the patient for any side effects or changes in efficacy is important.

15. What information should a patient have about digoxin?

A patient should receive verbal instruction and written drug information on the effects of the medication and discontinuation, the procedures for a missed dose, the signs and symptoms of toxicity, the other medications that can affect the blood level, the importance of not changing the brand without consulting with the prescriber, the necessity of taking the medication on an empty stomach, and the medications that should be taken at a different time. Most hospitals have electronic databases with wonderful patient drug education sheets that can be personalized. If these databases are not available, many websites provide this resource for free; **www.abouthf.org** by the HFSA and **www.americanheart.org** by the AHA are good resources.

16. What are the primary indications for IV inotropic agents?

- Symptomatic hypotension and evidence of organ hypoperfusion are the primary indications for inotropic therapy. In acute shock syndromes, dopamine is usually the first line of treatment to support the blood pressure (BP) until the cause is effectively treated. Acute decompensated heart failure (ADHF) with evidence of organ hypoperfusion may occur in the absence of significant hypotension. For maintenance of perfusion to more essential organs, blood flow is shunted from less essential organs to compensate for a chronic low output state. This has a far more discrete clinical presentation than that of the acute shock syndromes. ADHF may be the result of fluid volume overload, pump failure, or both. Therefore a two-step approach can classify the clinical presentation of ADHF and clarify the treatment approach:
  - Is there evidence of congestion? If yes, then the clinical status is classified as wet. If no, then the clinical status is classified as dry.

- Is there is evidence of inadequate tissue/organ perfusion? If yes, then the clinical status is classified as cold. If not, then the clinical status is classified as warm.
- Inotropes are reserved for cold clinical profiles, either with congestion (wet/cold) or without congestion (dry/cold). The least common hospital presentation of ADHF is the dry/cold clinical profile, and inotropic agents are the medicinal treatment of choice. Vasodilator or diuretic use in this clinical presentation can cause profound hypotension or irreversible organ damage or failure. Once the inotropic agent successfully augments the CO, concomitant use of vasodilators may be considered.
- A far more frequent hospital presentation of ADHF is the wet/cold clinical presentation, which can be corrected with IV diuretics because the cause of the low output state may be congestion. However, diuretics are often minimally effective or ineffective because of poor renal perfusion. In this scenario, concomitant administration of an inotrope can enhance renal perfusion so the IV diuretics can produce a more brisk diuresis.
- Essential to management of each of these clinical profiles is refined interviewing and assessment skills that can ferret out the more subtle signs and symptoms of low output. Most everyone can easily recognize the patient with congestion, but low output indicators are more discrete; they can be few and within just one organ. In fact, identification of an isolated sign or symptom (low serum sodium with fluid restriction or increased creatinine levels in a patient with euvolemia) can really affect outcomes by preventing organ failure. Actually, if the patient has numerous low output indicators that span multiple organ systems, cardiogenic shock may be imminent. Therefore honed assessment skills that recognize discrete low output indicators, accompanied by prompt tailored therapeutic interventions, can prevent organ failure and cardiogenic shock.

17. How do the signs and symptoms of low output differ from congestion?

To tailor the right therapy for the individual patient, differentiation of which signs and symptoms are related to congestion or low output is important. See the following table.

System	Congestion: "Wet"*	Low Output: "Cold"*
Cardiovascular	↑ Jugular venous distension (JVD), gallop, S_3, new onset or increased mitral regurgitation, + hepatojugular reflux, right ventricular heave. Hyperstatic (after standing for 3 min: blood pressure [BP] ↑ and heart rate [HR] ↓), ↑ central venous pressure (CVP) or right atrial pressure.	Absent JVD, ↓ systolic BP (usually <85 mm Hg or if symptomatic), positive orthostasis (after standing for 3 min: ↓ BP and ↑ HR), resting tachycardia, ↓ mean arterial pressure, narrow pulse pressure, ↑ systemic vascular resistance, ↓ temperature.

continued

System	Congestion: "Wet"*	Low Output: "Cold"*
Pulmonary	**Orthopnea, paroxysmal nocturnal dyspnea (PND), nocturnal cough**, dyspnea on exertion (DOE), **rales** (may be absent), wheezes, ↓ breath sound (BS), pleural effusions, ↑ respiratory rate (RR), ↓ O$_2$ saturations, fluid on chest radiograph (CXR); if absent, does not rule out congestion.	**Dyspnea without orthopnea or PND**, DOE with clear BS, ↑ RR, Cheyne-Stokes respirations, clear CXR, ↓ myocardial oxygen consumption and arterial O$_2$ saturations.
Gastrointestinal	**Hepatomegaly, ascites**, right upper quadrant (RUQ) tenderness, elevated liver function tests (LFTs), nausea, vomiting, diarrhea, and anorexia.	↑ **LFTs without hepatomegaly**, RUQ pain, nausea, vomiting, diarrhea, constipation, early satiety, anorexia, **bright red blood per rectum** with prolonged bowel ischemia.
Renal	Urinary output may be ↑ if oral intake ↑. Nocturia.	↑ Blood urea nitrogen (BUN), ↑ Creatinine (Cr). ↑ BUN:Cr ratio, oliguria, anuria (if acute ↓ output syndrome), ↔ if chronic low output.
Metabolic	**Excessive thirst, dry mouth.**	↓ **Serum sodium**, ↑ glucose intolerance, ↑ insulin requirements.
Neurologic	Can be normal or apprehensive.	Depression, confusion, **lethargy**, and **somnolence**.
Extremities	Warm; **pitting edema**; strong peripheral pulses, shoes and/or belt tightening.	**Cool**, absent or nonpitting edema, weak peripheral pulses.
General	Weight gain or stable weight with anorexia.	↓ Exercise capacity, **fatigue at rest**, weight loss, **cachexia, temporal wasting**.

*Indicators in bold are more classic hallmarks of the clinical profile.

18. What factors affect the choice of inotrope selection?

Many factors go into the inotrope selection. As previously stated, inotrope treatment should be reserved for the cold clinical profile. In the tailoring of therapy to each patient's unique clinical presentation, other important considerations are volume status, BP, pulmonary artery pressures, and current beta-blocker usage. Basically, milrinone can be the superior choice for the patient with the cold and wet profile without either orthostasis or hypotension (systolic BP [SBP], <90 mm Hg). In addition to its inotropic action, milrinone has greater vasodilatation properties than dobutamine, which provides better afterload reduction, and therefore more adequately lowers the pulmonary pressures. Milrinone is the better choice for the patient with ADHF on beta-blocker therapy because dobutamine's inotropic action is dependent on interfering with the beta1 receptors. However, if dobutamine is the preferred agent for another reason, it can be used in patients on beta-blocker therapy, but higher doses may be necessary to achieve the same desired effect and the side effects of inotropes are dose related.

In the patient with the cold/dry clinical profile and hypotension (SBP, <90 mm Hg), dobutamine is the drug of choice because it has less vasodilatory properties that can cause/exacerbate hypotension. Dobutamine and milrinone can be given together in the patient who is refractory to either treatment alone. For further information, see Question 20.

19. How are warm clinical presentations of ADHF treated?

These presentations are treated with increased dosage or frequency of oral diuretics, IV diuretics, or the addition of vasodilators.

20. What are common IV inotropes used in HF, and how are they used?

Agent		Indications	Dose Range	Primary Effect	Adverse Effects	Comments
Dopamine	Inotrope	Hypotensive shock states, symptomatic hypotension. Cold/dry clinical profile.	Renal perfusion range: 3 µg/kg/min No >20 µg/kg/min.	↑ Cardiac output (CO), ↑ stroke volume (SV), ↑ renal perfusion (only at doses <3/µg/kg/min).	↑ Heart rate (HR), ↑ arrhythmias, side effects dose related. ↑ systemic vascular resistance (SVR), ↑↑↑ cardiac damage and ↓ renal perfusion.	Not used in heart failure (HF) unless in cardiogenic shock or to ↑ renal perfusion at low doses. Can be used to temporarily treat bradycardia. Used only as adjunct agent when refractory to other inotropes.

continued						
Agent		**Indications**	**Dose Range**	**Primary Effect**	**Adverse Effects**	**Comments**
Dobutamine	Inotrope	Cold/dry or cold/ wet with hypotension.	≤6 µg/kg/ min is recommended because side effects are dose related.	↔ SVR, ↑ SV, ↑ CO ↑ cardiac index (CI) ↓ aortic impedance.	↑ HR, ↑ myocardial ischemia.	Tachyphylaxis: beta-blocker (BB) therapy, prolonged administration, or chronic HF. Proarrhythmic. Short half-life.
Milrinone	Inodilator: inotrope and vasodilator	Cold/wet: ideal therapy. Especially if ↑ pulmonary artery pressures (PAP), on BB, or with normotensive. Cold/dry if adequate blood pressure (BP).	*No bolus, start 0.1 µg/ kg/min titrate by 0.1 µg/kg/ min every 4 h and stop at 0.375-0.5 µg/ kg/min.	↓ SVR, ↓ pulmonary capillary wedge pressure ↓ pulmonary vascular resistance, ↑ SV ↑ CO, ↑ CI ↑ myocardial O₂.	Proarrhythmic: ↑ atrioventricular conduction, ↑ ventricular response in atrial fibrillation. Can cause ventricular tachycardia. Can cause sustained hypotension.	Orthostatics must be negative before starting. Long half-life means slow onset.

*Side effects are dose related; therefore lower doses than the packaging inserts purport are recommended.

21. What are the complications of IV inotropic therapy?

The possible complications of IV inotropic infusions are serious and are related to the infusion method, the length of infusion, the inotrope itself, and disease progression. Inotropes can cause profound hypotension and lethal arrhythmias and have been implicated in myocardial cell death. Prolonged indwelling IV access predisposes the patient to life-threatening infections. Infiltration into the periphery can cause tissue necrosis.

22. If the complications of IV inotrope therapy are serious, then why is there a trend to send patients home on long-term therapy?

There are two preferred circumstances in which patients may be considered for home IV inotropic therapy. The first is as a palliative measure for the patient with a formal do not resuscitate (DNR)/do not intubate (DNI) status. The goal of therapy is to improve quality of life, knowing that the quantity of life may be diminished.

The second reason home therapy may be considered is the patient who is transplant listed with a common blood type and body habitus. These patients are likely to require a lengthy waiting period and do not achieve priority status unless they are inotrope dependent or on a ventricular assist device. The traditional method to ensure safe passage for the patient who is inotrope dependent transplant listed has been a protracted hospitalization. Although this protects the patient physically, extended hospitalizations can have adverse psychological effects. Feelings of isolation, low self-esteem, loss of control, financial distress, depression, anxiety, and lost connectedness with friends and family affect outcomes. In addition, rising health care costs and acute care bed shortages make a suitable alternative attractive. The physical risks can be minimized with established written protocols and well-defined criterion.

23. What characteristics should the patient who is inotrope dependent (IDP) have to be considered for home therapy?

- First and foremost, the patient must be aware of the increased risk of sudden cardiac death (SCD), organ dysfunction, and sepsis (informed consent). An internal cardiac defibrillator minimizes this risk of SCD.
- The patient should have a history of adherence to medication and dietary regimes.
- The patient should show readiness, willingness, and capability to learn aseptic technique, how to run the infusion pump, and how to handle any pump malfunctions.
- The patient must have running water, electricity, and a telephone with long distance access.
- The patient should have a reliable household support system.
- The patient needs the capability and equipment necessary to monitor daily weights and twice daily BP, HR, and temperature.
- The patient should have reliable transportation to make biweekly (and even weekly if needed) clinic visits.
- The patient needs a home health agency for dressing changes and weekly lab sampling that is well versed on the specific care needs of the patient with HF (proper orthostatic measurements, the importance of fluid status evaluation, signs or symptoms of low output and sepsis).
- If the patient is more than 1 hour from the clinic:
  - he/she should have a local cardiologist who is willing to see the patient in a pinch.
  - he/she needs a local emergency department that transfers the patient to a tertiary center when needed
- The candidate for home inotrope therapy must have hemodynamic stability.

24. Exactly what constitutes stability?

Stability should be well defined by your institution and should not conflict with the institutional protocols, policies or procedures that are written to ensure safe management of the inpatient requiring inotrope infusions. An example follows. Within the past 2 weeks, the patient must show:

- Stable medication management without IV diuretics and only slight adjustments in oral diuretics determined by weight gain or symptomatology consistent with typical congestion.
- Stable rhythm; no new onset, hemodynamically significant arrhythmias, atrial or ventricular.
- Stable creatinine level: Each institution should establish a maximum rise in creatinine level (e.g., 0.4) that requires titration of the inotrope therapy.
- Stable potassium supplementation: no IV infusions to maintain a safe range or hyperkalemia requiring any potassium-lowering treatments.
- No IV fluid boluses to rescue BP or renal function.
- No increase in supplemental oxygen needs.
- The importance of fluid status evaluation, signs or symptoms of low output and sepsis.

25. What are the controversies surrounding the treatment of HF with inotropes?

Recent findings from the OPTIME study compared outcomes of patients treated with milrinone with those receiving placebo:

- Despite significant hemodynamic improvement with milrinone versus placebo, milrinone did not have a significant decrease in hospitalization days nor did it assist in maximizing oral medications that improve long-term prognosis.
- Sustained hypotension and new onset atrial fibrillation (AF) occurred more in the milrinone group than in the placebo group but did not translate into longer hospitalizations, increased readmissions, or mortality.
- Patients admitted for exacerbation of HF, without evidence of hypoperfusion, did not derive any added benefit over placebo.

The evidentiary lack of long-term benefit of milrinone therapy over placebo has appropriately lead researchers and practitioners to question the practice of using milrinone simply for symptom abatement. Increasing myocardial contraction in a weak heart is hypothesized to stimulate myocardial cell death, possibly sacrificing quantity for quality of life. Therefore the assumption is often adopted that the stronger the inotrope, the greater the myocardial damage. However, essential to incorporating research results into practice is a clear understanding of the study population characteristics that ensure that the patient being treated may achieve similar results. Although the OPTIME subjects were described as having "severe" HF they were also described as "not requiring IV inotrope" and had a mean SBP of 120 mm/Hg, a serum sodium level of 138, a serum creatinine level of 1.5, and BUN of 11.5—all indicative of a warm presentation of HF. Therefore OPTIME tells us that in the warm presentation of HF, symptom abatement is not an indication for inotropic therapy. However, symptoms indicative of organ hypoperfusion, as in the cold clinical syndromes, were not addressed in this study.

Key Points

- The target serum digoxin level is 0.5 to 0.9 ng/mL.
- Serum digoxin levels should not be drawn before 6 hours after dosing.
- Jugular venous distension is the most sensitive sign of high filling pressures.
- A common adverse effect of milrinone is atrial fibrillation.
- Adverse effects of dobutamine include an increase in HR, increase in myocardial workload, and increase in ventricular dysrhythmias.

Internet Resources

National Institutes of Health: Medline Plus: Health Information:
www.nlm.nih.gov/medlineplus/

Cleveland Clinic Heart Center: Heart Failure Disease Management:
www.clevelandclinic.org/heartcenter/pub/heartfailure/hf_diseasemanagement.htm

GlobalRPh: Digoxin Dosing Calculator
www.globalrph.com/digoxinsub.htm

Heart Failure Society of America:
www.hfsa.org

American College of Cardiology Foundation: ACC/AHA Guidelines for the Evaluation and Management of Chronic Heart Failure in the Adult
www.acc.org/clinical/guidelines/failure/hf_index.htm

Bibliography

Adams KF, Baughman KL et al: HFSA guidelines for the management of patients with heart failure caused by left ventricular systolic dysfunction: pharmacological approaches, *J Card Fail* 5(4):357-383, 1999.

Adams KF Jr, Gheorghiade M, Uretsky BF et al: Clinical benefits of low serum concentrations in heart failure, *J Am Coll Cardiol* 39(6):946-953, 2002.

Adams KF, Gheorghiade M, Uretsky BF et al: Patients with mild heart failure worsen during withdrawal from digoxin therapy, *J Am Coll Cardiol* 30(1):42-48, 1997.

Cohn JT: Heart failure. In Willerson JT, Cohn JN, editors: *Cardiovascular medicine,* New York, 1998, Churchill Livingstone, pp 947-979.

Gheorghiade M, Hall VB, Jacobsen G et al: Effects of maintenance dose of digoxin on left ventricular function and neurohormones in patients with chronic heart failure treated with diuretics and angiotensin-converting enzyme inhibitors, *Circulation* 92(7):1801-1807, 1995.

Grady KL, Dracup K, Kennedy G et al: Team management of patients with heart failure: a statement for healthcare professionals from the Cardiovascular Nursing Council of the American Heart Association, *Circulation* 102:2443-2456, 2000.

Greenberg BH, Hermann DD: *Contemporary diagnosis and management of heart failure,* Newton, Pa, 2002, Handbooks in HealthCare, pp 1-266.

Hunt SA, Baker DW et al: ACC/AHA guidelines for the evaluation and management of chronic heart failure in the adult: a report of the American College of Cardiology/American Heart Association Task Force on Practice Guidelines (Committee to Revise the 1995 Guidelines for the Evaluation and Management of Heart Failure), *Circulation* 104:2996-3009. 2001.

Hunt SA, Baker DW et al: ACC/AHA guidelines for the evaluation and management of chronic heart failure in the adult: executive summary: a report of the American College of Cardiology/American Heart Association Task Force on Practice Guidelines (Committee to Revise the 1995 Guidelines for the Evaluation and Management of Heart Failure), *J Am Coll Cardiol* 38:2101-2013, 2001.

Krum H, Bigger T, Goldsmith RL et al: Effect of long-term digoxin therapy on autonomic function in patients with chronic heart failure, *J Am Coll Cardiol* 25(2):289-294, 1995.

Newton GE, Tong JH, Schofield AM et al: Digoxin reduces cardiac sympathetic activity in severe congestive heart failure, *J Am Coll Cardiol* 28(1):155-161, 1996.

Williamson KM, Thrasher KA, Fulton KB et al: Digoxin toxicity, *Arch Intern Med* 158:2444-2448, 1998.

Young JB, Gheorghiade M, Uretsky BF et al: Superiority of "triple" drug therapy in heart failure: insights from PROVED and RADIANCE trials, *J Am Coll Cardiol* 32(3):686-692, 1999.

Young JB: *Chronic heart failure management in cardiovascular medicine,* Philadelphia, 1998, Lippincott-Raven.

Chapter 34

Antiarrhythmic Agents

Claudia A. Irmiere

1. What is an antiarrhythmic drug?

Antiarrhythmic drugs are pharmacologic agents used to treat cardiac arrhythmias. These medications are intended to restore or maintain normal sinus rhythm. They may also suppress life-threatening arrhythmias. These pharmacologic agents have a direct effect on cardiac muscle tissue, changing the physiologic properties and actions of cardiac tissue at the cellular level. These medications alter different phases of the cardiac cycle to suppress arrhythmias from recurring. With that definition in mind, nurses must be vigilant in assessing for expected responses and the potential complications this category of medication may create.

2. What effect do these medications have on the cardiac muscle?

Cardiac muscle tissues possess four unique properties that other types of body tissues do not. These properties are automaticity, excitability, conductivity, and contractility. Automaticity is the ability of the cell to generate an electrical impulse spontaneously. Cardiac cells have the ability to respond to an electrical stimulus (excitability). Once the impulse is generated, the cells can transmit the electrical impulse to other cells, known as conductivity. The transmission of energy within the cells can create a contraction of the myocardial tissue. All of these properties occur because of the changes in the electrical action potential of the cardiac cell.

The four phases of the action potential of cardiac cells are created by shifts of the intracellular ions sodium (NA), potassium (K), and calcium (CA). Any change in the relationship between the ions causes a change in the phase of the cardiac cellular potential. The length of the various phases is altered with the changes in the relationship of the intracellular ions. Antiarrhythmic drugs change the relationship of the ions by either prolonging or shortening the phases of the action potential. Alteration in timing of the action potential phases may create beneficial or deleterious effects.

3. How are antiarrhythmic drugs classified?

The Vaughan Williams classification system is the most popular and commonly used method to subdivide antiarrhythmic medications into four broad classes.

These classes divide the medications by their mechanism of action at the cellular level. Similar side effects, or toxicities, can also be grouped within each class. One shortcoming of the Vaughn Williams classification is that many of the pharmacologic agents have multiple mechanisms of action, making placement of the medication in only one category difficult. See the following table for the Vaughn Williams classification of antiarrhythmic agents.

Vaughn Williams Classification of Antiarrhythmic Pharmacologic Agents	
Class I (Rhythm Control)	Blocks fast sodium ion channels.
IA	Slows conduction velocity and prolongs cellular repolarization.
IB	Shortens repolarization and slows conduction velocity.
IC	Decreases conduction velocity and has variable effects on repolarization.
Class II (Rate Control)	Beta-adrenergic antagonist that blocks beta receptors at sinus node and atrioventricular node.
Class III (Rhythm Control)	Prolongs repolarization, specifically effective refractory period and action potential.
Class IV (Rate Control)	Blocks calcium entry into cell, which slows rate.

4. What does proarrhythmia mean?

Proarrhythmia is an undesirable or untoward effect on the cardiac rhythm from antiarrhythmic drugs. Proarrhythmia can be broadly defined as an aggravation of an existing arrhythmia or the development of a new arrhythmia during antiarrhythmic drug therapy. Proarrhythmia can manifest itself as bradycardia, tachycardia, or an increase in premature atrial/ventricular beats, torsades de pointes, ventricular tachycardia, or ventricular fibrillation leading to sudden death. Nurses need to be vigilant for any changes from the baseline cardiac rhythm with the initiation of antiarrhythmic medications. Before therapy is started, baseline electrocardiographic (ECG) measurements should be obtained, including the P-R, QRS duration, QT interval, and heart rate. These measurements should be monitored on a routine basis during the initiation of drug therapy and on subsequent visits, or as an inpatient, via continuous telemetry monitoring.

5. What factors need to be considered in selection of medications for atrial arrhythmias?

Numerous factors need to be considered in choosing the best medication for patients with atrial arrhythmias. The most important factor to take into consideration is the presence or absence of structural heart disease. Structural heart disease determines which antiarrhythmic agents can be used safely.

Other factors include the patient's age, comorbidities, symptoms, and previous antiarrhythmic drugs used.

6. What is structural heart disease?

Structural heart disease is any change or alteration in the normal function of the heart, including depressed left ventricular function with an ejection fraction of less than 40%, hypertension with left ventricular hypertrophy, the presence of congestive heart failure, valvular heart disease, congenital heart disease, or coronary artery disease.

7. What is the goal of antiarrhythmic therapy in the treatment of atrial arrhythmias?

Goals of therapy include:
- Ventricular rate control to minimize comorbidities (such as worsening heart failure) and symptoms.
- Maintenance of normal sinus rhythm.
- Prevention of recurrent episodes of paroxysmal atrial arrhythmias.

All adverse effects need to be considered before and during drug therapy. The best drug therapy for patients is the one that ultimately maintains quality of life and minimizes adverse drug effects. Finding and maintaining that best therapy is a difficult goal to accomplish.

8. Are there any other concomitant medications that should be considered for persons with atrial arrhythmias?

Anticoagulation therapy needs to be considered for persons with atrial arrhythmias. There is a four-fold to six-fold increase in the risk of stroke in persons with atrial arrhythmias, which is related to the presence of atrial stasis and the formation of thrombi. Whenever clinically indicated, anticoagulants should be combined with antiarrhythmic treatment.

9. What is the nurse's role with the initiation of antiarrhythmic medications?

Before the first dose of the antiarrhythmic drug is administered, the nurse should review the patient's medications. Many antiarrhythmic medications have numerous drug-drug interactions. For example, any antiarrhythmic that causes QT prolongation should be used with caution with other medications that may cause QT prolongation. This includes antiinfective, antifungal, and allergy medications. The nurse must be sure to note whether the patient is on anticoagulant therapy. If not, there should be consideration to starting therapy if the patient has had atrial fibrillation or atrial flutter. Special consideration should be taken in those persons with a contraindication for anticoagulation therapy. (See Chapter 29, Chronic Anticoagulation, for a review of anticoagulation therapy.) The following tables review the numerous antiarrhythmic agents available for use. As always, one should refer to the manufacturer's drug insert for a full description and prescribing information for each pharmacologic agent listed.

	Indications	Dosage	Nursing Implications
Class IA Agents	Slow conduction velocity and prolong cellular repolarization.		
Disopyramide (Norpace)	Off-label use in treatment of atrial arrhythmias.	400-800 mg by mouth every 6 hr.	Normal left ventricular (LV) function. No history of congestive heart failure. Dry mouth, constipation. Urinary retention: use with caution in men with prostate disease.
Procainamide hydrochloride (procainamide, Procanbid, Procan SR)	May be used in acute and long-term setting for atrial arrhythmias.	Acute setting: intravenous (IV) bolus of 20 mg/min to total of 17 mg/kg. Should be followed by infusion of 1-4 mg/min. Long term: Oral dose of 250 mg every 6 hr or 500 mg sustained release every 12 hr.	During bolus and infusion, measure QT interval every 5 min. Stop if QTc >50% baseline or hypotension. Side effects: thrombocytopenia, joint pain, and joint inflammation. With presence or sudden onset of joint pain, drug should be discontinued. Caution in patients with renal disease or failure as drug may accumulate and cause toxicity. Blood work, including chemistries and drug levels, should be monitored. Procainamide hydrochloride and NAPA (the metabolite of drug) levels should be drawn to assist in adjustment of medication dosage and early detection of toxicity. Careful measurement of QT interval: excessive QT prolongation predisposes patient to torsades de pointes. A 12-lead electrocardiogram (ECG) should be performed with subsequent follow-up visits. During follow-up visits, patients should be questioned about any history of syncope or palpitations. Presence of wax coating on medication in its sustained release form. Wax coating may be excreted in stool in undigested form.

continued

	Indications	Dosage	Nursing Implications
Quinidine (Quinaglute, Quinidex, quinidine sulfate)	One of oldest agents used to treat atrial arrhythmias. Quinidine depresses all phases of cardiac cell action potential.	324-648 mg orally every 12 hr	QT prolongation is concern. Not for use in persons with poor LV function. Monitor renal and liver functions. Side effects include drug interaction with numerous medications that may create toxicity. Drugs include digoxin, warfarin, phenothiazines, amiodarone, and anticholinergics. During follow-up, careful attention needs to be paid to symptoms of syncope, dizziness, or lightheadedness as these may indicate proarrhythmic effects of drug. Quinidine has many side effects including diarrhea, gastrointestinal irritation. If these occur, consideration in lowering dose should be taken.
Class IB and IC Agents			
IB	Shortens repolarization and slows conduction velocity.	Not generally used for persons with atrial arrhythmias.	
IC	Decreases conduction velocity and variable effects on repolarization.		
Flecainide acetate (Tambocor)	Available only in oral form in United States. Flecainide acetate and encainide hydrochloride were two of agents used to compare antiarrhythmic treatment in persons with benign ventricular ectopy in Cardiac	Initially 100 mg every 12 hr; titrate by 50 mg at 4 dose intervals. Maximum 400 mg daily.	In persons with history of ischemia or poor LV function, notable increased risk of sudden death was seen with these pharmacologic agents. Thus flecainide acetate is safe for use only in persons with normal LV function. May cause blurry vision, headaches, vertigo, and central nervous system (CNS) depression. Patients have described feeling "heady" or "intoxicated" from CNS side effects of drug. Dosage should be reduced if patient has these side effects.

Continued

continued

	Indications	Dosage	Nursing Implications
	Arrhythmia Suppression Trial (CAST). CAST study showed risk of treating benign ventricular ectopy is more dangerous than not.		On drug initiation, individuals should be counseled about driving and operating heavy machinery as drowsiness may occur. These symptoms are usually alleviated with long-term use or development of tolerance to medication. Dosages should be adjusted in persons with impaired renal and hepatic function. Flecainide acetate levels should be drawn to adjust medication dosage accordingly.
Propafenone hydrochloride (Rythmol)		150 mg by mouth every 8 hr, to total maximum dose of 300 mg every 8 hr.	For use in persons with no structural heart disease. Should not be used in persons with atrioventricular (AV) block. If fever or decrease in white blood cell count occurs, patient should undergo evaluation for agranulocytosis. Side effects include dizziness, elevated anti–nuclear antibody (ANA) titer, palpitations, and constipation.
Class II Agents			
Beta-blockers (acebutolol, atenolol, esmolol hydrochloride, metoprolol, propranolol, timolol maleate)	Beta-adrenergic antagonists block beta receptors at sinus and atrioventricular node.	Dosage varies, dependent on medication used.	Provides excellent rate control as they slow cardiac conduction. Useful in stabilizing cardiac cells and thus providing protection against arrhythmias in persons who have had myocardial infarction and ischemia. Patients should be monitored to detect severe bradycardia and AV block. Beta-blockers should not be abruptly withdrawn because rebound tachycardia and hypertension may occur. Hypotension may also occur. If beta-blockers are used with other agents that lower blood pressure, patients should stagger doses to prevent sudden drops in blood pressure.

	Indications	Dosage	Nursing Implications
continued			
			Caution should be used in patients with pulmonary disease, notably asthma, because bronchospasm may be exacerbated. Cardioselective agents are available, namely acebutolol (Sectral). Side effects include fatigue and lack of energy when beta-blockers are initiated. Gentle support and encouragement should be provided to patient as these symptoms improve over time. Common symptoms of patients on beta-blockers are cold fingertips and hands.
			Patients may report sleep disturbances, including nightmares, with beta-blockers. This usually resolves with changing from one medication to another. If this symptom does not improve, stopping medication should be considered.
			Impotence is commonly reported side effect of beta-blockers. Dose adjustment or changing pharmacologic agent should be considered.
			Drug should be titrated downward before discontinuation to prevent difficulty in drug withdrawal. (See Chapter 31.)
Class III Agents			
Amiodarone (Pacerone, Cordarone)	Off-label use in treatment of atrial arrhythmias. Most potent antiarrhythmic agent that is available in United States today. Possesses characteristics of beta, calcium, and K+ channel blockers.	In acute setting, 150 mg IV bolus in 100 mL D5 W over first 10 min followed by continuous infusion of 60 mg/hr over next 6 hr. Then maintenance infusion of 30 mg/hr (0.5 mg/min) over next 18 hr.	Amiodarone is distributed throughout body in fatty tissues; thus loading dose is required. Distribution into body fat tissues provides drug with long half-life of approximately 90-120 d, which is important to remember when switching medication regimens from one agent to another. Drug levels can be drawn to measure whether drug and its active metabolite des-ethyl amiodarone are present.

Continued

continued

	Indications	Dosage	Nursing Implications
		Can be used for up to 3 weeks. IV infusions should be covered to minimize light exposure. Oral loading dose of 1200 mg daily in divided doses for 5 d, with dose reduction to 400 mg twice daily for 2 wk followed by maintenance dose of 400 mg daily. Consideration must be given to reducing dose to 200 mg daily to help in reducing potential side effects.	Amiodarone ideally should be started as inpatient; however, it may be started as outpatient with frequent visits for ECG monitoring during first few weeks of therapy. Potentiates digoxin, Dilantin, and warfarin; thus levels need to be monitored carefully to prevent toxicities. Careful attention needs to be paid to other pharmacologic agents patient is on to prevent or minimize drug-drug interactions. Be sure to find out what over-the-counter or complementary medications patient presently takes. See Question 10 for more information.
Sotalol hydrochloride (Betapace, Betapace AF)	Conversion to and maintenance of sinus rhythm.	80 to 240 mg every 12 hr.	See Question 11.
Dofetilide (Tikosyn)	Newest agent for use in conversion and maintenance of sinus rhythm.	125 mcg up to 500 mcg every 12 hr.	See Questions 12 to 16.
Class IV Agents			
Calcium channel blockers (Covera HS, Calan, Calan SR, Isoptin, verapamil hydrochloride, Verelan)	Calcium channel blockers slow rate of conduction through sinus and atrioventricular node.	In acute monitored setting, IV bolus of 2.5 to 5 mg over 2 min may be given. Second dose of 5 to 10 mg may be given in 15 to 30 min for total dose of 30 mg.	Should not use in with patients with depressed LV function or heart failure. Hypotension occurs with IV administration of this drug as it causes peripheral vasodilatation. Use with caution in persons with AV block or Wolff-Parkinson-White syndrome. Educate patients about gastrointestinal side effects of this class of drugs, namely constipation. Education

continued

	Indications	Dosage	Nursing Implications
		Oral doses range up to 360 mg daily.	about increasing dietary fiber and fluid intake to overcome drug side effect should be included with each visit.
Diltiazem hydrochloride (Cardizem, Cardizem CD, Cardizem SR, Dilacor XR)	Provides excellent rate control of ventricular response in persons with sudden onset of atrial arrhythmias.	In acute monitored setting, bolus of 15 to 20 mg IV over 20 min. May be repeated after 15 min if adequate heart rate response was not achieved with initial bolus. Bolus dose should be followed with maintenance infusion of 5-15 mg/h. Oral dose ranges from 30 mg to 360 mg, with daily maximum dose of 360 mg.	Can be used with caution in persons with LV dysfunction. Less gastrointestinal side effects than other class IV agents, thus is better tolerated.

10. **What are the potential side effects and related nursing responsibilities with amiodarone?**

   - Cardiac:
     - Electrocardiographic changes may include atrioventricular (AV) block, bradycardia, and QT prolongation.
     - A baseline ECG should be obtained for comparison on subsequent visits for early detection of side effects.
   - Pulmonary:
     - Has the patient had breathlessness or shortness of breath at rest? Has the patient had difficulty catching his/her breath? Careful auscultation of lung sounds should be performed with each visit.
     - A chest radiograph and pulmonary function tests should be obtained because amiodarone has the potential to cause irreversible pulmonary toxicity and fibrosis. Chest radiographs should be repeated every 6 months to rule out pulmonary fibrosis.

- Gastrointestinal:
  - Amiodarone is metabolized by the liver; consequently, liver function studies and chemistries should be measured at baseline and every 6 months thereafter.
  - Any change more than 20% from baseline laboratory values should prompt a dose reduction or drug discontinuation.
  - The patient's weight should be documented.
  - Occasional symptoms of gastrointestinal disturbances, including nausea and a lack of appetite, occur with amiodarone. Patients should be encouraged to eat frequent small meals to alleviate this problem.
- Thyroid:
  - Amiodarone is an iodide base and is readily absorbed by the thyroid gland.
  - Thyroid function studies should be monitored for early detection of thyroid abnormalities.
  - Any significant weight gain or loss should be explored because it may be related to thyroid dysfunction.
  - Any change in laboratory values 20% from baseline should prompt the health care provider to reduce or stop the medication.
- Ocular:
  - Documentation of the patient's last eye exam should be noted because amiodarone can cause permanent ocular changes including optic neuritis, which may lead to blindness.
  - Commonly, amiodarone crystals deposits can be seen on the cornea.
  - During follow-up visits, the nurse should question patients for any changes in their vision or visual capacity.
- Integumentary:
  - Sun sensitivity is an important side effect about which patients should be educated to prevent harmful sunburns and poisoning.
  - Stressing the use of sunscreen with the strongest sun-blocking agent available is important with patients on amiodarone.
  - Sunscreen should be applied to the ear tips and hairline and to the rest of the body. A hat and eye protection should be worn to prevent damage.
- Patients may also have the "amiodarone blues" develop. The amiodarone blues are a bluish discoloration of the skin, especially the nose and fingertips. If this physical assessment finding is present, drug dosage should be adjusted.

11. What is the role of sotalol hydrochloride in the treatment of patients with atrial arrhythmias?

Sotalol hydrochloride contains both characteristics of nonselective beta-blockers and K+ channel blockers. It is used in the maintenance of sinus rhythm. As with the initiation of beta-blockers, caution should be used when starting this drug in persons with depressed left ventricular function and heart failure. Manufacturers' recommendations include drawing baseline chemistries because the drug is renally excreted. Electrolyte imbalances, especially hypo-kalemia and hypomagnesemia, need to be corrected before drug initiation. Lower doses need to be considered in persons with abnormal baseline renal function. Drug initiation should be in a monitored setting because QT prolongation and torsades de pointes are of concern. The drug effect is observed as the patient's heart rate is slowed and stabilized with observation of the 24-hour heart rate trend. Serial 12-lead ECGs should be obtained for accurate QTc interval measurement. If the QTc interval increases more than 550 ms, the dose should be reduced or the drug discontinued. Sotalol hydrochloride should not be used simultaneously with other antiarrhythmic medications. Any medications that may cause QT prolongation need to be assessed for potential interaction with sotalol hydrochloride. On subsequent follow-up visits, patients should have a 12-lead ECG to measure the QTc interval. Patients should be questioned about whether they have had any syncope because this may be a symptom of torsades de pointes. Common side effects of sotalol hydrochloride are similar to those of beta-adrenergic blockers, namely fatigue, dizziness, and bradycardia. Patients should be counseled about these side effects and should sit, rest, and gauge daily activities to alleviate them or prevent them from occurring.

12. What precautions should be taken when dofetilide (Tikosyn) is prescribed?

Dofetilide should only be prescribed by those who have received appropriate dosing and initiation education. Before the initiation of dofetilide, previous antiarrhythmic therapy should be withdrawn for a minimum of three half-lives. Amiodarone should be held for at least 3 months or have a level below 0.3 µg/mL before dofetilide initiation. Because of potential life-threatening side effects, verapamil hydrochloride, cimetidine, trimethoprim, ketoconazole, prochlorperazine, and megestrol acetate need to be discontinued before dofetilide is started. Digoxin levels should be obtained to ensure that they are within normal range. Serum K levels need to be within normal limits before the first dose of the drug. Telemetry monitoring is required either for a minimum of 3 days or for 12 hours after the conversion to sinus rhythm, whichever is longer. A baseline 12-lead ECG, serum creatinine level measured in mg/dL, and patient's body weight in kilograms are needed to calculate the appropriate dose of dofetilide. Dofetilide is contraindicated if the baseline QTc is more than 440 ms.

13. How do you calculate creatinine clearance to figure out the correct dose of dofetilide?

The following formulas are used to calculate the patients' creatinine clearance:

$$\text{Creatinine clearance (male)} = \frac{(140 - \text{age}) \times \text{body weight (kg)}}{72 \times \text{serum creatinine (mg/dl)}}$$

$$\text{Creatinine clearance (female)} = \frac{(140 - \text{age}) \times \text{body weight (kg)} \times 0.85}{72 \times \text{serum creatinine (mg/dl)}}$$

If the calculated creatinine clearance is less than 20 mL/min, dofetilide is contraindicated. If the calculated creatinine clearance is between 40 mL/min and 60 mL/min, the appropriate dose of dofetilide is 250 mcg twice a day (bid). If the calculated creatinine clearance is between 20 and 40 mL/min, the appropriate dose of dofetilide is 125 mcg bid.

14. What should the nurse do after the first dose of dofetilide?

After the first dose of dofetilide, a 12-lead ECG should be obtained. If the QTc increases to more than 15% above the baseline measurement, the dose of dofetilide should be decreased by half. Twelve-lead ECGs should be obtained before each subsequent dose of dofetilide for the first four doses. QTc measurements should be performed by the nurse every 2 to 4 hours during the drug initiation phase. The risk of torsades de pointes is dose related with dofetilide. It is important to emphasize that dofetilide be given every 12 hours, at the same time every day.

15. What are important considerations on hospital discharge for patients on dofetilide therapy?

Before hospital discharge, the prescribing physician or his/her designee should contact the mail-order pharmacy to place the outpatient prescription. At this time, the medication is only available by mail order to a limited number of pharmacies. The appropriate paperwork provided by the pharmacy needs to be completed along with a prescription to ensure prompt delivery of the medication. The patient should be discharged with a 7-day starter pack from the hospital pharmacy in the final dosage strength. Included with this packet are numerous educational materials for the patient and the primary care provider. A video, written materials, and identification card in English and Spanish are useful resources to help maintain patient compliance with dofetilide. The patient needs to understand that if more than two doses are missed, rehospitalization is required to restart the drug.

16. What medications are used to treat ventricular arrhythmias?

Medications used in the treatment of ventricular arrhythmias are used to suppress or prevent arrhythmic episodes. The drug of choice depends on the patient's underlying cardiac condition and the penultimate goal of therapy. Listed in the box on page 393 are the pharmacologic agents used for persons with ventricular arrhythmias. Please refer to the descriptions listed in the table in Question 9 for those previously discussed.

17. Can antiarrhythmic medications be used in conjunction with cardiac devices?

In individuals with implantable cardiac devices—pacemakers and ICDs—these medications can be safely used to decrease the frequency of tachyarrhythmias. Implantable cardiac devices may help to alleviate some drug side effects, for example, bradycardia. Should the patient have an "electrical storm" develop in which incessant ventricular tachycardia or fibrillation occurs, antiarrhythmic medication prevents the patient from receiving numerous ICD shocks. The patient's ICD should be retested in the appropriate setting to ensure an adequate safety margin is maintained after initiation of antiarrhythmic therapy.

Class IA Agents
Quinidine
Procainamide hydrochloride

Class IB Agents
Lidocaine
Dosage: 1.0 to 1.5 mg/kg intravenously (IV). For refractory ventricular fibrillation (VF), an additional 0.5 mg to 0.75 mg/kg IV push may be given and repeated in 5 to 10 minutes for a maximum total dose of 3 mg/kg. A continuous infusion of 1 to 4 mg/min should follow the bolus doses. Signs of toxicity include slurring of speech, confusion, seizure, and decreased level of consciousness. A decrease in dosage resolves these symptoms.

For many years, lidocaine was used as a first-line drug in advanced cardiac life support (ACLS) protocol for treatment of ventricular arrhythmias. Research has shown that its efficacy is poor in treatment of ventricular arrhythmias. Amiodarone is now considered the first-line treatment for life-threatening arrhythmias. Lidocaine should not be used prophylactically in the treatment of ventricular arrhythmias in patients with acute myocardial infarction. Mexiletine hydrochloride: Dosage: Initial dose of 200 mg by mouth every 8 hours. The dose may be adjusted in 2-day to 3-day intervals at 50-mg increments. A daily maximum dose of 900 mg should not be exceeded. The lowest possible dose that is effective is recommended for use in treatment of the patient's condition. Mexiletine hydrochloride should not be used with persons in cardiogenic shock or high-grade AV block. Mexiletine hydrochloride must be taken with food or antacids because it is known to cause gastrointestinal upset. Patients with liver dysfunction need to be carefully monitored while on this agent to prevent hepatotoxicity. Dizziness, tremor, nervousness, and blurry vision are common side effects of mexiletine hydrochloride. A dose adjustment usually alleviates these central nervous system side effects.

Class II Agents
Beta-blockers
Beta-blockers are effective in decreasing total mortality in patients after myocardial infarction, prevention of sudden death, and treatment of recurrent tachyarrhythmias.

Class III Agents
Amiodarone
The AVID (Antiarrhythmic versus Implantable Defibrillators) research trial showed that after implantable cardioverter defibrillator (ICD) therapy, amiodarone was the drug of choice in the treatment of life-threatening ventricular arrhythmias. Drug efficacy is listed as 85% in preventing or suppressing arrhythmias. Amiodarone is used in conjunction with ICDs in patients with frequent, uncontrollable ventricular ectopy.

Sotalol hydrochloride
Sotalol hydrochloride is the only Class III agent approved for use in the treatment of atrial and ventricular arrhythmias. Refer to question 11 for recommended dosage and administration information.

18. Why are some patients admitted to a telemetry/hospital setting for antiarrhythmic medications to be initiated?

Antiarrhythmic agents are used to alter the patient's cardiac conduction system. The greatest drug effect can be documented on the patient's ECG; therefore continuous monitoring in the most appropriate lead should be available. At the time of drug initiation, many patients may already be hospitalized for symptoms from the arrhythmia. The patient's underlying heart disease may also be used as a guide. If the patient has structural heart disease or the presence of congestive heart failure or is on numerous medications, admitting the individual to a monitored setting is advisable to prevent harm. Early detection of side effects assists in preventing permanent damage from the medications. Many medications carry manufacturers' recommendations and guidelines that require patients to be in a monitored setting before drug initiation because of the deleterious effects of QT prolongation. As always, patient safety is the priority. Patients with documented ventricular arrhythmias should be hospitalized if antiarrhythmic medications need to be changed. During the transition from one medication to the next, the patient may not be protected against recurrent arrhythmia. The patient should be provided with continuous monitoring for early detection of ventricular tachycardia or fibrillation. The medications most commonly started as an inpatient are class I and III agents.

19. Are there any controversies in the field of antiarrhythmic therapies?

Controversies persist over the best treatment of atrial arrhythmias. Results of the AFFIRM (Atrial Fibrillation Follow-Up Investigation of Rhythm Management) trial released in March 2002 showed no difference in mortality and morbidity rates between two groups of patients randomized to rate control versus rhythm control after a mean follow-up period of 3.5 years. The Pharmacologic Intervention in Atrial Fibrillation (PIAF) study did not show any significant difference in primary endpoint between the rate control group and the rhythm control group. Strategies for Treatment of Atrial Fibrillation (STAF) trial results also did not show any difference between the two treatment strata. All of the studies agreed that the use of anticoagulation therapy with therapeutic international normalized ratio (INR) levels reduced the risk of stroke, a major complication of atrial fibrillation. In the electrophysiology community, the use of pharmacologic and nonpharmacologic means of treating atrial arrhythmias has been under investigation. Radiofrequency catheter ablation for the modification of cardiac tissue to provide rate control or maintain sinus rhythm is being considered as a feasible method for treatment of atrial arrhythmias. Until a firm scientific conclusion is made, patients should be treated on an individual basis to minimize symptoms, prevent medication side effects, and maintain quality of life.

A second point of controversy is the prophylactic use of antiarrhythmic agents in persons with ICDs. No definitive studies have been conducted observing the use of antiarrhythmic agents to prevent or reduce the number of arrhythmic episodes in persons with ICDs. Prevention of the arrhythmia ultimately reduces the number of therapies or shocks that a person receives. Theoretically, this prolongs the life of the ICD. The OPTIC (Optimal Therapy for ICD patients) study is an ongoing trial investigating which oral antiarrhythmic agent is best in combination with ICD placement. The three treatment arms include beta-blocker alone (with metoprolol, carvedilol, or bisoprolol), sotalol hydrochloride, or amiodarone plus beta-blocker. Information is being collected on the number of therapies (shocks) a patient receives while taking optimal doses of these antiarrhythmic agents.

20. What does the future hold in the field of antiarrhythmic agents?

Future research is exploring:
- Pharmacologic agents that target specific phases of the action potential.
- Development of cardioselective medications to minimize effect on other organ systems.
- Development of more effective agents to treat paroxysmal episodes of arrhythmias.
- Comparison of drug efficacy for treatment of various arrhythmias of market available drugs.

Key Points

- Treatment goals for the use of antiarrhythmic agents include either restoration/maintenance of sinus rhythm or suppression of life-threatening arrhythmias.
- The Vaughn Williams classification system separates antiarrhythmic medications into classes, depending on mechanism of action on a cellular level.
- Class I and III agents maintain or restore sinus rhythm.
- Class II and IV agents provide AV node blocking properties.
- Baseline ECG measurements, especially the QT interval, are important to obtain before the initiation of antiarrhythmic medications.
- Antiarrhythmic medications have numerous drug-drug interactions. Therefore a review of the patients' medication list before starting any antiarrhythmic medications is important.

Internet Resources

NASPE Heart Rhythm Society:
www.naspe.org

Guidant.com: Information for Medical Professionals and Patients and Families:
www.guidant.com

American Heart Association:
www.americanheart.org

St. Jude Medical: AF Suppression:
www.aboutatrialfibrillation.com

ACC/AHA/ESC Guidelines for the Management of Patients With Atrial Fibrillation:
http://www.acc.org/clinical/guidelines/atrial_fib/af_index.htm

Continued

Internet Resources   *continued*

Patient Health International:
www.patienthealthinternational.com

Information on Atrial Fibrillation (choose from the drop-down menu):
www.pfizer.com

Information on Atrial Fibrillation and other arrhythmias
www.medtronic.com

Bibliography

Albers GW: The value of anti-thrombotic therapy in atrial fibrillation: who should be treated? *Today in Cardiology* 3: 7-9, 2002.

American Heart Association in collaboration with International Liaison Committee on Resuscitation: Guidelines 2000 for cardiopulmonary resuscitation and emergency cardiovascular care: International consensus on science, part 3: adult basic life support, *Circulation* 102(suppl I):I22-I59, 2000.

Antiarrhythmics Versus Implantable Defibrillators (AVID) investigators: A comparison of antiarrhythmic-drug therapy with implantable defibrillators in patients resuscitated from near-fatal ventricular arrhythmias, *N Engl J Med* 337:1576-1583, 1997.

CAST Investigators: Preliminary report effect of encainide and flecainide on mortality in a randomized trial of arrhythmia suppression after myocardial infarction, *N Engl J Med* 321:406-412, 1989.

Diaz A, Clifton GD: Dofetilide: a new class III antiarrhythmic for the management of atrial fibrillation, *Prog Cardiovasc Nurs* 16(3):126-129, 2001.

Levy S: Pharmacologic management of atrial fibrillation: current therapeutic strategies, *Am Heart J* 141(2):S15-S21, 2001.

Murphy JL, editor: *Monthly prescribing reference (MPR)*, New York, 2002, Prescribing Reference Inc.

Naccarelli GV et al: Proarrhythmia, *Med Clin North Am* 85(2):503-526, 2001.

Roden DM: Antiarrhythmic drugs: from mechanisms to clinical practice, *Heart* 84:339-346, 2000.

Vaughn Williams EM: Classification of antiarrhythmic actions, *Handbook Experimental Pharmacol* 89:45-62, 1989.

Wyse DG: Antiarrhythmic strategies for management of atrial fibrillation, *Today Cardiol* 3:4-6, 2002.

Wyse DC et al: A comparison of rate control and rhythm control in patients with atrial fibrillation, *N Engl J Med* 347(23):1825-1833, 2002.

Section VI

Cardiovascular Risk Reduction

Smoking Cessation

Jane S. Kaufman

1. Why is smoking detrimental to health, especially with cardiovascular (CV) disease?

- Nicotine itself has harmful effects on blood vessels via catecholamine release and vasoconstriction and likely causes atherosclerosis progression.
- Smokers are likely to have hyperlipidemia and hypertension develop.
- Women who smoke and use oral contraceptives greatly increase the risk of coronary heart disease (CHD) and stroke.
- Smokers have double the risk of ischemic stroke.
- Graft occlusion in coronary artery bypass grafting (CABG) and angioplasty failure are exceptionally high in those who continue to smoke.
- Thirty percent of cases of CHD and approximately 90% of cases of peripheral vascular disease (PVD) can be attributed to cigarette smoking in the nondiabetic adult population.

2. Does smoking cessation actually normalize physiological alteration and risks of disease/death?

Some positive changes of smoking cessation occur in the short term and can be emphasized. For example:
- Within 2 hours of smoking cessation, the blood pressure (BP) and pulse normalize.
- Within 4 hours after smoking or inhaling cigarette smoke, the carbon monoxide (CO) level of the blood returns to normal. (CO is the same poison in exhaust fumes from cars.)

Long-term changes also occur with smoking cessation. For example:
- Benefits from quitting are seen even after years of heavy smoking.
- The decreased risk to CHD mortality occurs relatively soon after smoking cessation.
- As reported by Burns, after 15 years of smoking cessation, the risk of a new myocardial infarction (MI) or death from CHD is similar to that in those who never smoked.
- Persons with diagnosed CHD have as much as 50% reduction in risk of reinfarction, sudden cardiac death, and total mortality if they quit after the first infarction.

3. **When a patient history is taken, what issues about smoking are important to assess?**
   - Ask the number of years smoked and the number of packs per day during those years to determine pack year history to determine cumulative exposure to smoke (years smoked × packs per day = pack year history).
   - Ask how long after awakening is the first cigarette smoked. (If it is within 30 minutes on awakening, the patient likely has nicotine addiction.)
   - Review family history and who else in the household smokes; this gives a clue as to challenges to quit.
   - Is there a history of any smoking-related diseases, such as chronic obstructive pulmonary disease (COPD), CHD, or PVD, including intermittent claudication and cancer?
   - Are there any smoking-related symptoms, such as cough, sputum production, shortness of breath, or recurrent respiratory infections?

   Concerning intent to quit, what questions formulated from evidence-based research should be asked at every healthcare visit?
   - Every health care visit should include a screening for smokers. This brief intervention takes only about 3 minutes. (See the following question adapted from Clinical Practice Guidelines.) The "5 As" in Question 4 (Ask, Advise, Assess, Assist, and Arrange) can be implemented to assess willingness to quit.

4. **Concerning intent to quit smoking, what are the "5 As" that should be included in every health care visit?**
   - **Ask** about the patient's smoking habits and intentions to quit.
   - **Advise** in a clear, strong, personalized manner; urge the patient to stop smoking now. Clear advice might be: "I believe it is important for you to quit smoking now, and I can help you." A strong statement would be: "You need to know that quitting smoking is the most important action you can take to protect your current and future health. We have ways to help you." A personalized statement emphasizes how smoking cessation improves the health of the person and others in the household, especially children, who are exposed to secondhand smoke. The statement could also point out the expense involved in smoking.
   - **Assess** the willingness to quit now. If the answer is "yes," proceed to the "assist" step. If the person is clear about not wanting to quit, provide a motivational intervention via the "5 Rs" in Question 9.
   - **Assist** the person willing to quit with counseling and pharmacotherapy resources.
   - **Arrange** follow-up contact, preferably within the first week after the quit date.

5. **Should the nurse perform any particular physical assessments that correlate with long-term tobacco use?**
   - Elevated BP.
   - Increased hemoglobin.
   - Tachycardia.
   - Inflammation of ears, nose, sinuses, mouth, or pharynx from irritation of tobacco smoke.
   - Leukoplakia, especially under the tongue.

- Barrel chest or increased anterior/posterior lung diameter.
- Morning cough.
- Crackles or rhonchi in the chest.
- Staining of nicotine on the fingers of the dominant hand. Note: If the person is a heavy drinker, then the staining is on the nondominant hand. A person drinks with the dominant hand but then smokes with the nondominant.
- Clubbing of the fingers/toes.
- Evidence of PVD, including a history of intermittent claudication.
- Premature aging of the skin.

6. What advice can the nurse give a patient who is "thinking about stopping smoking?"

The nurse should give the clear, strong, personalized answer as noted in Question 1 relating to "advise." According to a well-known theory of change developed by Prochaska et al, people with addictive behaviors move in a spiral, up and down through stages as they are seeking to change. (Stages are pre-contemplation—no intention to change; contemplation—person knows there is a problem that needs changing; preparation—intention to take action to change in the near future; action—behavior is modified; and maintenance—work to modify behavior and prevent relapse that lasts at least 6 months.)

7. What stages do people go through as they are seeking change?

In the previous question, the patient is contemplating change. According to Prochaska et al, the nurse should seek to move the patient to the next stage, which is preparation for change. The nurse should suggest some small change that the person could make that would be helpful (e.g., smoking fewer cigarettes). Then he/she can move on to the action stage where the behavior is altered and the goal is no cigarettes.

8. What if someone has made the decision to stop smoking and is ready to do it now?

This person is in the action stage from 1 day to up to 6 months before moving to a maintenance stage. The "assist" aids the patient in quitting by the following strategies (adapted from Clinical Practice Guidelines). See the following table.

Action	Strategies for Implementation
Help patient with quit plan.	Patient's preparations for quitting: Set a quit date, ideally within 2 weeks. Tell family, friends, and coworkers about quitting and request understanding and support. Anticipate challenges to quit attempt, especially during the first few weeks. These include nicotine withdrawal symptoms.

Continued

continued	
Action	**Strategies for Implementation**
	Remove tobacco products from the environment. For example, clean out the car and buy a fragrance to block the smell of smoke. Before quitting, avoid smoking in places where you spend a lot of time (e.g., work, home, car). You need to break the cycle that reminds you of smoking. For example, if you always smoke after breakfast while reading your paper at the kitchen table, move to the den to read your paper.
Provide practical counseling (problem solving/training).	Abstinence: total abstinence is essential—not even one puff after the quit date. Past quit experience: identify what helped and what contributed to relapse in past attempts. Anticipate triggers or challenges and how the person will successfully overcome them. Alcohol: consider limiting/abstaining from alcohol while quitting because alcohol can cause relapse. Other smokers in the household: encourage housemates to quit or not smoke in their presence because other smokers in the same house make quitting more difficult.
Provide intratreatment social support.	Provide a supportive clinical environment while encouraging the person in the quit attempt. Continue to assure the person that you or the office or ward staff will assist them.
Help patient obtain extratreatment social support.	Help person develop social support for the quit attempt by asking spouse/partner, friends, and coworkers for support.
Recommend use of approved pharmacotherapy, except in special circumstances.	Recommend the use of first-line therapies, such as nicotine replacement or bupropion SR (sustained release). Explain that these medications increase smoking cessation success and reduce withdrawal symptoms.
Provide supplementary materials.	Provide information about local and national agencies that are the type appropriate for them.

9. What should the nurse do if the patient is not interested in stopping smoking?

The nurse should record in the chart the status of the patient's smoking and the lack of interest in stopping now. If there are others who smoke in the household, record in the chart "exposed to passive smoke." If the patient is unwilling to quit, a brief intervention seen in the following table should be implemented to motivate smoking cessation. The patient may be motivated to quit with the "5 Rs" noted in the Clinical Practice Guidelines in the table.

Relevance	Be as specific as possible in pointing out why the person would benefit from smoking cessation. For example, relate smoking cessation to the current disease and to family members whose health would benefit. Persons who have undergone coronary artery bypass grafting have higher rates of occlusion if they continue smoking, and persons who have had an angioplasty have higher rates of failure if they continue smoking.
Risks	Ask the patient to list short-term and long-term risks with continued smoking. Emphasize that smoking low-tar/low-nicotine cigarettes or using other forms of tobacco does not eliminate these risks.
Rewards	Ask the patient to identify potential benefits of stopping smoking. You might add the following: Food will taste better. They will save money. They will feel better about themselves and feel better physically. Blood pressure will be lower. Home, car, clothing, and breath will smell better. They will set a good example for children, and they will be healthier. They will see reduced wrinkling/aging of the skin. Their heart will not be stressed as much. Lung function will not decline nearly as fast.
Roadblocks	Ask the patient to list barriers to stopping and what treatments might address these barriers. Typical barriers might be: withdrawal symptoms, fear of failure, weight gain, lack of support, depression, enjoyment of smoking, lack of money to buy supplies, and other household members who continue to smoke.
Repetition	Repeat the previous messages each time the patient visits the clinic. Tell patients that most people make repeated attempts before they are successful.

10. When are patients likely to relapse, and what strategies might prevent relapse?

- A study by Hays et al reported that after successful intervention for smoking cessation three fourths of persons relapse within 6 to 12 months. However, relapse may occur within 3 months and even years after quitting.
- Relapse prevention interventions are vital for the person who has recently quit. Abstinence after week 1 is a strong predictor of 12-month abstinence. Nurses should stress this predictor in the patient's initial attempts at quitting.

11. What strategies might prevent relapse?

The person can be seen in the outpatient clinic or receive supportive telephone calls from the nurse. The nurse can emphasize the "assist or 5 Rs." Also, the patient should be encouraged to report any difficulty promptly (e.g., side effects of medications) while he/she continues to quit. If the patient has a specific problem that might cause relapse, then the nurse should approach the problem carefully and specifically. A study by Hays et al reported that in persons who were able to stop smoking with 7 weeks of bupropion (Zyban), an additional 12 months of bupropion (Zyban) delayed smoking relapse and resulted in less weight gain.

12. What are common reasons that patients' attempts to quit smoking are threatened, and what can be done about the problems?

Problems	Responses
Lack of support for quitting attempt	Schedule follow-up visits or telephone calls with the patient. Help the patient to identify sources of support in his/her setting. Refer the patient to an age, gender, and culturally appropriate resource/organization.
Negative mood or depression	Try counseling or refer to a provider that further counsels and provides medication if indicated. Be sure that clinical depression is treated because this is frequently found in smokers.
Strong or prolonged withdrawal symptoms	Refer to the provider who might consider extending the use of an approved smoking cessation medication or therapy or adding/combining other medications to control the symptoms.
Weight gain	Encourage increased physical activity and not strict dieting. Some weight gain after quitting is expected, but most persons gain <10 lb. Emphasize eating a healthy diet. Maintain the patient on therapies known to delay weight gain (e.g., bupropion SR, nicotine replacement therapies, especially gum). Stress that the health risks of weight gain are small when compared with the risks of continued smoking.
Feeling deprived	Reassure the patient that these feelings are common. Recommend rewarding activities. Inquire to be sure the patient is not smoking periodically. Emphasize that even one puff increases urges and makes quitting more difficult; encourage patients to be abstinent!

13. What pharmacological products are on the market to aid in smoking cessation?

In addition to counseling, all patients attempting to quit smoking should be encouraged to use effective pharmacotherapies for stopping smoking, except in the presence of special circumstances. Multiple randomized controlled clinical studies have shown the effectiveness of pharmacotherapies. The likelihood of relapse may be lessened with long-term use of the previously mentioned therapies. The US Food and Drug Administration (FDA) has approved five first-line and two second-line medications that have a consistent body of scientific evidence to support their use. (Note: Cost from national chain drugstore, February 2003). See the following table.

Drug and Cost	Precautions	Dosage/Duration	Adverse Effects	Prescribing Instructions
First-Line				
Bupropion SR (Zyban): (prescription only) helps reduce withdrawal symptoms and urge to smoke. $3.80 twice daily (bid) dosing.	Pregnancy and lactation, cardiovascular (CV) diseases. Contraindicated: history of seizure or eating disorder, use of another form of bupropion or monooxidase inhibitor in last 14 days.	150 mg every morning for 3 d, then 150 mg bid. Start 1-2 wk before quit date. Take 7-12 weeks after quit date, and may continue for up to 6 mo.	Insomnia; dry mouth	
Nicotine gum (Nicorette and Nicorette Mint— over-the-counter [OTC]). Generic brands. Nicorette 2 mg: $6.25/10 pieces. Nicorette 4 mg: $5.40/10 pieces. Generic: 2 mg: $3.89/10 pieces. 4 mg: $4.54/10 pieces.	Pregnancy and lactation, CV diseases.	Smokers using <25 cigarettes/d = 2 mg gum up to 24 pieces/d. Smokers >25 cigarettes/d = 4 mg gum up to 24 pieces/d. Use up to 12 wk.	Mouth soreness, dyspepsia, hiccups, jaw aches.	Gum should be chewed until "peppery" taste, then "parked" between cheek and gum to allow nicotine absorption. Chew and park about 30 min or until taste disappears. Do not eat or drink (except water) 15 min before or during chewing.
Nicotine inhaler (prescription only). $10.95/10 cartridges. of therapy.	Pregnancy and lactation, CV diseases.	6-16 cartridges/d. Up to 6 mo. Taper during final 3 mo.	Local irritation of mouth and throat, coughing, rhinitis.	In cold weather, keep in inside pocket or warm area. Do not eat or drink (except water) 15 min before or during inhalation.
Nicotine nasal spray (Nicotrol NS) (prescription only). $11.04/12 doses.	Pregnancy and lactation, CV diseases. Do not use with severe reactive airway disease.	Initial dosing = 1/2 dose/hr, increasing as needed for symptom relief. Minimum of 8 doses/d, with maximum of 40 doses/d. Use 3-6 mo.	Nasal irritation.	Do not sniff, swallow, or inhale through nose. Tilt head slightly back when using.

Continued

continued

Drug and Cost	Precautions	Dosage/Duration	Adverse Effects	Prescribing Instructions
Nicotine patch (Nicoderm CQ, Nicotrol, Habitrol, Nictrol, generic—OTC; other patches—prescription). Nicoderm CQ (cost/patch) 21, 14, 7 mg = $3.57/patch Generic 21, 14 mg = $3 7 mg = $1.87	Pregnancy and lactation, CV diseases.	4 wk = 21 mg/ 24 hr; then 2 wk of 14 mg/24 hr; then 2 wk of 7 mg/24 hr (Nicoderm CQ) OR 8 wk of 15 mg/16 hr (Nicotrol)	Local skin reaction, insomnia.	Each patch should be placed on relatively hairless location. Apply as soon as patient awakens on quit day. If patient has sleep disturbances, remove 24-hr patch before bed or use 16-hr patch.
Second-Line				
Clonidine hydrochloride (oral or transdermal by prescription). 0.2 mg tab = $0.27. Transdermal = $0.25/patch.	Pregnancy and lactation. Rebound hypertension if dose is not gradually reduced over 2-4 d.	0.15-0.75 mg/d orally to 0.10 to 0/20 mg/d transdermal.	Dry mouth, drowsiness, dizziness, sedation, and constipation. Do not discontinue abruptly.	Initiate shortly before (up to 3 d) or on quit date. For transdermal, at start of week, patch should be placed on relatively hairless location between neck and waist.
Nortriptyline hydrochloride (prescription only). 75 mg = $0.65.	Pregnancy. Use with extreme caution with CV disease— arrhythmia risk.	Start at 25 mg/d orally. Increase dose to 75-100 mg/d for 12 wk.	Sedation, dry mouth, blurred vision, urinary retention, lightheaded- ness, shaky hands.	Risk of overdose.

14. Is one nicotine replacement more effective?

No clear evidence exists that any one delivery method is more effective.

15. Can the patient continue to smoke while using the nicotine patch or gum?

No. The incidence rate of adverse reactions is greater, and the development of angina and arrhythmias has been implicated if smoking continues.

16. May the previously mentioned pharmacotherapies be combined?

Yes. Evidence supports that combining the nicotine patch with either nicotine gum or nicotine nasal spray increases long-term abstinence rates when compared with the use of a single form of nicotine replacement therapy. Also, treatment with bupropion (Zyban) and a nicotine patch (or just bupropion alone) results in higher long-term abstinence rates than use of a nicotine patch.

17. What about acupuncture or hypnosis as therapy?

A review of studies to date shows acupuncture to be ineffective as a smoking cessation strategy. The reviewers for the Clinical Practice Guidelines were unable to find enough studies that were appropriately designed with the hypnosis method. The reviewers did site an independent review (Cochrane Group) of hypnotherapy, which was unable to show the effectiveness of hypnotherapy.

18. Are there contraindications to nicotine replacement with patients with CV disease?

The Clinical Practice Guidelines note that inaccurate media coverage has associated the use of the nicotine patch and CV risk. However, to date, CV risk with these medications has not been shown. However, it is recommended that (just as the nicotine from smoking would not be advisable during these periods) caution should be used in certain CV groups:
- Persons within 2 weeks of MI.
- Persons with serious arrhythmias.
- Persons with serious or worsening angina.

19. Can someone become addicted to the nicotine gum or patches?

The dependence is not as strong as with cigarettes and may be seen only after long-term (>12 months) use. Long-term use of these therapies does not present a known health risk.

20. What are some physiological and psychological symptoms of nicotine withdrawal, and how long do the cravings last after smoking cessation?

Most people who smoke more than 10 to 15 cigarettes per day for several weeks usually have some sort of physical or psychological dependence develop. Withdrawal symptoms may occur within 24 hours of last exposure to nicotine. Symptoms peak with 1 to 3 weeks and may last for days or weeks. Craving tobacco may last for years. See the following table.

Symptoms can include:

Headache	Sweating	Negative mood	Hostility
Increased appetite	Dizziness	Restlessness	Drowsiness

Continued

continued			
Decreased blood pressure and heart rate	Gastrointestinal disturbances, such as constipation	Urges to smoke or craving	Difficulty concentrating
Increased skin temperature	Anxiety	Insomnia	
Tremors	Irritability	Depression	

21. Is it better to go "cold turkey" or gradually stop?

Some people are able to go "cold turkey," but most people benefit from preparation to quit. With the "cold turkey" approach, they need to be prepared to fight the withdrawal symptoms. Most people need to move through the stages as outlined by Prochaska (see Question 7).

22. What strategies can help fight the cravings?

Strategies that help are taking slow deep breaths, doing something else, telling oneself "Don't give in. I can do this." Also helpful are sipping water, chewing sugarless gum, using a toothpick, moving around, and keeping the hands busy—with beads, paper clips, doodling, crossword puzzles. The nurse should prepare a list of activities that will genuinely distract the person and keep them busy. Drinking water also helps.

23. How long should counseling sessions for smoking cessation last, and how should they be conducted?

Counseling persons about quitting smoking does not need to take hours. Evidence shows that the more intense and longer the intervention, the more likely the patient is to stay smoke free. However, an intervention that lasts less than 3 minutes is effective. Therefore counseling can be performed as a brief treatment or an intensive treatment.

Evidence supports that proactive telephone counseling and group or individual counseling formats are effective and should be used in smoking cessation interventions. See the answers to Question 8.

24. What kind of support groups might help in smoking cessation?

Support groups do not have to be formal, but the nurse can educate the patient to solicit support from family, friends, and coworkers. Hotlines or help lines should be offered to the patient. Internet sites also offer programs and support. The nurse could mail letters to supportive others or phone them. If a formal smoking cessation program exists, the assigning of "buddies" provides for outside support.

25. Is use of chewing tobacco, snuff, pipes, or cigars as harmful as cigarette smoking for CV disease?

People who smoke cigars or pipes seem to have a higher risk of death from CHD, but the risk is not as great as for cigarette smokers, probably because cigar and pipe smokers are less likely to inhale the smoke. These other forms of tobacco use have the same effects as nicotine from cigarettes (i.e., tachycardia, vasoconstriction, acute increase in BP, and addiction).

26. What about the dangers of second-hand smoke related to CV disease?

Several studies document the health hazards posed by passive smoking (i.e., increased heart rate, BP, decrease in high-density lipoprotein (HDL) levels. The American Heart Association (AHA) noted that an epidemiological study by J. He shows that passive smoking increases the relative risk of CHD in men by 22% and in women by 24%. The AHA notes that about 40,000 people die of CV disease caused by other people's smoke each year. Children exposed to passive smoking are at risk for adverse lipid profiles and increased platelet aggregation and thus increased thrombotic potential.

27. For patients unwilling to stop smoking, is there an advantage to tobacco cessation short term, for example, quitting before surgery?

Yes. Some preliminary studies reported by Moller et al reported a trend that CV complications after surgery are decreased by 10% with a 6-week to 8-week smoking cessation or a 50% reduction in smoking for the same time period. In the same study, only 5% of patients who cut back or stopped smoking for 6 to 8 weeks had wound complications develop compared with 31% of patients who did not cut back.

28. What community/Internet resources exist for patients/nurses who want to know more about smoking cessation and actual online programs?

World Health Organization: **www.who.int.**

 Key Points

- Positive changes of smoking cessation exist in the short and long term for the person with CV disease.
- At every health care visit, a brief, even 3-minute, intervention can increase the success rate of smoking cessation. The "5 As" should be implemented: Ask, Advise, Assess, Assist, Arrange.
- Combination of the nicotine patch with either nicotine gum or spray or use of bupropion (Zyban) with the nicotine patch results in higher abstinence rates than use of a patch alone.
- Cardiovascular risk with nicotine replacement products has not been shown, but caution should be used with persons within 2 weeks of MI, with serious dysrhythmias, or with serious or worsening angina.

Internet Resources

Programs for smoking cessation:

American Cancer Society:
www.cancer.org.

American Lung Association:
www.lungusa.org

Nicotine Anonymous:
www.nicotine-anonymous.org

Quitnet (from Boston University):
www.quitnet.com

Quit Smart:
www.quitsmart.com

Smoke Enders:
www.smokenders.com

Smokestoppers:
www.smokestopppers.com

Other resources:

Agency for Healthcare Research and Quality:
www.ahrq.gov

American Heart Association:
www.amhrt.org

National Cancer Institute:
www.nci.nih.gov

National Center for Tobacco Free Kids:
www.tobaccofreekids.org

National Heart, Lung and Blood Institute:
www.nhlbi.nih.gov/index.htm

National Institute on Drug Abuse:
www.nida.nih.gov/NIDAHome1.html

Office on Smoking and Health at the Centers for Disease Control:
www.cdc.gov/tobacco

United States Surgeon General:
www.surgeongeneral.gov

Bibliography

Andrews J et al: Meeting national tobacco challenges: recommendations for smoking cessation groups, *J Am Acad Nurse Pract* 12:522-530, 2000.

American Heart Association: *Cigarette smoking and cardiovascular diseases: AHA scientific position,* available online: http://216.185.112.5/presenter.jhtml?identifier=4545.

Barton S, editor: *Clinical evidence,* ed 6, London, 2001, BMJ Publishing Group.

Burns DM: Nicotine addiction. In Braunwald E et al, editors: *Harrison's principles of internal medicine,* ed 15, New York, 2001, McGraw-Hill, pp 2574-2577.

Doering PL: Substance-related disorders, alcohol, nicotine, and caffeine. In DiPiro JO et al, editors: *Pharmacotherapy: a pathophysiologic approach,* ed 4, Stamford, Conn, 1999, Appleton, pp 1104-1107.

Fiore MC, Bailey WC, Cohen SJ et al: *Treating tobacco use and dependence: clinical practice guideline,* Rockville, Md, 2000, U.S. Department of Health and Human Services, Public Health Service.

Froelicher ES et al: Women's initiative for nonsmoking (WINS) IV: description of 277 women smokers hospitalized with cardiovascular disease, *Heart Lung* 31:3-14, 2002.

Gidding SS et al: *Active and passive tobacco exposure: a serious pediatric health problem: a statement from the Committee on Atherosclerosis and Hypertension in Children, Council on Cardiovascular Disease in the Young,* American Heart Association, 1994, available online: http://216.185.112.5/presenter.jhtml?identifier=1213.

Goolsby MJ: Treating tobacco use and dependence, *J Am Acad Nurse Pract* 13:101-105, 2001.

Hays J et al: Sustained-release bupropion for pharmacologic relapse prevention after smoking cessation: a randomized, controlled trial, *Ann Intern Med* 135:423-433, 2001.

He J et al: Passive smoking and the risk of coronary heart disease—a meta-analysis of epidemiological studies, *N Engl J Med* 340:920-926, 1999.

Jorenby DE: A controlled trial of sustained-release bupropion, a nicotine patch, or both for smoking cessation, *N Engl J Med* 340:685-691, 1999.

Koda-Kimble M, Young L: *Applied therapeutics: the clinical use of drugs,* ed 7, Philadelphia, 1998, Lippincott Williams & Wilkins.

Lindell KO, Reinke LF: Nursing strategies for smoking cessation, *Heart Lung* 28:295-302, 1999.

Moller AM et al: Effect of preoperative smoking intervention on postoperative complications: a randomised clinical trial, *Lancet* 359:114-117, 2002.

Ockene IR, Miller NH, for the AHA Task Force on Risk Reduction: Cigarette smoking, cardiovascular disease, and stroke: a statement for healthcare professionals from the AHA, *Circulation* 96:3243-3247, 1997; available online: http://www.americanheart.org/presenter.jhtml?identifier=1737.

Prochaska JO et al: In search of how people change: applications to addictive behaviors, *Am Psychol* 47:1102-1104, 1992.

Scheibmeir MS, O'Connell KA: Promoting smoking cessation in adults, *Nurs Clin North Am* 37:331-340, 2002.

Uphold CR, Graham MV: *Clinical guidelines in adult health,* ed 2, Gainesville, Fl, 1999, Barmarrae Books.

Chapter 36

Lipid-Lowering Strategies

Julie T. Ruch

1. What is cholesterol?

Cholesterol is a fatty substance that is normally found in the body as a component of cell membranes and neuron insulation and in some hormones. Cholesterol is produced by the liver and is also absorbed in the gut from ingested animal products. Cholesterol is transported through the blood by lipoproteins.

2. What affect does cholesterol have on heart disease?

High cholesterol is one of the major risk factors for atherosclerosis. Atherosclerosis involves the deposition of fatty plaques in the walls of the arteries. This plaque may contain a large amount of cholesterol and can tear or rupture, leading to clot formation that occludes blood flow. When this happens in the coronary arteries, ischemia or a myocardial infarction can occur.

3. What does a cholesterol panel consist of, and what do each of the parts mean?

The standard lipid profile consists of a direct measurement of:
- Total cholesterol (TC).
- High-density lipoprotein–cholesterol (HDL-C).
- Triglycerides (TGs).
- Low-density lipoprotein–cholesterol (LDL-C).

Total cholesterol is simply the total amount of cholesterol in the plasma. HDL-C is the most dense lipoprotein because it is comprised largely of protein (50% protein, 20% cholesterol, and 25% phospholipid). HDL-C facilitates the removal of cholesterol from the plasma and is thus considered the "good" cholesterol. An HDL-C level of more than 60 mg/dL is considered a negative risk factor because it has a protective effect on the heart. TGs are made up of fatty acids and glycerol and are used to store energy. The relationship of an elevated TG level to atherosclerosis is still inconsistent but is believed to be associated with an increase in heart disease. LDL-C, or "bad" cholesterol, is the major carrier of cholesterol in the blood and is comprised of 50% to 60% cholesterol, 25% protein, and 20% phospholipid. This level can be directly measured with ultracentrifugation, although it is usually calculated with the Friedewald equation:

$$LDL\text{-}C = TC - HDL\text{-}C - (TG/5)$$

Note that the TG level must be 400 mg/dL or less to prevent miscalculation of the LDL-C. Elevated levels of LDL-C significantly increase the risk of heart disease, and therefore LDL-C lowering is generally the focus of treatment.

4. What are the "normal" levels?

Total cholesterol	<200 mg/dL	Desirable
	200-239 mg/dL	Borderline high
	≥240 mg/dL	High
Low-density lipoprotein–cholesterol	<100 mg/dL	Optimal
	100-129 mg/dL	Near optimal/above optimal
	130-159 mg/dL	Borderline high
	160-189 mg/dL	High
	≥190 mg/dL	Very high
High-density lipoprotein–cholesterol	<40 mg/dL	Low
	>60 mg/dL	Negative risk factor
Triglycerides	<150 mg/dL	Normal
	150-199 mg/dL	Borderline high
	200-499 mg/dL	High
	≥500 mg/dL	Very high

Adapted from Executive Summary of the Third Report of the National Cholesterol Education Program (NCEP) Expert Panel on Detection, Evaluation, and Treatment of High Blood Cholesterol in Adults (Adult Treatment Panel III), *JAMA* 285(19):2486-2497, 2001.

5. How often should adults have a lipid panel done? At what age should initial screening begin?

According to the National Cholesterol Education Program's (NCEP) Adult Treatment Panel III (ATP III) guidelines, all adults over the age of 20 years should have a fasting lipoprotein panel (TC, TG, HDL-C, LDL-C) every 5 years.

6. Is fasting important for every lipid panel? For how long?

All lipid panels should be fasting. An accurate lipid panel can only be assessed after 12 hours of fasting. If the patient does not fast, only a TC and an HDL-C should be obtained. TGs are abnormally elevated postprandially and result in an inaccurately calculated LDL-C. If a nonfasting TC is 200 mg/dL or more or the HDL-C is less than 40 mg/dL, a fasting lipoprotein profile is needed to assess LDL-C.

7. What is the goal of treatment?

Low-density lipoprotein–cholesterol lowering is the primary goal of treatment. To determine LDL-C goal, the number of risk factors the patient has for coronary heart disease (CHD) must be considered.

- If the patient has known CHD, diabetes mellitus (DM), or other atherosclerotic diseases, including peripheral vascular disease (PVD), abdominal aortic aneurysm (AAA), or symptomatic carotid artery disease, the LDL-C goal is less than 100 mg/dL.
- If the patient does not have any known disease, the major independent risk factors must be added up first (see the following box).

Major Risk Factors (Exclusive of LDL-C) That Modify LDL Goals*

- Cigarette smoking.
- Hypertension (blood pressure [BP] ≥140/90 mm Hg or on antihypertensive medication).
- Low HDL-C (<40 mg/dL).[†]
- Family history of premature CHD (CHD in male first-degree relative <55 years; CHD in female first-degree relative <65 years).
- Age (men ≥45 years; women ≥55 years).*

Reproduced from Executive Summary of the Third Report of the National Cholesterol Education Program (NCEP) Expert Panel on Detection, Evaluation, and Treatment of High Blood Cholesterol in Adults (Adult Treatment Panel III), *JAMA* 285(19):2486-2497, 2001.

*In ATP III, diabetes is regarded as a CHD risk equivalent.

[†]HDL-C ≥60 mg/dL counts as a "negative" risk factor; its presence removes one risk factor from the total count.

- If the patient has two or more risk factors, their 10-year CHD risk should be calculated with the Framingham risk assessment. If the 10-year risk is 20% or more, the LDL-C goal is less than 100 mg/dL. If the 10-year risk is less than 20%, the LDL-C goal is less than 130 mg/dL (see the Framingham Risk Score on pages 416-417).
- If the patient has zero to one risk factor, the LDL-C goal is less than 160 mg/dL.

8. What is meant by therapeutic lifestyle changes (TLCs)?

Therapeutic lifestyle changes are what were traditionally known as lifestyle modifications. All patients with hyperlipidemia need to be educated to begin TLCs as a first-line of treatment, regardless of whether they are on pharmacologic therapy. TLCs include:

- Reduced intake of saturated fats (<7 % total calories) and cholesterol (<200 mg/d).
- Added intake of LDL-C–lowering plant stanols/sterols (2 g/d). Plant stanols and sterols are derived from soy and other plant sources and are found in spreads such as Benecol and Take Control. They inhibit the absorption of cholesterol into the body, resulting in an LDL-cholesterol reduction of as much as 10%.

Estimate of 10-Year Risk for Men (Framingham Point Scores)

Age (yr)	Points
20-34	−9
35-39	−4
40-44	−0
45-49	3
50-54	6
55-59	8
60-64	10
65-69	11
70-74	12
75-79	13

Total Cholesterol (mg/dL)	Points				
	Age 20-39 yr	Age 40-49 yr	Age 50-59 yr	Age 60-69 yr	Age 70-79 yr
<160	0	0	0	0	0
160-199	4	3	2	1	0
200-239	7	5	3	1	0
240-279	9	6	4	2	1
≥280	11	8	5	3	1

	Points				
	Age 20-39 yr	Age 40-49 yr	Age 50-59 yr	Age 60-69 yr	Age 70-79 yr
Nonsmoker	0	0	0	0	0
Smoker	8	5	3	1	1

HDL (mg/dL)	Points
≥60	−1
50-59	0
40-49	1
<40	2

Systolic BP (mm Hg)	If Untreated	If Treated
<120	0	0
120-129	0	1
130-139	1	2
140-159	1	2
≥160	2	3

Point Total	10-Year Risk Percentage
<0	<1
0	1
1	1
2	1
3	1
4	1
5	2
6	2
7	3
8	4
9	5
10	6
11	8
12	10
13	12
14	16
15	20
16	25
≥17	≥30

Estimate of 10-Year Risk for Women (Framingham Point Scores)

Age (yr)	Points
20-34	-7
35-39	-3
40-44	0
45-49	3
50-54	6
55-59	8
60-64	10
65-69	12
70-74	14
75-79	16

Total Cholesterol (mg/dL)	Points				
	Age 20-39 yr	Age 40-49 yr	Age 50-59 yr	Age 60-69 yr	Age 70-79 yr
<160	0	0	0	0	0
160-199	4	3	2	1	1
200-239	8	6	4	2	1
240-279	11	8	5	3	2
≥280	13	10	7	4	2

	Points				
	Age 20-39 yr	Age 40-49 yr	Age 50-59 yr	Age 60-69 yr	Age 70-79 yr
Nonsmoker	0	0	0	0	0
Smoker	9	7	4	2	1

HDL (mg/dL)	Points
≥60	-1
50-59	0
40-49	1
<40	2

Systolic BP (mm Hg)	If Untreated	If Treated
<120	0	0
120-129	1	3
130-139	2	4
140-159	3	5
≥160	4	6

Point Total	10-Year Risk Percentage
<9	<1
9	1
10	1
11	1
12	1
13	2
14	2
15	3
16	4
17	5
18	6
19	8
20	11
21	14
22	17
23	22
24	27
≥25	≥30

- Increased soluble fiber (10 to 25 g/d).
- Weight reduction.
- Increased physical activity.

9. What are the most common medical treatment options for hyperlipidemia?

Drug	Therapeutic Benefits	Adverse Effects
HGM-CoA reductase inhibitors (statins): atorvastatin calcium (Lipitor), fluvastatin (Lescol), lovastatin (Mevacor), pravastatin sodium (Pravachol), simvastatin (Zocor).	↓ Low-density lipoprotein–cholesterol (LDL-C; 18%-55%) and triglycerides (TGs; 7%-30%) by inhibiting cholesterol synthesis in liver. Also may ↑ high-density lipoprotein–cholesterol (HDL-C) by 5%-15%. Some have been shown to decrease coronary events and death.	Gastrointestinal (GI) disturbances. ↑ Liver enzymes. Myalgias, myopathies.
Bile acid sequestrants: cholestyramine, (Questran), colestipol hydrochloride (Colestid), colesevelam (WelChol).	↓ LDL-C (15%-30%) by absorbing bile in small intestine and increasing conversion of cholesterol to bile acid. May ↑ HDL-C by 3%-5%. Also, may ↑ TGs.	GI distress, constipation, bloating. Decrease absorption of other drugs.
Nicotinic acid: immediate-release and extended-release forms.	↓ LDL-C (5%-25%) by reducing liver's production of very LDL-C. Also ↑ HDL-C by 15%-35% and ↓ TGs by 20%-50%.	Flushing, itching. Hyperglycemia. Gout. Upper GI distress. Hepatotoxicity.
Fibrates: gemfibrozil (Lopid), fenofibrate (Tricor).	↓ TGs by increasing catabolism of TG-rich particles. Also ↑ HDL-C by 10%-20%. Variable effect on LDL-C.	Dyspepsia. Gallstones. Severe myopathy, especially when used with statins.
Cholesterol absorption inhibitor: ezetimibe (Zetia)	↓ LDL-C by inhibiting absorption cholesterol from small intestine. Monotherapy: ↓ LDL-C by 18%. Combined with statins: ↓ LDL-C by additional 25%. Therapeutic changes in TGs (↓) and HDL-C (↑).	Similar to placebo. ↑ Liver function tests in combination with statins.

10. What important patient teaching should be done for patients started on cholesterol-reducing medications for the first time?

First, assurance that the patient has already received thorough education on TLCs is important. Patients need to be reminded that they must continue to follow the TLC recommendations along with the medical treatment. Many patients once started on cholesterol-lowering medication think they no longer need to follow a low cholesterol diet. Second, as with other medications, patients need to be instructed of the side effects, the best time to take the medication, and the symptoms that necessitate a call to the physician or nurse practitioner. They also should be told the LDL-C goal and educated about the amount of cholesterol lowering expected with each dose. Forewarning that titration may be necessary prevents undue discouragement if the dose needs to be increased. Finally, patients should be instructed that follow-up lab tests are done periodically to assess the efficacy of medication and to monitor for liver dysfunction with some medicines.

11. What are the most common side effects of statins?

An elevated liver enzyme level is the most common side effect of statin therapy (1% to 2%). Therefore baseline liver function tests (LFTs) should be obtained before drug initiation. LFTs should be repeated at least once after the drug therapy has begun or the dose has been increased (see product insert for specific guidelines regarding frequency of liver function monitoring for a specific drug). Elevation of liver enzyme levels is dose dependent, and discontinuation of the drug should be done if LFTs are elevated three times the upper limit of normal on two separate occasions at least 1 week apart. The patient must understand that liver abnormalities are almost always reversible once the drug is stopped or reduced.

Other common side effects include gastrointestinal (GI) disturbances, diarrhea, nausea, or vomiting. A more rare but serious side effect of statins is rhabdomyolysis.

12. What is rhabdomyolysis?

Rhabdomyolysis is the acute breakdown of skeletal muscle that results in creatine kinase elevation 10 times greater than normal, associated muscle soreness, and weakness and myoglobinuria. The incidence rate in statin monotherapy is very low (0.1%), but the rate increases with combination with other agents such as cyclosporine, gemfibrozil, niacin, erythromycin, protease inhibitors, nefazodone hydrochloride, and the macrolide antibiotics. Patients should be instructed to notify their physician or nurse practitioner in the event of muscle pain, weakness, fatigue, or brown urine.

13. What is the metabolic syndrome?

The metabolic syndrome is a constellation of risk factors of metabolic origin that is closely linked to insulin resistance. The syndrome is found primarily in people with excess body fat and physical inactivity. The ATP III defines the metabolic syndrome as a combination of three or more of the following:
• Abdominal obesity (waist circumference: men, >40 in; women, >35 in).
• Triglycerides 150 mg/dL or more.

- High-density lipoprotein–cholesterol less than 40 mg/dL in men and less than 50 mg/dL in women.
- Blood pressure 130/85 mm Hg or more.
- Fasting glucose more than 110 mg/dL.

The management of the metabolic syndrome focuses primarily on TLCs to control weight and increase physical activity. Other goals are to treat elevated blood pressure and TGs and low HDL-C, which may require medication and TLCs.

14. How are elevated serum TGs treated?

Elevated serum TGs have been shown to be a risk factor for CHD, particularly in combination with low HDL-C. The pattern is usually found in patients with the metabolic syndrome. Other contributing factors include being overweight, physical inactivity, cigarette smoking, excess alcohol intake, high carbohydrate diets (>60% of caloric intake), type II diabetes, chronic renal failure, nephrotic syndrome, hypothyroidism, certain drugs, and genetic lipid disorders. When TGs are borderline high, the primary treatment is TLCs. For high TGs, a non–HDL-C goal (TC–HDL-C) should be set at 30 mg/dL higher than the LDL-C goal. To achieve this goal, either LDL-C lowering can be intensified with a statin or a second drug can be added for TG lowering (nicotinic acid or fibrate, or fish oil). Adjunct therapy should be used with caution because the incidence rates of myositis and elevated liver enzymes increase with combination therapy. Finally, if TGs are very high (500), the initial goal is to lower TGs to prevent pancreatitis.

15. Should low HDL-C be treated, and if so, how?

Low HDL-C is known to be a strong independent risk factor for CHD. This condition is primarily found in the metabolic syndrome but also in cigarette smoking and high carbohydrate diets and with certain drugs. A significant raise in HDL-C is difficult, and therefore the primary goal of therapy remains LDL-C. Once the LDL-C goal is achieved, attention should be given to the non–HDL-C goal (see previous question). Increasing activity, smoking cessation, and weight management are the best ways to raise HDL-C. Consideration can be given to nicotinic acid and fibrates for HDL-C-raising primarily in patients with CHD or CHD risk equivalents.

16. When is niacin used? How can the side effect of flushing be curbed?

Nicotinic acid is used in dyslipidemia to raise HDL-C, lower TGs, and moderately lower LDL-C. Nicotinic acid is fairly inexpensive, but proper education and slow titration is necessary to improve patient tolerance to the uncomfortable, although harmless, side effect of cutaneous flushing. Extended-release or sustained-release forms have also been shown to decrease incidence of flushing; however, the extended-release form has a lower incidence of LFT elevation. Patient instructions include:
- Take at bedtime.
- Avoid hot beverages and alcohol with administration.

- Take aspirin (80 to 325 mg) 30 minutes before taking nicotinic acid.
- Take with small, low-fat snack.

Other side effects of niacin include GI symptoms, increased incidence of gout, and worsening glucose control in patients with diabetes and conversion of insulin resistance to frank diabetes. In general, with proper education and encouragement, nicotinic acid is well tolerated and effective.

17. What affect does fish oil have on cholesterol?

Fish oils (eicosapentaenoic acid [EPA] and docosahexaenoic acid [DHA]), whether in fish consumption or dietary supplementation, have been associated with a significantly reduced risk of CHD. At the dose of 2 to 5 g per day, these omega-3 fatty acids decrease plasma levels of TGs by 20% to 30% and cause a modest rise in HDL-C. Side effects include mostly GI symptoms, therefore supplements should be taken with food.

18. What is LDL apheresis? When is it indicated?

Low-density lipoprotein apheresis is plasmaphoresis that specifically removes apoB-containing lipoproteins from the blood and is primarily performed in regional medical centers usually every 1 to 2 weeks. The US Food and Drug Administration (FDA) has approved LDL apheresis for patients with familial hypercholesterolemia who after a 6-month trial of dietary and medication therapy continue to have very high levels of LDL-C that are refractory to medication. For patients with CAD, LDL-C must be >200 gm/dL. For patients without CAD, LDL-C must be >300 mg/dL.

19. What are the current controversies/future directions of lipid management? Is "the lower the better" the answer?

The ATP III from NCEP has emphasized more aggressive LDL-C lowering based on the growing body of data that show that reducing LDL-C is associated with a reduced risk in coronary heart disease. The recently reported Heart Protection Study showed that statin therapy reduced cardiovascular events and mortality regardless of baseline LDL-C level. This suggests that patients at high risk should be treated with a statin even if LDL is optimal. Whether a low amount of LDL-C is best or whether it just needs to be lowered from baseline is still debatable, however, there are ongoing studies that hopefully will answer the question.

20. What is the evidence surrounding lipoprotein particle size and density, lipoprotein [a] (Lp[a]), C-reactive protein, and homocysteine?

Interest is growing in lipid particle size and density, or atherogenic dyslipidemia. Small, dense LDL-C is associated with the metabolic syndrome, which itself is associated with increased risk for CHD. Whether the increased CHD risk is from the small, dense LDL-C or simply the atherogenic metabolic syndrome has yet to be determined. Exercise, weight loss, and the use of niacin does increase particle size.

Lipoprotein [a] is identical to LDL-C except for the addition of apoprotein [a]. Some studies have shown an association between CHD risk and elevated Lp[a] but primarily in the presence of high LDL-C concentrations. Niacin can lower Lp[a], however, Lp[a] has been shown to lose its predictive value once LDL-C is significantly reduced.

High-sensitivity C-reactive protein (hs-CRP) is an acute phase reactant inflammatory marker that is an independent predictor of coronary artery disease. The Centers for Disease Control (CDC) and the American Heart Association (AHA) have recently recommended it for use in clinical practice, primarily in patients at intermediate risk. These are patients without known cardiovascular disease who have a 10% to 20% 10-year Framingham risk score. An elevated hs-CRP could be used to further guide therapy in primary prevention and possibly to motivate patients in TLCs. Hs-CRP should be drawn twice, 2 weeks apart, in a patient with a metabolically stable condition.

Elevated levels of plasma homocysteine have been linked to increased risk for CHD, PVD, and cerebrovascular disease. Homocysteine levels can be reduced with folic acid and vitamins B_6 and B_{12}. However, research is needed to show whether lowering homocysteine reduces CHD.

21. Do statins have other cardioprotective mechanisms other than lowering cholesterol?

Some studies suggest that lipid lowering alone is not enough to explain the significant reduction in coronary events from statin therapy. Therefore other cardioprotective mechanisms of statins are being proposed and investigated:
- Atherosclerotic plaque stabilization and repair.
- Decreased vascular inflammation.
- Improved coronary endothelial function.
- Antithrombotic effects.

22. What new lipid-lowering medications are on the horizon?

- Ezetimibe was approved by the FDA at the end of 2002 and represents a totally new class of cholesterol medication. It is a selective inhibitor of dietary and biliary cholesterol absorption from the small intestine. Ezetimibe can be used in monotherapy or in combination with statins to lower TC and LDL-C. It also has therapeutic changes on TGs and HDL-C. This medication is proving useful in achieving LDL goals for patients with very elevated LDL-C levels and for those who do not tolerate statin therapy.
- Medications that raise HDL-C are currently in development and under clinical investigation.
- Rosuvastatin, or Crestor, was approved by the FDA in September 2003. While similar to other statins, rosuvastatin offers greater efficacy in LDL-C reduction.

Key Points

- Lowering the LDL is the goal of therapy for both primary and secondary prevention of coronary artery disease.
- Statins are the mainstay of therapy for risk reduction.
- For patients at intermediate risk, the Framingham risk score should be calculated to further risk stratify the patient.
- All patients with high cholesterol should be taught the recommendation for TLCs.

Internet Resources

National Heart, Lung, and Blood Institute: National Cholesterol Education Program: Third Report of the Expert Panel on Detection, Evaluation, and Treatment of High Blood Cholesterol in Adults (Adult Treatment Panel III):
http://www.nhlbi.nih.gov/guidelines/cholesterol/index.htm

Preventive Cardiovascular Nurses Association:
http://www.pcna.net/

The National Lipid Association:
http://www.lipid.org/

American Heart Association: Cholesterol:
http://www.americanheart.org/presenter.jhtml?identifier=1516

Bibliography

Braun L, Davidson M: Cholesterol-lowering drugs bring benefits to high-risk populations even when LDL is normal, *J Cardiovasc Nurs* 18(1):44-49, 2003.

Executive summary of the Third Report of the National Cholesterol Education Program (NCEP) Expert Panel on Detection, Evaluation, and Treatment of High Blood Cholesterol in Adults (Adult Treatment Panel III), *JAMA* 285(19):2486-2497, 2001.

Forrester J et al: The aggressive low density lipoprotein lowering controversy, *J Am Coll Cardiol* 36(4):1419-1425, 2000.

Gagne C et al: Efficacy and safety of Ezetimibe added to ongoing statin therapy for treatment of patients with primary hypercholesterolemia, *Am J Cardiol* 19(10):1084-1091, 2002.

Gotto A: Statins: powerful drugs for lowering cholesterol, *Circulation* 105:1514-1516, 2002.

Gotto A, Pownall H: *Manual of lipid disorders: reducing the risk for coronary heart disease,* ed 2, Baltimore, 1999, Williams & Wilkins.

Gotto A: *Contemporary diagnosis and management of lipid disorders,* ed 2, Newtown, Pa, 1999, Handbooks in Healthcare.

Heart Protection Study Collaborative Group: MRC/BHF Heart Protection Study of cholesterol lowering with simvastatin in 20,536 high-risk individuals: a randomized placebo-controlled trial, *Lancet* 360:7-22, 2002.

Hu FB et al: Fish and omega-3 fatty acid intake and risk of coronary heart disease in women, *JAMA* 287(14):1815-1821, 2002.

Kuncl N, Nelson K: Getting the skinny on lipid-lowering drugs, *Nursing* 30(7):52-53, 2000.

Lamendola C: Hypertriglyceridemia and low high-density lipoprotein: risks for coronary artery disease? *J Cardiovasc Nurs* 14(2):79-90, 2000.

McCormick J, Deeg M: Pharmacologic treatment of dyslipidemia, *Am J Nurs* 100(2):55-60, 2000.

Pearson T et al: Markers of inflammation and cardiovascular disease: application to clinical and public health practice: a statement for healthcare professionals from the Centers for Disease Control and Prevention and the American Heart Association, *Circulation* 107:499-511, 2003.

Piskur J, Stone N: Statins as cardioprotective agents, *Am J Managed Care* 8(9 suppl):25-29, 2002.

Pradka L: Lipids and their roles in coronary heart disease: what they do and how to manage them, *Nurs Clin North Am* 35(4):981-991, 2000.

Stone N, Blum C: *Management of lipids in clinical practice,* ed 4, Caddo, Ok, 2002, Professional Communications, Inc.

Physical Activity

Rebecca Gary

1. What are some noted benefits of physical activity?

Although physical activity has not shown the independent ability to prevent the progression of coronary artery disease (CAD), it does have known antiatherogenic effects. Less severe CAD, larger coronary artery lumens, and decreased atherosclerosis progression are associated with regular physical activity. In addition, physical activity reduces the amount of adipose tissue, lowers elevated blood pressure, reduces elevated triglycerides and low-density lipoprotein (LDL), and increases high-density lipoprotein (HDL) cholesterol levels. Randomized clinical trials show that regular physical activity reduces on average the systolic blood pressure by 10 mm Hg and the diastolic pressure by 7.5 mm Hg. A number of studies concluded that physical activity reduces total cholesterol by 6.3%, LDL cholesterol by 10.1%, and total/HDL cholesterol by 13.4% and increases HDL by 5%. However, when diet modifications and increased physical activity are combined, the total reductions in total and LDL cholesterol have been much greater, up to 30% in some instances.

Cardiac workload is reduced through an improved balance of oxygen supply and demand. The training effect of regular physical activity is a lower heart rate (HR) and systolic blood pressure, reducing myocardial oxygen demands and coronary artery blood flow requirements. In other words, the person can stay active longer or at greater intensity levels while demanding less work from the cardiovascular system. These changes benefit individuals with cardiovascular disease, who after exercise training may achieve a higher level of physical activity before myocardial ischemia.

An improvement in insulin sensitivity and glucose usage occurs with increased levels of physical activity. The Diabetes Prevention Program reported that the loss of 15 lb and participation in 30 minutes of daily physical activity reduced diabetes incidence by 58% and decreased cardiovascular risk significantly.

The effects of physical activity on weight loss are variable. The "dose" of physical activity to produce weight loss is not well understood but is thought to represent more vigorous levels than are currently recommended. Evidence shows that when diet and physical activity are combined more positive outcomes for weight loss occur.

Physical activity has shown effectiveness in improvement in a sense of well-being, mood, self-confidence, and quality of life in persons with cardiovascular disease. Exercise has also been shown to reduce some type A behaviors in addition to attenuating cardiovascular and neurohormonal responses to mental stress.

2. What is the current recommendation for physical activity for health benefits, including cardiovascular risk reduction?

Adequate levels of physical activity significantly reduce the risk of cardiovascular disease and all-cause mortality. Physical activity performed for 30 minutes to 1 hour at moderate intensity on most days of the week is adequate for health benefits, including cardiovascular risk reduction.

3. What percentage of US adults does not receive adequate amounts of physical activity?

Seventy percent of US adults are estimated to not meet minimal requirements for physical activity. As a result, physical inactivity has become a national health priority and is now identified as a significant, modifiable risk factor for heart disease.

4. Define physical activity and describe subcategories that should be taken into consideration in advising patients.

Physical activity refers to any voluntary movement produced by skeletal muscle that results in energy expenditure. Physical activity and exercise are often used interchangeably, but differences do exist. Physical activity is multidimensional as evidenced by efforts to define the dose (frequency, duration, and intensity) in relation to morbidity, mortality, and quality of life outcomes in specific patient populations.

In addition, the type of activity (e.g., endurance, resistance, or flexibility) has different outcomes related to disease and physical function. For example, cardio-respiratory outcomes are improved to a greater extent by endurance activities rather than strength training.

The several subcategories of physical activity include occupational physical activity (OPA), leisure-time physical activity (LTPA), and exercise. For persons who are employed, OPA, or activities that take place within the workplace during a conventional 8-hour workday, should be considered in discussion of physical activity level. Creative exercises or short bouts of walking during the day may be the most useful in this situation. Unless an individual spends a minimum of 30 minutes per day walking during their workday, their activity level should be supplemented with leisure time exercise.

Free-time activities that are based on personal interests and needs (i.e., gardening, exercise programs, sports, dance) are considered LPTA. Women tend to describe housework as physical activity and generally use less leisure time activities than men. When advising women with cardiovascular disease, encouraging activities that can be incorporated into their everyday activities is recommended. For example, walking to a neighbor's house, or several short 10-minute bouts per day, may be preferable to one continuous 30-minute activity.

Exercise, a subcategory of LPTA, is defined as planned, structured, and repetitive bodily movement performed to maintain one or more components of physical fitness. Physical fitness is related to specific attributes people have or obtain to perform physical activity. Health-related fitness collectively represents cardio-respiratory function, body composition (bone, muscle, fat, and water), and muscle strength and endurance.

5. In general terms, what does moderate physical activity mean in relation to physical activity level for healthy adults and those with cardiovascular disease?

Moderate intensity is equivalent to walking at a brisk pace at 3 to 4 miles per hour for healthy individuals. For patients with cardiovascular disease, the moderate intensity level may be much lower depending on age, health status, and level of physical conditioning. Identification of routine activity in a 24-hour period on a weekday and weekend can be useful for estimating general level of physical activity and the type of activity that would be appropriate to consider for persons with cardiovascular disease.

6. Can any health benefit be achieved with routine activities of daily living?

According to the new guidelines, health benefits can be achieved with moderate intensity physical activities of daily living, such as house and yard work, and with occupational and leisure activities. These guidelines emphasize all types of activities that are more compatible with the multiple roles and responsibilities in everyday life.

These recommendations reflect the benefits derived with some type of physical activity at moderate intensity on a regular basis, at least three to four times per week.

7. Does intermittent physical activity provide any health benefits?

Intermittent bouts of physical activity have the same health benefits as continuous activity. For those persons with busy schedules and in the early phases of beginning a new activity program, intermittent sessions may provide a greater incentive for maintaining adequate levels of physical activity.

Depending on the health status and level of physical conditioning, short activity sessions can be accomplished by walking up and down stairs instead of taking the elevator, walking instead of driving relatively short distances, parking at a greater distance when shopping, using the stationary bicycle or treadmill while watching television, gardening projects, carrying groceries instead of having them carried, walking a 9-hole golf course instead of riding in a cart, hanging out clothes instead of using a dryer, or washing the car; these activities could all be used to reach the daily activity goal of 30-minutes. Emphasizing that joining a health club or buying equipment is not necessary for a successful program of physical activity that satisfies current recommendations is important.

8. What are the risks associated with physical activity?

If CAD is present, an exercise test is highly recommended before any physical activity program is started. Otherwise, for apparently healthy adults, exercise tests are recommended but not required. Age, presence of heart disease, and the intensity of physical activity are the most important factors to consider in assessment of individual risk factors for activity participation and potential for adverse events. However, a number of other considerations should be taken into account that may also influence the individual degree of risk associated with physical activity, such as medical history and the presence of comorbid illnesses, current treatment methods, and routine activity level.

Sudden cardiac death under the age of 40 years is most often to the result of congenital heart disease and over the age of 40 years is more likely the result of CAD. Vigorous activity is more likely to result in sudden cardiac death in persons with CAD versus healthy individuals. Among outpatient programs, the risk of cardiovascular mortality is estimated to be 1 per 116,400 hours of exercise to 1 per 784,000 hours of exercise (Williams, 2001).

Importantly, among physically inactive persons, the relative risk of an acute myocardial infarction (AMI) is reported to be 107 times that of baseline, whereas individuals who participate in regular activity five times per week have a 2.4 chance of an AMI compared with baseline. It is important to remember that the least active individuals have the greatest risk of an AMI and must be advised to begin physical activity slowly, increasing duration and frequency of activity before intensity level.

Musculoskeletal injuries, including bruises, sprains, and joint and back pain, are by far the most common injuries that are likely to occur. Higher impact activities, such as running and step aerobics, are associated with more stress on the hips, knees, ankles, and feet and have a higher risk of associated injury. High-impact physical activities are not recommended for persons over the age of 50 years because of increased risk of orthopedic injuries. Low-impact exercises, such as walking, cycling, Tai Chi, or water aerobics, are the safest and are suitable for most individuals, including those with osteoarthritis and adults more than 50 years of age.

9. Are there any contraindications to participation in physical activity?

- Unstable angina.
- Uncompensated heart failure.
- Severe aortic stenosis.
- Active myocardial infections.

- Recent embolisms and thrombophlebitis.
- Uncontrolled sinus tachycardia (>120 bpm).
- Uncontrolled atrial or ventricular arrhythmias.
- Third-degree atrioventricular block (no pacemaker).
- Uncontrolled hypertension during rest.
- Orthostatic systolic hypotension.
- Acute illness.
- Unstable neurological disorders.
- Uncontrolled metabolic diseases, such as diabetes mellitus.
- Severe electrolyte imbalances.

10. Should physical activity be initiated in patients hospitalized with an acute cardiovascular event?

Patients who are admitted to the hospital for an acute cardiac event are often placed on bed rest for 24 to 48 hours. During this time, physical activities should be aimed at self-care activities, low-resistance range of motion, and flexibility exercises with the goal of avoiding complications associated with bed rest. Activity should progress gradually from lying, to sitting, to standing, with hemodynamic response to these position changes monitored. How rapidly a patient progresses in activity status depends primarily on clinical status, medical history, and current symptoms, such as angina and dyspnea.

11. How should exercise be progressed during hospitalization?

With first ambulation, monitoring and recording of activity tolerance is essential for determination of how activity should progress during the remainder of hospitalization. Vital signs before, during, and after the first activity session and telemetry monitoring for arrhythmias are important baseline assessments that should be recorded. In addition, the nurses' presence may provide some reassurance to the patient during the first several activity sessions. The level of exertion during physical activity should not exceed 12 to 13 on the rate of perceived exertion scale (6 to 20 scale). For patients after AMI, the HR should be kept within 20 beats of the resting HR during walking sessions, unless otherwise instructed. The initial duration on physical activity is largely dependent on patient ability, clinical status, and discretion, but generally no longer than 5 minutes is advised during the first few activity sessions. If the patient's condition is stable and early mobilization and ambulation are warranted, then activity three to four times per day up to 20 minutes per day should be encouraged. The goal at discharge should be for the patient to be able to ambulate continuously for 5 to 10 minutes at a low-intensity to moderate-intensity level. Walking is the recommended activity unless physical limitations prevent this mode.

12. Why should warm-up and cool-down periods be considered part of the physical activity program?

The purpose of the warm-up period is to increase blood flow to the muscles and surrounding ligaments, increase muscle temperature, and prepare the cardiopulmonary system for an increase in physiological stress. Warm-up activities should be 5 to 10 minutes in length ideally and should consist of stretching, range of motion, and flexibility exercises. A warm-up period that is too brief can result in soreness, stiffness, and injury to the muscles, joints, and ligaments.

The cool-down period is designed to allow for a gradual decrease in the heat load and peripheral vasodilatation experienced during increased physical activity. Venous pooling and hypotension may occur if the cool-down period after physical activity is too short. The amount of time recommended for cool-down is 5 to 10 minutes with slow walking, stretching, and range of motion exercises. In older adults, warm-up, cool-down, and rest between activities, depending on age and level of conditioning, may require a longer period of time.

13. What type of physical activity is recommended for persons with cardiovascular disease?

Endurance activities have the greatest potential for increasing oxygen consumption and improving cardiovascular fitness. Maximal aerobic fitness refers to the ability of the body to maximally transport and use oxygen in the cells (VO_{2max}). Walking, cycling, swimming, and stair stepping are common endurance-building activities. However, walking should be routinely advised at a low-intensity to moderate-intensity level until exercise testing is conducted or a safety level is established.

14. Do cardiac medications influence exercise response?

Beta-blockers may blunt exercise HR response and lower blood pressure. Vasodilators, angiotensin-converting enzyme (ACE) inhibitors, and calcium channel blockers may also decrease blood pressure response to exercise. Hydralazine, in particular, may cause a reflex elevation in HR (reflex tachycardia) that may occur during exercise. Certain antiarrhythmics, such as amiodarone, may result in a significant decrease in HR during exercise and in increases in QRS duration. Diuretics typically have little influence on cardiac response during exercise. However, because of a reduction in plasma volume or electrolyte depletion, muscle fatigue, ventricular ectopy, and hypotension may occur in response to increased physical activity.

15. What are the basic principles that are important to include when advising cardiovascular patients concerning endurance activities?

Three specific areas of instruction should be emphasized when advising patients about endurance activities: frequency, duration, and intensity of physical activity.
- Frequency includes the number of sessions the person is advised to perform during a specific time period. The frequency of physical activity in persons beginning an endurance-training program should be 3 to 5 days a week

preferably. Increasing frequency in the early weeks of the program to several times per day for short intermittent periods of time may also serve to encourage behavioral change and adherence to a regular pattern of physical activity.

· Duration is the amount of time the person engages in the activity. It is imperative to begin slow and increase duration gradually, 2 to 3 minutes per session up to a goal of 30 minutes or longer per session as tolerated. Duration of activity is based on individual tolerance level and is always increased before intensity level.

· Intensity generally refers to a percentage of maximal oxygen consumption (VO_{2max}) during performance of the activity. When results from an exercise test are available, the HR reserve method with Karvonen's formula is often used for prescribing a specific level of intensity during physical activity. Low-intensity to moderate-intensity levels (40% to 60%) should be used during the first weeks of a new physical activity program. For example, a 40% intensity (low) level would be calculated as follows: [(maximal HR – resting HR) × 40%] + resting HR. Intensity levels can be determined at any level with this method. If feasible, the person should obtain a wrist-worn HR counter (cardiotachometer) for the purpose of keeping HR within the prescribed range. Cardiotachometers can be purchased at most sporting equipment stores for $40 to $60 and are accurate for monitoring HR during activities such as walking. If this is not feasible, then the person should be instructed how to manually count the pulse.

If an exercise test is not available, the rating of perceived exertion (RPE) may be used to estimate intensity level. The Borg RPE scale is a well-known measure of subjective exertion during activity (see the following table) that ranges from 6 (extremely light) to 20 (very, very hard or maximal intensity). Initially the RPE

Borg Rating of Perceived Exertion (6 to 20 version)	
Category Scale	Verbal Anchor
6	Rest
7	Very, very light
8	—
9	Very light
10	—
11	Fairly light
12	—
13	Somewhat hard
14	—
15	Hard
16	—
17	Very hard
18	—
19	Very, very hard
20	Maximal exertion

should be kept between 11 and 13 to ensure the intensity level is around 40% to 60% of maximal oxygen consumption (VO_{2max}). The person should be given a copy of the RPE scale and instructed how to use it to maintain a safe intensity level of activity. The "talk test" can also be used to estimate intensity level. In other words, the patient should be able to carry on a normal conversation or recite a favorite poem without becoming short winded.

16. Should resistance exercise be recommended to patients with cardiovascular disease?

Resistance training is relatively safe for cardiovascular patients. The major benefits of resistance training are an increase in muscle mass, strength, and basal metabolic rate. Both healthy individuals and cardiac patients must be screened for musculoskeletal and orthopedic conditions that could result in injury during resistance exercise.

In the early weeks of resistance training, and particularly for older cardiac patients, the use of elastic tubing is recommended. Different colors of elastic tubing represent different levels of resistance. The tubing can be purchased in most sporting goods stores. From elastic tubing, patients can progress to dumbbells and stationary weights. Patients can also use 1-lb or 2-lb bags of rice initially to exercise upper body areas. The importance of starting slow with low weight resistance and increased number of repetitions is important to reduce the chance of injury. Contraindications for resistance training are similar to those used for aerobic training.

17. Are flexibility activities appropriate to recommend for physical activity programs for patients with cardiovascular disease?

The benefits of Tai Chi and yoga for relaxation and improving flexibility and balance have been reported in cardiovascular patients.

18. When should patients be advised to stop or slow down physical activity?

Patients should stop or slow down physical activity with these signs:
- Chest pain or upper extremity or trunk discomfort.
- Atypical chest pain, such as shoulder, neck, and jaw.
- Dizziness, lightheadedness.
- Increased dyspnea or severe fatigue.
- Increased dyspnea, wheezing, or greater than a 5-minute recovery period.
- Appearance of back or joint pain (may be indicative of musculoskeletal injury).
- If chest pain persists after stopping activity, the person should be advised to call 911 and take nitroglycerin and aspirin if available.

The activity regime should be completed with adequate energy to carry out the rest of the day's routine. Occasional nausea or faintness may occur after physical activity. If this occurs, the patient should extend the cool-down period and reduce the intensity level. In the initial weeks of beginning activity, muscle soreness may occur. However, stiffness and difficulty moving suggest too much exercise and indicate a reduction in duration or intensity of exercise.

19. What are some general guidelines for recommending physical activity in cardiovascular patients?

- Physical examination and exercise stress test before beginning program.
- Set personal goals to accomplish on a daily or weekly basis.
- Do not engage in activity when ill or when getting over an illness.
- Drink fluids before, during, and after activity sessions of 30 minutes or longer.
- When temperature is more than 80° F, be prepared to exercise indoors.
- Walk in an area that is flat, especially in the first 4 to 6 weeks.
- Use HR, RPE scale, or talk test to estimate intensity level.
- Wear comfortable shoes and clothing.
- Wear loose-fitting clothes that are climate appropriate.
- Wait approximately 2 hours after eating a heavy meal to engage in activity.
- Enjoy the activity!

 Key Points

- Moderate-intensity endurance activities performed intermittently or continuously on most days of the week have a wide range of positive health benefits for patients with cardiovascular disease with few adverse effects reported.
- Sedentary individuals have a much greater risk of AMI compared with those who are physically active.
- Cardiovascular patients who are hospitalized should be encouraged to begin a physical activity regime as soon as their condition is stabilized, with close hemodynamic monitoring performed by the nurse.
- With low-intensity exercise based on HR and exertion level, the nurse can slowly increase frequency, duration, and intensity level of physical activity to a total of 10 to 15 minutes daily before discharge.

 Internet Resources

National Heart, Lung, and Blood Institute: Check Your Physical Activity & Heart Disease IQ:
http://www.nhlbi.nih.gov/health/public/heart/obesity/phy_act.htm

American Heart Association: Exercise (Physical Activity):
http://www.americanheart.org/presenter.jhtml?identifier=4563

U.S. Department of Health and Human Services: Physical Activity Fundamental to Preventing Disease:
http://aspe.os.dhhs.gov/health/reports/physicalactivity/physicalactivity.pdf

Continued

Internet Resources   *continued*

Johns Hopkins Bayview Medical Center: Exercise and Heart Disease:
Centerhttp://www.jhbmc.jhu.edu/CARDIOLOGY/rehab/exercise.chd.html

National Coalition for Women With Heart Disease:
http://www.womenheart.org/

The Physician and Sportsmedicine: Preventing Coronary Heart Disease:
http://www.physsportsmed.com/issues/2001/02_01/lee.htm

The U.S. Department of Health and Human Services: Physical Activity Fundamental to Preventing Disease
http://aspe.os.dhhs.gov/health/reports/physicalactivity/

National Women's Health Information Center: Heart and Cardiovascular Disease:
http://www.4woman.gov/faq/heartdis.htm

Bibliography

American College of Sports Medicine: *ACSM's guidelines for exercise testing and prescription,* ed 6, Philadelphia, 2001, Lippincott Williams & Wilkins.

Diabetes Prevention Program Research Group: Reduction in the incidence of type 2 diabetes with lifestyle intervention or metformin, *N Engl J Med* 346:393-403, 2002.

Eakin EG, Glasgow RE, Riley KM: Review of primary care-based physical activity intervention studies: effectiveness and implications for practice and future research, *J Fam Pract* 49(2):158-168, 2000.

Fletcher GF, Balady GJ, Amsterdam EA et al: Exercise standards for testing and training: a statement for healthcare professionals from the American Heart Association, *Circulation* 104:1694-1740, 2001.

Howley ET: Type of activity: resistance, aerobic and leisure versus occupational physical activity, *Med Sci Sports Exerc* 33(6):S364-S369, 2001.

Lamonte MJ, Ainsworth BE: Quantifying energy expenditure and physical activity in the context of dose response, *Med Sci Sports Exerc* 33(6):S370-S378, 2001.

McArdle WD, Katch FI, Katch VL: *Exercise physiology: energy, nutrition, and human performance,* ed 4, Baltimore, 1996, Williams & Wilkins.

Williams MA: Exercise testing in cardiac rehabilitation: exercise prescription and beyond, *Cardiol Clin* 19(3):415-431, 2001.

Chapter 38

Cardiac Rehabilitation

Jason Barnes Harrell and Leslie Davis

1. What is cardiac rehabilitation (rehab)?

Cardiac rehab is a program that combines prescriptive exercise training with education about coronary risk factor modification. The Agency for Healthcare Research and Quality (AHRQ) defines cardiac rehab as "a comprehensive long-term service involving medical evaluation; prescribed exercise; cardiac risk factor modifications and education; counseling and behavioral intervention." Patient perception of the importance of cardiac rehab is influenced by nurses' attitudes and input. Therefore nurses must support rehab by encouraging physicians to prescribe rehab and by influencing patients to actively participate.

2. What are the key goals of cardiac rehab?

- Enhance functional status.
- Decrease symptoms.
- Provide information needed to assume responsibility for self-care and lifestyle modifications (smoking cessation, dietary modification, weight loss).
- Teach skills needed to ensure achievement and maintenance of optimal health.
- Decrease cardiac risk.
- Manage the disease (i.e., atherosclerosis, hypertension, diabetes).
- Maintain psychosocial health (addressing sexual function, social relationships, depression, anger, hostility).
- Adapt to limitations imposed by the disease process (changing roles in the family, vocation, hobbies, and recreational activities).

3. Who can benefit from cardiac rehab?

Many people can benefit from cardiac rehab; however, it is not necessarily for everyone and is costly. Rehab is for patients who need physician supervision, which is why payers only cover rehab for a select few diagnoses (see Question 4). Patients who are frequently referred for rehab include those who:

- Are at risk for myocardial infarction (MI) or have already had one.
- Have had coronary artery bypass graft (CABG) surgery.
- Have coronary artery disease.
- Have had heart valve surgery.
- Have congestive heart failure.
- Have had coronary intervention (angioplasty or coronary stent).
- Have peripheral vascular disease.

4. What are the requirements for reimbursement from Medicare and other third-party reimbursements?

- Physician order with appropriate diagnostic codes for MI, CABG, or stable angina.
- Additional precertifications may be required.

Diagnoses not covered by Medicare are:
- Coronary artery disease with intervention (i.e., percutaneous coronary intervention).
- Congestive heart failure.
- Heart valve surgery.
- Peripheral vascular disease.
- Patients with multiple risk factors for heart disease.

5. What documented positive effects has cardiac rehab shown for patients?

- Increased functional capacity.
- Increased compliance with the medical treatment plan.
- Increased high-density lipoprotein (HDL).
- Smoking cessation.
- Decreased emotional distress.
- Increased quality of life (QOL).
- Decreased cardiovascular mortality.
- Mitigation of cardiac symptoms (i.e., decreased exercise intolerance, fatigue).
- Promotion of reversal of atherosclerosis.

6. What are the barriers for patients to participation in cardiac rehab?

- Lack of physician understanding of the benefit; therefore patient is not referred.
- Poor motivation from the patient.
- Poor logistical support (i.e., transportation, location of facility, and hours of operations, particularly for those patients who are employed).
- Cost for those who do not have insurance.
- Educational materials used in cardiac rehab. The materials may be at too high of a reading level. The average reading level in the United States is grade 7, but 1:7 adults read below a fourth grade level.

7. When should rehab start?

Patients with uncomplicated conditions after MI or CABG usually begin phase one rehab while they are still inpatients, within the first day or two after the event (or surgery). This early ambulation is the first step toward formalized cardiac rehab.

8. What benefits are there for starting cardiac rehab as an inpatient versus later as an outpatient?

The benefits for starting early are mainly noncardiac. Patients often get deconditioned after long periods of bed rest. Early rehab helps prevent deconditioning.

It also helps decrease anxiety and depression and improves functional status of the patient at the time of discharge. However, patients should not actually start inpatient rehab (phase I) without a risk stratification to assess the risk of mortality and morbidity during exercise. Encouragement to start rehab as an inpatient also shows that rehab is important and valued by the entire health care team.

9. What are the phases/steps of rehab?

- Phase I: Inpatient setting. During this phase, education regarding diet, coronary anatomy, and disease management occurs. Physically, the patient is able to ambulate.
- Phase II: Patient participation in supervised exercise or education program after discharge or from the date of the cardiac event through 12 weeks after the event. During this phase, patients are monitored for electrocardiographic (ECG) changes, chest pain, and tolerance during the supervised exercise.
- Phase III: During this phase, the patient is still supervised yet has intermittent or no ECG monitoring done during the exercise. This is a variable-length program that progresses to maintenance therapy up to 1 year past the cardiac event.
- Phase IV: No ECG monitoring, with limited supervision during exercise. During this phase, the patient is basically on maintenance therapy in a facility outside the health care/rehab setting.

10. What is the recommended continuum of care for cardiac rehab services?

- 0 to 2 weeks: inpatient post–cardiac event pathway.
- 1 to 6 weeks: transitional care, subacute facility, possibly home training/care.
- 1 to 12 weeks: formal cardiac rehab program.
- 4 weeks and beyond: maintenance and continued lifestyle changes and exercise regimen at local facility or at home.

11. Once an exercise activity has begun, what adverse responses would lead to discontinuation of the exercise?

- Extremes of baseline heart rate (>130 bpm or <30 bpm).
- Diastolic blood pressure (BP) of 110 mm Hg and above.
- Decrease in systolic BP by 10 mm Hg.
- Significant ventricular arrhythmias (such as nonsustained ventricular tachycardia) or atrial arrhythmias (such as atrial fibrillation or flutter).
- Second-degree or third-degree heart block.
- Signs or symptoms of exercise intolerance, including angina pectoris and marked dyspnea.

12. What important information is needed to help risk stratify patients before cardiac rehab is started?

- Current medical history: medical or surgical profile (or both) including complications, comorbidities, and other pertinent medical history.

- Physical examination.
- Resting 12-lead ECG to rule out ongoing ischemia and arrhythmias and to be used as a baseline comparison.
- A stress test may or may not be included.
- Current medications, including dose and frequency.
- Cardiac disease risk profile including:
  - Use of tobacco products.
  - History of hypertension.
  - Lipid profile including total cholesterol, HDL, and low-density lipoprotein (LDL; before the event or 6 weeks after the event).
  - Nutritional assessment, especially dietary fat, saturated fat, cholesterol, and calories.
  - Body composition analysis.
  - Fasting blood glucose or hemoglobin A1c.
  - Physical activity status.
  - Stress level.
  - Psychological history, particularly evidence of depression.
  - Family history.
  - Age.
  - Gender (and menopausal status if female).

13. How is risk stratification used in the cardiac rehab setting?

Risk stratification helps determine the optimal dosage of exercise. The rating of perceived exertion (RPE) along with heart rate are used to gauge exercise intensity. If the risk stratification does not include a stress test, the following formula is used to determine the patient's exercise tolerance:

Heart rate at rest + 30 bpm or onset of symptoms (i.e., chest pain).

14. What are the levels of risk?

	Lowest Risk	Moderate Risk	Highest Risk
Ventricular function	No significant left ventricular (LV) dysfunction (ejection fraction [EF], >50%).	Moderately impaired LV dysfunction (EF 40% – 49%).	Documented LV dysfunction (EF <40%).
Exercise tolerance	No resting or exercise-induced complex dysrhythmias.	Signs/symptoms including angina at moderate levels of exercise (5-6.9 metabolic equivalents [METs]) or in recovery.	Complex ventricular dysrhythmias at rest or with exercise.

continued

	Lowest Risk	Moderate Risk	Highest Risk
Severity of cardiac event and treatment of that event	Uncomplicated myocardial infarction (MI); coronary artery bypass grafting; angioplasty; arthrectomy or stent; absence of congestive heart failure (CHF) or signs/symptoms (s/s) indicating postevent ischemia.	Not applicable.	MI or cardiac surgery complicated by cardiogenic shock, CHF, or s/s of postprocedure ischemia.
Hemodynamic status	Normal hemodynamics with exercise or recovery.	Normal hemodynamics	Abnormal hemodynamics with exercise (especially flat or decreasing systolic blood pressure or chronotropic incompetence with increasing workload).
Symptomatic/ asymptomatic	Asymptomatic including absence of angina with exertion or recovery.	Not applicable	Signs/symptoms including angina pectoris at low levels of exercise (<5.0 METs) or in recovery.
Functional status	Functional capacity ≥7.0 METs.	Not applicable	Clinically significant depression.
Level of risk	Lowest risk classification assumed when each of risk factors in category is present.	Moderate risk is assumed for patients who do not meet classification of either highest risk or lowest risk.	Highest risk classification is assumed with presence of any one of risk factors included in category.

15. What is the purpose of stress testing before a patient's entry into cardiac rehab?

Stress testing combined with a medical evaluation is essential to identify limitations to exercise participation. Stress testing helps determine the level of exercise at which symptoms or cardiac ischemia are induced. This information helps establish the patient's cardiovascular disease risk factors and identify goals/expected outcomes for the patient and staff.

16. When should stress testing be repeated?

Stress testing should be repeated any time symptoms or clinical changes are seen or in follow-up assessment of exercise training program.

17. What are the contraindications to exercise training?

Cardiac rehab is not just an exercise program; it is also an education and behavior modification program for risk factor management. So, even if the patient cannot exercise, he/she could participate in the education sessions. See the following table.

Absolute Contraindications	Relative Contraindications
Acute myocardial infarction (within 2 d).	Severe arterial hypertension.
Unstable angina.	Electrolyte abnormalities.
Uncontrolled cardiac arrhythmia causing symptoms or hemodynamic compromise (i.e., atrial or ventricular arrhythmias, third-degree atrioventricular block [without pacemaker]).	Asymptomatic tachyarrhythmias or bradyarrhythmias.
Symptomatic severe aortic stenosis (peak systolic pressure gradient >50 mm Hg with aortic valve orifice area <0.75 cm^2 in average-size adult) or other forms of outflow obstruction.	Moderate stenotic valvular heart disease.
Decompensated heart failure.	Left main coronary artery stenosis.
Acute pulmonary embolism or pulmonic insufficiency.	Mental or physical handicap.
Acute myocarditis or pericarditis.	
Acute aortic dissection.	
Uncontrolled diabetes (resting blood sugar >400 mg/dL).	

18. Do education and behavior management work?

Yes, if the patient stays with the changes. However, the odds are that greater than 50% of the participants discontinue the healthy changes within 1 year.

19. Can patients with heart failure benefit from cardiac rehab?

Patients with moderate to severe left ventricular dysfunction can improve functional capacity and QOL and reduce symptoms, mortality, and hospital readmission rates by participating in a well-planned physical conditioning program.

20. How does the rehab program differ for patients with heart failure?

First, the selection criteria:
- Patients must have hemodynamically stable conditions (stable baseline BP; i.e., systolic BP >90 mm Hg) with a stable medication regimen (medications at a stable dose, not being titrated upward).

- Patients must have an appropriate chronotropic response to exercise (i.e., heart rate is appropriately responsive to exercise).
- Patients must have the capacity of more than 3 metabolic equivalents (METs; a MET is the amount of energy used by the body while performing activities of daily living or exercise routines). At rest, the average person has an oxygen consumption of 1 MET (or 3.5 ml/kg-min). MET values increase when more strenuous body movement is performed.
- Patients cannot participate if they have an absolute contraindication such as acutely decompensated heart failure, obstruction to the left ventricular outflow tract, or life-threatening arrhythmias.

Second, the exercise regimen:
- The regimen should be based on a symptom limited treadmill or cycle ergometer evaluation and ancillary study data like an exercise echocardiogram (to help determine what exercise intensity produces ischemic wall motion abnormalities).
- Warm-up and cool-down phases should be a minimum of 10 to 15 minutes.
- The exercise sessions should be initially brief (10 to 20 minutes) with training sessions of 2 to 6 minutes separated by 1 to 2 minutes of rest. Resistance training can be used to complement the program 2 to 3 days a week.
- Workload targets or heart rate have to be changed to perceived exertion and dyspnea to assess the quality of the exercise session.

21. What are some of the concerns regarding cardiac rehab for heart transplant recipients?

Because the transplant surgeons do not reconnect the autonomic nervous system to the donor heart, different cardiorespiratory, hemodynamic, and neuroendocrine responses to rest and exercise exist. The heart transplant patient has a delayed increase in heart rate, but once the metabolic demand and subsequent catecholamine levels rise, the cardiac output increases along with the heart rate and stroke volume. The same is true of rest after exertion. The heart is delayed in its response to decrease metabolic demand. The exercise regimen is similar to that of the heart failure patient, with the exception that the focus is on resting and exercise BPs and possible adverse side effects of the immunosuppressive agents and evidence of graft rejection.

 Key Points

- Patient perception of the importance of cardiac rehab is influenced by the nurses' attitude and input.
- Documented positive effects of cardiac rehab include: increased functional capacity, increased compliance with medical treatment plan, decreased emotional stress, and decreased cardiovascular mortality.

Continued

Key Points   *continued*

- Cardiac rehab should start when the patient is still in the hospital as an inpatient 1 to 2 days after the event, if the MI is uncomplicated.
- Absolute contraindications to post-MI exercise include: acute MI within 2 days, unstable angina, uncontrolled cardiac arrhythmias or third-degree heart block, uncontrolled diabetes (blood sugar, >400 mg/dL), and decompensated heart failure.
- Education and behavior management work if the patient stays with the changes. However, the odds are that greater than 50% of the participants discontinue the healthy changes within 1 year.

 Internet Resources

Cardiovascular & Pulmonary Rehabilitation:
www.aacvpr.org

Scottish Intercollegiate Guidelines Network:
www.sign.ac.uk/guidlines/fulltext/57

New York University Cardiac Rehab:
www.med.nyu.edu/cardiacrehab

UK National Electronic Library for Health: Cardiac Rehabilitation:
www.nelh.nhs.uk/nsf/chd/nsf/chapter7/chapter7.htm

Canadian Association of Cardiac Rehab:
www.cacr.ca/rd/education.htm

Iowa University Virtual Hospital:
www.vh.org/adult/patient/internalmedicine/champs/#toc

American College of Sports Medicine:
www.acsm.org

Bibliography

ACC/AHA 2002 guideline update for exercise testing: Summary article: a report of the American College of Cardiology/American Heart Association Task Force on Practice Guidelines (Committee to Update the 1997 Exercise Testing Guidelines), *J Am Coll Cardiol* 40(8):1531-1540; 2002.

American Association of Cardiovascular and Pulmonary Rehabilitation: *Guidelines for cardiac rehabilitation and secondary prevention programs,* Champaign, Ill, 1999, Human Kinetics Publishers.

American College of Sports Medicine: ACSM's guidelines for exercise testing and prescription, ed 6, Philadelphia, 2000, Lippincott Williams & Wilkins, pp 165-196.

Balady GJ, Ades PA, Comoss P et al: Core components of cardiac rehabilitation/secondary prevention programs: a statement for healthcare professionals from the American Heart Association and the American Association of Cardiovascular and Pulmonary Rehabilitation writing group, *Circulation* 102:1069, 2000.

Cardiac rehabilitation: a national clinical guideline, pub no 57, Jan 2002, Scottish Intercollegiate Guidelines Network.

Grundy SM, Pasternak R, Greenland P et al: Assessment of cardiovascular risk by use of multiple-risk-factor assessment equations: a statement for healthcare professionals from the American Heart Association and the American College of Cardiology, *Circulation* 100:1481-1492, 1999.

Smith SC, Blair SN, Crigqui MH et al: Preventing heart attack and death in patients with coronary disease, *Circulation* 92:2-4, 1995.

Wenger NK, Froelicher ES, Smith LK et al: *Cardiac rehabilitation,* Clinical Practice Guideline no. 17, U.S. Department of Health and Human Services, Public Health Service, Agency for Health Care Policy and Research and the National Heart, Lung, and Blood Institute, Rockville, Md, AHCPR pub no. 96-0672, October, 1995.

Chapter 39

Psychosocial Considerations

Valerie H. Lunsford

1. What does the term *psychosocial* mean?

Psychosocial denotes the combination of psychological factors and social and cultural factors. This combination provides a context, or background, for evaluation of a patient's physiological and emotional responses to illness and some understanding of how the patient may have become ill in the first place.

2. What are some of the psychosocial issues that may affect the development, expression, and recovery from coronary heart disease (CHD)?

Psychosocial issues related to CHD can be divided into the following four categories: mood states, social factors, personality factors, and stress (see the following table).

Categories	Issues
Mood states	Depression
	Anxiety
Social factors	Socioeconomic status
	Race
	Gender
	Social isolation
	Social support
Personality factors	Type A personality
	Hostility
Stress	Life events
	Daily hassles

3. Identified risks for CHD include physiological and behavioral factors (smoking, inactivity, diabetes, hypertension, hypercholesterolemia, and obesity), but what is the role of psychosocial factors?

In trying to understand behavioral and physical risk factors and their relationship to CHD, scientists discovered that these risk factors did not explain all the cases of CHD. In fact, these factors explained less than half of the cases of CHD. In evaluation of the other possible contributing factors, a cluster of factors was identified that incorporated certain psychosocial issues. However, these psychosocial issues, when added to the physical and behavioral risk factors, still did not explain all the cases. It became evident that an interaction of physical and behavioral risk factors with psychosocial factors explained many more cases of CHD. This perspective, which examines the interactions of physical, behavioral, psychological, and social factors, is called a biopsychosocial model and is used in much research related to prevention and treatment of CHD and in understanding why and in whom CHD occurs.

4. How do emotions and environment affect the occurrence of a heart attack or recovery from one?

Explanations of this are still in the theory stages, but a few examples include such associations as:

- The experience and expression of certain emotions with the release of stress-related hormones, such as cortisol and epinephrine, which in turn are related to immunosuppression, arrhythmias, and increases in blood pressure and heart rate.
- The experience of social disadvantages with poor health behaviors leading to higher levels of physiological risk.
- The perception and experience of social support with changes in blood pressure.
- The experience of depression or anxiety with high levels of stress hormones and blood pressure, cardiac rhythm, or coronary blood vessel flow or with health behaviors leading to physiological risk.
- Many biopsychosocial theories guide research of these complex interrelationships. The accumulated findings support a strong link between the mind and the body that influences health maintenance or development of disease.

5. Are findings the same for men and women?

Most earlier research has been conducted with men, and results have been generalized to women. Over the last several decades, there has been a growing awareness that multiple gender differences exist in the development, expression, experience, recovery, and adjustment to CHD. Although more research has been undertaken to better understand CHD in women and to include them in clinical trials, limitations remain. Women tend to be more difficult to recruit and retain in studies, the number of those participating is often small, women's data is not analyzed separately from men's data, and scant numbers of ethnically and culturally diverse women participate. Evidence is beginning to accumulate that women tend to have more psychosocial distress after CHD than do men. However, women in general report having more distress throughout life. Thus the findings related to psychosocial distress and CHD are more difficult to interpret.

6. How does socioeconomic status (SES) affect CHD?

The relationship between CHD and SES is complex, representing the interactions of many factors. The concept of SES includes not only education and income but age, race, and gender as well. CHD is more prevalent in men until about age 50 years when women begin to catch up. The high incidence rate of CHD in this decade of life may be particularly potent for women because of the context and experiences related to aging (women may be living on a fixed income, caring for an ill spouse, be socially isolated, and have more comorbidities). Their resources, both social and economic, may be more restricted, limiting their access to up-to-date acute care and to follow-up care and cardiac rehabilitation. Some evidence suggests that SES and gender combine to create a bias in the diagnosis and treatment of CHD in women. SES may be related to the development of and recovery from CHD through less favorable patterns of lifestyle and biomedical risk factors and through less favorable psychosocial patterns, such as social isolation, racism, powerlessness, and unemployment. It has even been suggested that low SES may be the mechanism by which anxiety is generated, leading to anxiety's subsequent deleterious effects on the heart.

7. The influence of SES on CHD sounds like a societal problem. What can nurses do about it?

Obviously social inequities cannot be undone, but nurses can work with their patients to devise mechanisms to decrease CHD risk within the context of the social and cultural environment. The nurse can obtain referrals for needed services and tailor education to better meet the needs and realities of patients' lifestyles. The suggestion that the patient increase the intake of fruits and vegetables may be meaningless to someone whose local grocer carries little in the way of these foods or to someone who is unable to shop because of a lack of transportation. The important thing is to work with them and to be aware of and direct them to community resources that may help them achieve a more heart healthy lifestyle.

8. What is social isolation, and what impact does it have on CHD?

Findings support the relationship of social support to recovery from CHD measured in functional and emotional outcomes. Social isolation, or the lack of social support, is more closely related to death and disability. Social support functions more effectively to enhance and support recovery versus prevent disease. However, the relationship of social isolation to the incidence and occurrence of CHD is much less clear. Individuals who report a lack of emotional support after a myocardial infarction (MI) have a three times greater risk of dying. The mechanisms by which social factors influence CHD recovery differ between men and women. The relationship is thought to be more complex in women. The popular assumption that women would be more responsive to social support than men led to most of the previous research on social support being conducted with women. However, today, findings support that men may, in fact, be more responsive to social support. Men who reported social isolation and a lack of social support had a much higher risk of dying after MI than did women or men with social support. Intervention studies that test the effects of social and emotional support have found that those most in need benefit the most.

9. What interventions can nurses offer patients with CHD who experience social isolation?

A nurse can provide encouragement to the patient to participate in cardiac rehabilitation programs. These programs provide education, physical training, counseling, and informal social support. Participation in stress management programs offers an alternative to traditional cardiac rehabilitation programs. Encouragement of participation in activities works well for those who are able to participate, but those who lack the resources to participate should be referred for available assistive services to alleviate the sense of social isolation. Family should be made aware of the patient's need for social and emotional support as recovery progresses and assisted to provide these resources.

10. What evidence relates depression to the risk for the development and expression of CHD?

Evidence is strongly suggestive that depression is a potent risk factor for the development and expression of CHD. Men who reported having an episode of major depression had more than twice the risk of development of CHD. Even milder symptoms of depression limited to 2 weeks were associated with double the risk of development of CHD. Multiple studies have confirmed these findings. One way in which depression is thought to influence CHD is by the effect of the stress hormone epinephrine on heart rate. People with depression tend to have higher heart rates and also have shown less of the adaptive responses of the heart to various demands, such as stress or changes in the environment. Other proposed mechanisms by which depression influences CHD is that individuals with depression have higher blood pressures and a higher tendency to have atherosclerotic plaques develop because of "stickier" platelets.

11. Does depression affect the recovery from or the reoccurrence of CHD?

Depression is more prevalent in women and the elderly. One third of patients after cardiac events report symptoms of depression. Multiple studies with patients after MI have shown that individuals with depression have significantly higher death rates than those who are not depressed, even after accounting for severity of cardiac status. Recent findings indicate that depression is a potent risk factor for cardiac death in older adults, even in those free of CHD at study entry. However, support for the link between depression and poor recovery after cardiac event has been inconsistent. Three recent studies found that depression predicted poor quality of life, not mortality, after MI. Another study found depression predictive of death in men but not in women. The disparities in these findings could result from the use of different measures of depression from clinical depression as determined by skilled interviewers to self reports of depressive symptoms. With death, disability, or dissatisfaction, depression increasingly appears related to the incidence of and the recovery from CHD.

12. What are symptoms of depression?

The symptoms of depression—difficulty sleeping, loss of interest and pleasure in activities, lethargy, difficulty concentrating, and worry—are similar to the symptoms one would normally see after an MI but need to be monitored if associated with high levels of distress or if they persist for longer than 2 weeks. Recognition allows awareness of the patient's emotional state and more appropriate interpretation and response to behaviors. Beta-blockers, which are frequently prescribed for patients with CHD, can contribute to symptoms of depression or mimic those symptoms. Treatment with beta-blockers has been associated with fatigue, difficulty in concentration, loss of mental alertness, insomnia, nightmares, and sexual dysfunction. Calcium channel blockers may cause palpitations, mimicking symptoms of anxiety, and antilipid agents may cause fatigue.

13. Is there evidence of a relationship between anxiety and CHD?

Anxiety, manifested as a transient reaction to something perceived as threatening, is considered to be a state or temporary condition. Anxiety that represents a perspective in which the environment and relationships are a constant source of threat is a trait, or part of the personality. Researchers and counselors often identify anxiety as a counterpart to depression because they often occur simultaneously. Anxiety is characterized as a negative affect, whereas depression is a negative affect combined with a lack of a positive affect. Although women are more likely to have anxiety compared with men, most research conducted has been with white, middle-class men.

Anxiety has been identified as a risk factor for the development of CHD and as a triggering mechanism for plaque rupture and subsequent MI. These findings have been supported through estimation of risk in large population studies and in experimental clinical studies. A number of theories link anxiety to the risk for development of CHD through various mechanisms including deleterious lifestyle behaviors, development of atherosclerotic plaques or hypertension, and electrical instability of the heart's rhythm, leading to potentially fatal arrhythmias.

14. How do depression and anxiety affect the nursing care of patients with CHD?

Although research has not established the same strength of relationship between depression, anxiety, and CHD as has been established between smoking and CHD, these psychosocial issues still exert a profound influence on the patient's recovery and well being and the patient's family. Recognition of depression or anxiety facilitates communication with the patient about fears, concerns, and feelings of hopelessness. The nurse can let the patient know that after a heart attack people often have feelings of depression but that these feelings need to be monitored carefully and reported if prolonged or worsened. This information should be provided to all patients and families.

15. What effect do type A personality and the specific component of hostility have on CHD?

Type A personality was the seminal concept that sparked an interest in the relationship of psychosocial factors to CHD. Early anecdotal observations suggested that a certain type of man was more prone to MI and death from it. These men were characterized as aggressive, impatient, and often hostile. As the concept was more fully investigated and refined, impatience and aggression became less relevant and the focus of investigations became hostility. Recent research conducted with women indicates that women also are susceptible to the effects of hostility on CHD, not just men. The concept of hostility continues to be further specified and investigated.

Individuals who display more hostility have also displayed exaggerated hemodynamic and cardiovascular responses to social and behavioral stressors, suggesting a link whereby hostility may be associated with CHD.

Observation of the cardiac patient and reporting of evidence of high hostility to the physician or nurse practitioner (NP) may assist in getting the patient treatment for this behavioral risk factor. Individuals can be effectively counseled or can participate in behavioral or cognitive therapies to learn to more effectively moderate hostile tendencies.

16. Does increased stress cause CHD?

Multiple associations exist between the experience of stress and the incidence of CHD. Whether the major stressors in one's life, such as death of a loved one, loss of a job, or divorce, or the small irritants, or daily hassles, of day-to-day life are most strongly associated with CHD remains unclear. Anecdotal evidence has shown that the person who has just lost a life partner is more likely to die of MI within 6 months than is someone who remains partnered. On the other hand, how a person approaches the daily hassles of life may indicate a general disposition to be more cardiac-disease prone. Perhaps more important is the fact that many people attribute CHD or heart attack to stress, not to lifestyle choices or genetics. Belief plays an important part in how a person responds to and manages an illness, and if they firmly attribute CHD to factors outside of themselves, they may be less amenable to behavioral lifestyle changes.

In providing care and education to the patient, one should incorporate all the evidence relating CHD to physiological and psychosocial risks. How multiple factors may influence the disease process and, more importantly, that they may interact for a more pervasive impact should be emphasized.

17. **Most of the treatment given to cardiac patients is related to medicines and interventions. What can the nurse do to promote awareness of psychosocial issues and incorporate the treatment of these problems into the plan of care?**

Psychosocial distress is becoming increasingly recognized for deleterious effects on health and behavior. As this awareness grows, so do the options for treatment. Today depression, anxiety, and other areas of psychosocial distress are more frequently screened and the patient is more often referred for treatment. This treatment often occurs in the hospital but is also recognized in the outpatient setting. Family members often report the signs and symptoms of psychosocial distress and request intervention. The nurse should support the patient and family dealing with psychosocial distress and report this information to the physician, NP, and other members of the health care team. Through recognition and effective multidisciplinary treatment, morbidity, mortality, and dissatisfaction with quality of life after MI can be improved for men and women of all groups and ages.

Key Points

- Evidence strongly suggests that depression is a potent risk factor for the development and expression of CHD.
- Recognition of depression or anxiety facilitates communication with the patient about fears, concerns, and feelings of hopelessness.
- The nurse should let the patient know that after a heart attack people often have feelings of depression but that these feelings need to be monitored carefully and reported if prolonged or worsened.
- The nurse should support the patient and family dealing with psychosocial distress and report this information to the physician, NP, and other members of the health care team. Through early recognition and effective multidisciplinary treatment, morbidity, mortality, and dissatisfaction with quality of life after MI can be improved for men and women of all groups and ages.

Internet Resources

ENRICHD: Enhancing Recovery in Coronary Heart Disease:
http://www.bios.unc.edu/units/cscc/ENRI/enridesc.html

Depression and Heart Disease:
http://www.nimh.nih.gov/publicat/depheart.cfm

Stress and Heart Disease:
http://www.americanheart.org/presenter.jhtml?identifier=4750

Bibliography

Barrick CB: Sad, glad, or mad hearts? Epidemiological evidence for a causal relationship between mood disorders and coronary artery disease, *J Affect Disord* 53:193-201, 1999.

Dixon T et al: Psychosocial experiences of cardiac patients in early recovery: a community-based study, *J Adv Nurs* 31(6):1368-1375, 2000.

Ferketich A et al: Depression as an antecedent to heart disease among women and men in the NHANES I study, *Arch Intern Med* 160:1261-1268, 2000.

King KB: Psychologic and social aspects of cardiovascular disease, *Ann Behav Med* 19(3):264-270, 1997.

Knox SS: Hostility, social support, and carotid artery atherosclerosis in the National Heart, Lung, and Blood Institute Family Heart Study, *Am J Cardiol* 86(10):1086-1089, 2000.

Krantz DS, McCeney M: Effects of psychological and social factors on organic disease: a critical assessment of research on coronary heart disease, *Annu Rev Psychol* 53:341-369, 2001.

Kubzansky LD et al: Anxiety and coronary heart disease: a synthesis of epidemiological, psychological, and experimental evidence, *Ann Behav Med* 20(2):47-58, 1998.

Lane D et al: Effects of depression and anxiety on mortality and quality-of-life 4 months after myocardial infarction, *J Psychosom Res* 49(4):229-238, 2000.

Mayou RA et al: Depression and anxiety as predictors of outcome after myocardial infarction, *Psychosom Med* 62:212-219, 2000.

Penninx BW et al: Depression and cardiac mortality, *Arch Gen Psychiatry* 58:221-227, 2001.

Section VII

Special Patient Populations

C h a p t e r 40

Cardiovascular Disease and Women

Valerie H. Lunsford

1. Do men and women experience heart disease differently?

Many differences are seen, including:

- Disease incidence and prevalence.
- Risk factors.
- Signs and symptoms.
- Diagnosis and management.
- Recovery issues.

However, many of these differences were unrecognized until the 1980s. Before that decade, most research was conducted with men and the outcomes were assumed to be the same for women. It is now apparent that heart disease has been viewed and treated as a "man's disease" and that much remains to be known about the differences women experience.

2. Do men and women have the same morbidity and mortality rates associated with coronary heart disease (CHD)?

Heart disease is the leading cause of death in the United States for women and men. More people die of CHD than die of all forms of cancer. Men have more heart attacks, both fatal and nonfatal, than women do in the earlier years. After menopause, the incidence changes and women start having heart attacks at nearly the same rate as men. The highest death rate from CHD in all groups occurs in black women in the South, with 553 deaths per 100,000 reported annually, compared with 400 white women per 100,000. It is estimated that 6.5 million women are living with some form of CHD.

Women have higher levels of morbidity and mortality once CHD is manifested. The higher morbidity and mortality rates experienced by women after age 60 years have been associated with older age at first myocardial infarction (MI), a higher number of comorbidities, living alone, caring for an ill spouse, failure to recognize and seek treatment for symptoms, failure to recognize symptoms by health care providers, lack of aggressive treatment, social inequities, and higher levels of psychosocial distress.

3. What risk factors for CHD differ between women and men?

Many of the risk factors for CHD identified with men are also present in women. However, certain risk factors may be more prevalent in women, or more potent. Also, some risk factors are unique to women. Interestingly, research conducted with women after MI showed that many women did not consider themselves to be at risk for CHD, even though documentation in the medical record indicated they had multiple risk factors for CHD.

- Shared risk factors:
  - Family history is a risk factor for women but is a more potent risk factor for men.
  - Current evidence suggests that obesity may be a more potent risk factor for women, particularly central obesity. A further association of the presence of central obesity and the occurrence of type 2 diabetes may exist.
  - Diabetes is associated with a higher risk of CHD in women as compared with men.
  - Women who smoke are more likely to have MI and are more likely to die of the MI than are women who do not smoke. Smoking is a much more potent risk factor for women than for men, especially for women who concurrently take oral contraceptives (OCPs). Evidence suggests that smoking negates the natural protection conferred by estrogen before menopause through the mechanisms of decreased endogenous estrogen levels, increased levels of low-density lipoproteins (LDLs), and decreased levels of high-density lipoproteins (HDLs). Moreover, low HDL levels have been found to be the most significant predictor of CHD risk in women.
  - Elevated triglycerides may be more predictive of CHD risk, and triglycerides increase more rapidly with age in women than in men.
- Unique risk factors:
  - These unique risk factors are related to women's reproductive hormones. During women's childbearing years, an increased risk of CHD is associated with the use of OCPs; cigarette smoking further potentiates this risk.
  - Menopause is a unique risk factor that signals the end of women's childbearing capacity and the decrease of endogenous estrogen levels. Before menopause, estrogen is thought to have a cardioprotective effect. Menopause becomes an independent risk factor for CHD with the decrease in estrogen levels at menopause. Decreased estrogen is associated with changes in lipoprotein levels, specifically increased LDL and decreased HDL. Research suggests that the risk of CHD associated with menopause may be attenuated by walking briskly 3 hours per week.
  - Multiple large cohort studies investigated the role of hormone replacement therapy (HRT) in prevention of coronary events. The Heart and Estrogen/ Progestin Replacement Study (HERS) and the Women's Health Initiative (WHI) found no protective effects of HRT in prevention of coronary events. Moreover, HRT was associated with significant risks of venous thromboembolism, gallbladder disease, and breast cancer.

4. How do the signs and symptoms of MI differ in women?

- The onset of MI is most often associated with crushing substernal chest pain and diaphoresis, although women may have different symptoms.

- Noncardiac chest pain. Research indicates that many women have the "typical" chest pain and that many women have noncardiac chest pain, such as abdominal pain, jaw or neck pain, and back pain. The noncardiac pain may be present over several weeks to a month, unlike the abrupt onset of typical cardiac chest pain, and is often associated with profound fatigue and a general sense of "not feeling well."
- Atypical symptoms. Women have had episodes of chest pain while at rest, during sleep, and with mental stress. Generally, men do not manifest chest pain in these circumstances, and until recently, conventional wisdom has not incorporated atypical symptoms into the list of symptoms diagnostic of MI. Women also manifest a condition called syndrome X, in which they have chest pain but the coronary arteries are normal during angiography. A theory of why women's symptoms and experiences of MI differ from men's suggests that women's smaller diameter coronary vessels and less developed collateral coronary circulation may be partly responsible.
- Other symptoms. MI is traditionally associated with the symptoms of crushing substernal chest pain, perhaps radiating to the jaw or down the left arm, diaphoresis, nausea and vomiting, and shortness of breath. These symptoms are predominant in men. Women may have nausea and vomiting and shortness of breath, but they may also have symptoms of indigestion, palpitations, dizziness, loss of appetite, flushing, fatigue, and syncope.

5. What are the differences in CHD diagnosis and treatment for women and men?

Diagnosis. Although improvements in diagnosis and advances in technology continue to be made, diagnosis of MI or CHD in women may be delayed because of several factors.

- Women may not recognize the symptoms as significant and may delay seeking treatment. Any delay in treatment may result in more myocardial damage and dysfunction.
- Clinicians may fail to recognize women's symptoms as an indication of MI or the presence of CHD, leading to delayed treatment.
- The electrocardiogram (ECG) shows lower sensitivity for correct identification of MI in women than in men and reveals more false-positive and false-negative changes, leading to a higher number of unrecognized MIs.
- Exercise-induced ST segment depression of more than 1 mm, noted during ECG stress testing, has a lower diagnostic accuracy in women as compared with men, especially in younger women. The inclusion of additional parameters in the exercise test, such as heart rate index or presence of angina during exercise, improves predictive estimates. Sensitivity and specificity of the stress test for diagnosis of CHD in women are enhanced with stress perfusion imaging, stress echocardiography, pharmacologic stress testing, and electron beam computed tomography.
- Selection of the first noninvasive diagnostic test for a woman includes consideration of the women's age, symptoms, risk-factor profile, body habitus, and functional capacity.

Treatment. Once recognized, women are admitted for treatment at the same rates as are men. However, differences exist in the treatments used.

- Women are less likely to undergo diagnostic cardiac catheterization. Although female gender is considered the main factor influencing referral for angiography, other important considerations include age, comorbidities, and other factors that may increase the risk for surgery.
- Women have fewer revascularization procedures (angioplasty or bypass surgery), which may be because of age, comorbidities, and a more unstable clinical profile at diagnosis. Women tend to have a higher cardiac surgical mortality than men.
- Women are less likely to receive thrombolytic therapy, and they realize fewer benefits than men.
- Women are less likely to be prescribed beta-blockers or angiotensin-converting enzyme (ACE) inhibitors. The pharmacologic agents provide similar benefit in women and men, but why prescriptions for women are limited remains unanswered.
- Women are less likely to be referred to phase II cardiac rehabilitation, less likely to participate when referred, and more likely to drop out before completion.

6. What are the differences in recovery/adjustment?

Some aspects of the adjustment process are similar, but some important differences also exist. Compared with men:

- During the first year after diagnosis of CHD, women have a greater risk of death, cardiac distress, and reinfarction.
- Women may continue to have angina after revascularization procedures because of graft occlusion, which may occur as the result of smaller coronary vessel diameter.
- Women have more congestive heart failure (CHF) than men, although women have a better prognosis but a worse quality of life (QOL).
- Women are less physically, sexually, and socially active and return to work less often.
- Women have multiple stressors in living with CHD as a chronic illness, including inability to carry out daily activities, problems in dealing with treatment and symptoms, changes in roles, restricted social activities, and apprehension about the future.
- Women have higher levels of depression and anxiety after CHD diagnosis, and they have more cardiac symptoms and report lower levels of satisfaction with social support during recovery.
- Women's participation in cardiac rehabilitation programs is estimated to be as low as 5% to 6%, even though women participating in rehabilitation realize comparable or even greater improvements in functional capacity, QOL, psychosocial well being, and CHD risk factors.
- Women often do not perceive themselves to be at risk for CHD, even after MI, so they may not be prepared to enact lifestyle changes necessary to prevent disease progression.

7. What are the nursing implications of these gender differences in CHD?

The most central implication of these differences is the critical need for education about CHD in women for women of all ages.

- Risk factors. Nurses can begin educating women about risk factors for CHD starting at an early age, even starting the education in their own homes. Obesity and physical inactivity represent an ever-increasing problem, with the number of obese American adults and children on the rise. Education about the cardiovascular risks of obesity and inactivity can begin in the home and at school. Smoking is a significant risk factor for CHD. The segment of the population that shows the largest increase in numbers of smokers is adolescent girls. This provides another opportunity for nurses to provide education in the home, the schools, and the community. Nurses can counsel women about the increasing risks of CHD throughout the lifespan, highlighting significant risk factors for specific age groups. Risk factor education can be provided through informal conversations with female friends, acquaintances, and patients.
- Signs and symptoms. Nurses can increase their knowledge and awareness of how women's symptoms of MI or CHD may be different than what has been traditionally recognized. Nurses can then provide a much broader and more inclusive perspective on women's symptoms to other health care workers, thereby increasing their awareness and sensitivity to gender differences in presenting symptoms. Nurses can also provide education to other women, and to their families, so that treatment seeking is not be delayed.
- Management and treatment. Nurses can become more familiar with the differences in the long-term management and specific treatments for CHD in women so they are better able to communicate these regimens to their female patients and their families. Nurses can advocate for their female patients by offering the suggestion to physicians that women are more likely to participate in a program of cardiac rehabilitation if their participation is strongly recommended by their physician and supported by their children.
- Recovery/adjustment.
  - Depression and anxiety exert a profound influence on the patient's recovery and well being and on the patient's family. Recognition of depression or anxiety facilitates communication with the patient about fears, concerns, and feelings of hopelessness. The nurse can let the patient know that people often have feelings of depression after a heart attack but that these feelings need to be monitored carefully and reported if prolonged or worsened. This information should be provided to all patients and their families. Symptoms of depression include difficulty sleeping, loss of interest and pleasure in activities, lethargy, difficulty concentrating, and worry. These symptoms are similar to the symptoms one would normally see after MI but need to be monitored if associated with high levels of distress or if they persist for longer than 2 weeks.
  - The nurse can work with patients to identify mechanisms to decrease CHD risk within the context of social and cultural constraints. Patients should be educated about all the evidence relating CHD to physiological and psychosocial risks, with emphasis on how multiple factors may influence the disease process, and more importantly, that they may interact for a more pervasive impact.

- The nurse can obtain referrals for needed services and can tailor education to better meet the needs and realities of the women patients' lifestyles.
- The nurse can encourage female patients to participate in cardiac rehabilitation programs, which provide education, physical training, counseling, and informal social support. Women who lack the resources to participate should be referred for available assistive services in an effort to alleviate the sense of social isolation. Family should be made aware of the patient's need for social and emotional support as recovery progresses and assisted to provide these resources.

Key Points

- Cardiovascular disease is the number one killer of women as well as men. However, many women remain unaware of this statistic, which suggests a critical need for education about CHD in women for women of all ages.
- Women have some unique risk factors related to reproductive hormones that put them at higher risk of cardiovascular disease at certain times in their lives.
- Many aspects of cardiovascular disease differ between men and women. These include differences in:
  - Disease incidence and prevalence.
  - Risk factors.
  - Signs and symptoms.
  - Diagnosis and management.
  - Recovery issues.

Internet Resources

The National Coalition for Women with Heart Disease:
http://www.womenheart.org/

Women and Heart Disease: An Atlas of Racial and Ethnic Disparities in Mortality:
http://www.cdc.gov/cvh/womensatlas/index.htm

The Heart Truth: A National Awareness Campaign for Women about Heart Disease:
http://www.nhlbi.nih.gov/health/hearttruth/index.htm

Bibliography

Deaton C, Kunik C, Hachamovitch R et al: Diagnostic strategies for women with suspected coronary artery disease, *J Cardiovasc Nurs* 15(3):39-53, 2001.

DeVon H, Zerwic J: Symptoms of acute coronary syndromes: are there gender differences? A review of the literature, *Heart Lung* 31:235-245, 2002.

Fleury J, Cameron-Go K: Women's rehabilitation and recovery, *Crit Care Nurs Clin North Am* 9(4):577-587, 1997.

Giardina EV: Heart disease in women, *Int J Fertil* 45(6):350-357, 2000.

King KB: Emotional and functional outcomes in women with coronary heart disease, *J Cardiovasc Nurs* 15(3):54-70, 2001.

King K, Quinn J, Delehanty J et al: Perception of risk for coronary heart disease in women undergoing coronary angiography, *Heart Lung* 31:246-252, 2002.

Low K: Recovery from myocardial infarction and coronary artery bypass surgery in women: psychosocial factors, *J Women's Health* 2(2):133-139, 1993.

McSweeney J, Cody M, Crane P: Do you know them when you see them? Women's prodromal and acute symptoms of myocardial infarction, *J Cardiovasc Nurs* 15(3):26-38, 2001.

Oliver-McNeil S, Artinian N: Women's perceptions of personal cardiovascular risk and their risk-reducing behaviors, *Am J Crit Care* 11(3):221-227, 2002.

Richardson L: Women and heart failure, *Heart Lung* 30:87-97, 2001.

Chapter 41

Cardiovascular Disease and the Elderly

Cindi A. Sullivan and Leslie Davis

1. What age is considered a cardiovascular risk factor for adults?

Age is the major risk factor for coronary heart disease (CHD). Specifically, women aged 55 years or greater and men aged 45 years or greater are at higher risk for CHD. In general, men are at a higher risk for CHD in the early to middle adult years. By age 65 years, the number of deaths from CHD in women surpasses death in men by 11%. After menopause, women face a two to three times greater risk of CHD development than before menopause. Cardiovascular disease (CVD), including stroke and CHD, remains a leading cause of death for Americans over the age of 65 years. CHD is clearly a problem of major proportions in the elderly. In octogenarians, 27% of men and 17% of women have overt coronary disease. More than 50% of those older than 65 years of age die of coronary artery disease (CAD).

2. How does a family history of premature CHD as a risk factor relate to age?

A family history of premature CHD as a risk factor is defined as CHD in a male first-degree male relative less than 55 years or CHD in a female first-degree relative less than 65 years of age.

3. What are "normal" aging changes in the cardiovascular system and implications for assessment?

- It has been increasingly apparent that factors that relate to lifestyle (e.g., physical activity or nutritional habits) and the environment in which aging occurs have a substantial impact, not only with respect to the exponential occurrence of CVD later in life but also with respect to the rate of aging in the absence of disease. Whether some of the cardiovascular changes that accompany age are simply caused by deconditioning rather than by an aging process has been debated.
- Cardiovascular and autonomic aging. The left ventricular (LV) wall thickness increases with age, largely from an increase in the size of cardiac myocytes accompanied by focal increases in collagen. Less significant changes include gradual myocyte death without replacement. With advancing age, large arteries dilate. These large arteries' walls become thickened, and the media exhibit an increased collagen content and frayed elastin. Stiffening of the arteries typically leads to systolic hypertension (HTN).

- The most prominent and consequential change is the decrease in the response to beta-receptor stimulation. In the elderly, blood pressure (BP) is higher at rest and shows more of an increase during exercise than in young adults. During exercise, the increase in heart rate is blunted at all levels.
- Other observable changes include systolic HTN, ventricles that contract with good strength but more slowly than in young hearts, a poor tolerance of hypovolemia, and a diminished chronotropic and inotropic response to anything that involves beta-receptor stimulation, including exercise, exogenous catecholamine administration, or baroreflex.
- Inotropic changes. A gradual increase is seen in cardiac weight (i.e., an increase in LV mass and wall thickness, left atrial enlargement, and aortic root dilatation). Cardiac output and stroke volume decrease by approximately 0.5% yearly after midlife, and cardiac index falls linearly with age. Altered diastolic dysfunction (or compliance) has been shown in experimental models but has been hard to reproduce in humans because of the difficulty in diagnosing diastolic dysfunction (see Chapter 11, Heart Failure). An increased stiffness is associated with morphologic changes in the aging heart.
- Chronotropic changes. The resting heart rate changes little with age; however, the heart loses the ability to raise its maximal rate in response to stress or exercise. Maximal heart rate declines about 1 beat/y because of diminished (or blunted) beta-adrenergic responsiveness. The aging heart compensates by increasing end-diastolic and stroke volumes to preserve cardiac output.
- The vasculature. The veins contain at least 75% of the blood volume and are responsible for maintaining a relatively constant central blood volume (lungs and heart) despite changes in posture or changes in blood volume. Arterial stiffening may explain the overall increase in systolic BP with age. Loss of elastin, changes in collagen, and an increased rate of atheromatous calcification of the aorta and major arteries are associated with increased age.
- Electrical conduction system changes. With age, a decrease is seen in the number of pacing myocytes in the sinoatrial (SA) node and the atria, which are replaced by fibrosis and fatty infiltration. The atrioventricular (AV) node, bundle of His, and other bundle branches also undergo progressive cell loss. Combined with microcalcification of the conduction system, these changes place the elderly at an increased risk for altered conduction. For all organ systems, age is associated with a loss of physiological reserve that increases the vulnerability to disease and decreases the ability to compensate for stress.

4. What are the most common cardiovascular conditions for which the elderly are most at risk?

- Hypertension. BP progressively rises with increased age. Approximately 60% of those aged 65 years and older have HTN, with the prevalence being higher in women than in men. In Americans older than age 60 years, 60% of whites, 71% of blacks, and 61% of Hispanics have HTN. Systolic HTN is a better predictor of both mortality and morbidity from cardiovascular-related events; however, diastolic HTN is also an independent risk factor. Isolated systolic HTN (systolic BP, >140 mm Hg) increases by 7% in those older than 70 years of age and by 25% in those older than 80 years. HTN is known to be the most modifiable risk factor for stroke.

- Arrhythmias. These occur more frequently in the elderly because of an increased incidence of CAD and HTN. Bradyarrhythmias and heart block are more common in the elderly because of conduction system changes (see Question 2). Atrial fibrillation (AF) prevalence doubles with each advancing decade of age, from 0.5% at age 50 to 59 years and to 10% at age 80 to 89 years. Ventricular arrhythmias increase in frequency with age.
- Valvular heart disease. The cause of valvular heart disease primarily is degenerative disease. Senile degeneration and calcification of the aortic valve results from aortic stenosis (AS), which affects approximately 4% to 6% of those older than 65 years. However, a more common condition, aortic sclerosis, occurs in about one third of those older than age 65 years. Aortic valve replacement is the procedure of choice for symptomatic older persons with severe AS. Added heart sounds and systolic murmurs, such as mitral regurgitation, are normal variant findings in the elderly population.
- Congestive heart failure (CHF). The incidence of CHF is more prevalent in the elderly, mostly as a result of end-stage CAD, HTN, or valvular heart disease. CHF is the most common reason for hospitalization in the United States for those 65 years and older. Age-related changes in the organ system can impair the ability of older persons to compensate for HF. Older patients are more likely to have other conditions that produce symptoms and signs compatible with HF.

5. How does the presentation of CVD in the elderly differ from that in other age groups?

Presenting symptoms of elderly patients may be different than those of younger patients. The following table summarizes unique manifestations that occur in the elderly with various cardiac conditions.

Cardiac Condition	Subjective Symptoms	Objective Signs
Coronary artery disease or acute myocardial infarction	Dyspnea (especially on exertion) more frequent than pain. Silent ischemia common. Chest, arm, or "atypical" pain.	Added heart sounds or mitral regurgitation more common. Arrhythmias may be presenting sign.
Hypertension	Usually asymptomatic.	Isolated systolic hypertension common. Orthostasis common.
Arrhythmias	Palpitations. Lightheadedness.	Abnormal heart rate/electrocardiogram. Nonaccidental falls; syncope or presyncope.
Valvular heart disease	Feeling weak or tired.	Murmur, click, abnormal heart sounds.
Congestive heart failure	May attribute symptoms to "getting older."	Weight gain. Decreased exercise tolerance. Shortness of breath (dyspnea) at rest or exertion. Pedal edema (elderly are generally less active; prolonged sitting).

6. Should diagnostic testing for CVD conditions differ in the elderly?

- Exercise testing. The elderly need particularly close evaluation before exercise testing is ordered. The occurrence of fatigue and lightheadedness from muscle weakness and reconditioning, vasoregulatory abnormalities, and difficulty with gait are important concerns to be considered as possible problems with exercise testing completion.
- Cardiac catheterization. Angiographic success rates are similar for all age groups, but complication rates are higher for older patients (>80 years of age). Decreased renal function must be considered. The elderly have a 10% decline in creatinine clearance per decade after the age of 40 years.
- Electrophysiology (EP) test. Indications for EP testing are similar in older and younger adults. Closer monitoring of respiratory status for the older adult undergoing interventional procedures is a consideration. Careful monitoring of amnesic drugs and sedation is a concern because of increase sensitivity to medications.

7. Does treatment/disease management for various types of CVDs differ for elders?

- Coronary artery disease. Morbidity and mortality rates are higher in older patients. Relative contraindications to thrombolytic therapy for acute myocardial infarction (AMI) increase with age. Some octogenarians are functional and live independently with few serious medical issues; therefore some elderly persons may derive benefit from an aggressive interventional approach to AMI, treatment such as direct angioplasty.
- Hypertension. All types of HTN (systolic, diastolic, isolated systolic, and combined systolic/diastolic) increase in prevalence with age. People with borderline isolated systolic HTN have an increased risk for all CVD, CHD, stroke, transient ischemic attack, heart failure, and mortality from CVD.
- Several large randomized trials have shown the benefits of BP control in the elderly. Treatment reduced the incidence rate of CHD by 19% and of stroke by 13%. Recommendations for treatment include nonpharmacological methods such as:
  - Dietary modifications.
  - Weight loss.
  - Consistent exercise.
  - Sodium restrictions.
  - Reduction in alcohol consumption.
- Blood pressure targets are the same for the elderly as for middle aged and younger individuals (140/90 mm Hg). The Systolic Hypertension in the Elderly Program (SHEP) showed that morbidity rates are reduced when patients older than 60 years with isolated systolic HTN above 160 mm Hg are effectively treated with diuretics or diuretics and beta-blockers.
- Arrhythmia. The rate of stroke is 10 times higher in older than in younger patients with AF. Solid evidence shows that the risk of bleeding from appropriately dosed and monitored warfarin does not rise with age alone. The elderly are also at an increased risk for sinus and AV nodal dysfunction. Pacemaker implantation can be performed with light anesthesia with few

complications. Quality and length of life can be improved; therefore age is not a contraindication for pacemaker implantation.

- Valvular heart disease. Valvular disease is common in patients older than 65 years of age. Diagnosis can be accomplished with echocardiography. Surgical intervention in the management of valve disease is only affected by an increased intraoperative surgical risk and any concomitant age-related conditions, such as CAD.
- Congestive heart failure. CHF as a manifestation of end-stage ischemia, HTN, or valvular heart disease is as high as two million patients in the United States. The mortality rate is 50% within 5 years of the diagnosis. It is the number one reason for hospitalization and rehospitalization in the United States in the Medicare population. Despite the fact that mortality and morbidity in CHF is significantly improved with angiotensin-converting enzyme (ACE) inhibitor and beta-blocker therapy, these therapies are less often used in the elders. The bias among physicians is that the elderly have more side effects with the use of beta-blockers and ACE inhibitors. Beta-blockers may have higher plasma levels in the elderly than in young subjects. Many elderly have some degree of impaired renal function, which would affect dosing of both beta-blockers and ACE inhibitors.
- Hyperlipidemia. More evidence suggests that the use of statins in older adults reduces the risk of a first cardiovascular event or death from any cause. The Cardiovascular Health Study (CHS) lends support to the recommendation for screening and treatment of high cholesterol in elderly men and women in the same manner as middle-aged individuals are treated and screened.

8. Does nutritional treatment for CVD differ for elders?

About 90% of Americans of more than 65 years of age have one or more nutrition-related cardiovascular risk factor. A direct independent association has been shown between nutrition-related risk factors (increased low-density lipoprotein–cholesterol [LDL-C], HTN, and diabetes), morbidity, and health care expenditures in older people. Nutrition-based interventions have been shown to improve dietary control and reduce the need for medication in older persons with diabetes and HTN. Most estimates show that more than 20 million persons older than 65 years have elevated LDL-C, diabetes, or HTN. Individuals would benefit from nutritional therapy as part of the routine management. Older blacks are more likely than white persons to have these conditions.

9. What common side effects from cardiac medications are the elderly most likely to have?

- Beta-blockers. The negative inotropic and chronotropic effects reduce their suitability in older patients, as does their tendency to suppress conduction system activity. The incidence rate of postural hypotension is higher in the elderly.
- ACE inhibitors. Dose response may be lower in older patients. Adverse effects, such as coughing, and contraindications are more numerous than in younger adults.

- Calcium channel blockers. These are the vasodilator of choice in patients with low renin activity. Gastrointestinal (GI) symptoms, such as constipation, are common. These may cause cardiac conduction delay in the elderly.
- Diuretics. Side effects include their primary physiological effect on cardiac preload and the potential for precipitating hypokalemic.
- Polypharmacy is an issue for elders. In fact, the risk of adverse medication reactions increases from 6% when two medications are used to 50% when five medications are prescribed and 100% when eight or more medications are combined.
- As with the initiation of any therapy in the elderly, it is advisable to "start low and go slow."
- Compliance is the most important aspect of patient and family education. The nurse should attempt to minimize complications by teaching patients how to take medications, when to take them, and what combinations of medications are best not to take at the same time. Nurses should write out all medication names and dosages clearly in layman's terms. In addition, they should instruct patients about what to expect and how to treat side effects.

10. What are the current controversies in regard to treatment of CVD and elderly patients?

The three areas of controversy that exist in regard to treatment offered to the elderly include:

- Whether statin therapy is beneficial in the elderly. The CHS reports that the reduction in risk for people younger than 74 years who are taking statins is similar to that of people aged 74 years and older, yet many prescribers do not offer statins to the elders.
- Whether thrombolytic therapy is the treatment of choice for AMI for those patients aged more than 75 years. Thrombolytic therapy has not been adequately studied in patients over age 75 years. Careful assessment of risk and benefit of reperfusion for each elderly patient with AMI should be done by an experienced physician. Future studies are needed to determine benefit. (See Chapter 10, Myocardial Infarction.)
- Whether invasive procedures (percutaneous coronary intervention [PCI] or coronary artery bypass grafting [CABG]) should be offered to the elderly. Overall use of interventional cardiac procedures in the elderly has been increasing proportionally over time. However, currently, about one in five PCIs and CABG procedures in the United States are performed on patients aged 75 years and older. As surgical techniques have improved, so have the outcomes for the elderly without coexisting morbidity.

Key Points

- The normal aging process is associated with physiologic and cellular changes of the cardiovascular system.
- In treatment of the elderly, chronological age should not be the determining factor. One should look at the whole patient.
- A classic presentation of symptoms should not be expected in the geriatric patient.
- Medical care is aimed at preservation of cardiac function.
- Economics is a real consideration related to compliance with medications.

Internet Resources

Open Directory Project: Geriatrics:
http://dmoz.org/Health/Medicine/Medical_Specialties/Geriatrics/

Clinical Geriatrics (Monthly Journal):
http://www.mmhc.com/cg/

Ohio State University Extension Program: Senior Series:
http://ohioline.osu.edu/ss-fact/0127.html

Merck Manual of Geriatrics:
http://www.merck.com/pubs/mm_geriatrics/contents.htm

Bibliography

Cuttingham S: Health promotion and disease prevention: high blood pressure. In Woods S, Frelichen ESS, and Motzer SU. *Cardiac nursing,* ed 4, Philadelphia, 2000, Lippincott, pp 405-406, 802.

Etrlinger T, Pollock H, Appel L: Nutrition-related cardiovascular risk factors in older people: results from the Third National Health and Nutrition Survey, *J Am Geriatr Soc* 48(10):1486-1489, 2000.

Hutt E: Heart disease in the elderly. In Adair OV: *Cardiology secrets,* ed 2, Philadelphia, 2000, Hanley & Belfus, pp 188-191.

Kroll C, Ohman M: Should reperfusion strategies in myocardial infarction be modified for the very elderly? *Am Heart J* 143:374-375, 2002.

Laird RD, Studenski SS: Management of hypertension for stroke prevention in older people, *Clin Geriatr Med* 15(4):663-684, 1999.

Lakatta EG: Cardiovascular aging in health, *Clin Geriatr Med* 16(3):419-444, 2000.

Lakatta EG: Age-associated cardiovascular changes in health: impact on cardiovascular disease in older persons, *Heart Failure Rev* 7:29-49, 2002.

Lewis S: Cardiovascular disease in post menopausal women: myth and reality, *Am J Cardiol* 89(suppl):5E-11E, 2002.

Nixon JV: The aging heart. In Alpert JS: *Cardiology for the primary care physician,* ed 3, Philadelphia, 2001, Current Medicine, Inc, pp 401-410.

Rich M: Cardiovascular risk factors. In Gerstenblith G: *Acute coronary syndrome,* Chapter 12 syllabus in Adult Clinical Cardiology Self-Assessment Program V, American College of Cardiology 9-31, 2002.

Roberts B, Eastman L: Care of the older adult. In Beare PG, Myers JL: *Adult health nursing,* ed 3, St Louis, 1998, Mosby, pp 411, 494.

Sabatini T, Frisoni G, Barbisoni P et al: Atrial fibrillation and cognitive disorders in older people, *J Am Geriatr Soc* 48:387-390, 2000.

Saxon S, Etten M: *Physical change & aging: a guide for helping professions,* ed 3, New York, 1994, Tiresias Press, pp 129, 136-139.

Ueda-K: Longitudinal studies in geriatric medicine, *Nippon Ronen Igakkai Zasshi* 35:343-352, May 1998.

Whetstone G, Boswell S: The geriatric heart, *Am J Nurs* 102(9 suppl):22-24, 2002.

Chapter 42

Cardiovascular Disease and Ethnicity

Brenda S. Thompson

1. What facts show the prevalence of cardiovascular diseases among black Americans and other minorities?

The American Heart Association published "Heart Facts 2002," which reveals that cardiovascular disease is still the number one killer of Americans, claiming more than 40% of 2.4 million deaths each year. Cardiovascular disease has been the number one killer of Americans every year since 1900, except for 1918. Cardiovascular disease claims almost as many lives as the next seven leading causes of death each year. Approximately 62 million Americans have cardiovascular disease, which includes the diagnosis of coronary heart disease, hypertension, heart failure, congenital heart defects, arteriosclerosis, and diseases of the circulatory system.

The following table depicts the prevalence of cardiovascular disease among the various ethnic groups based on gender.

Ethnic Group	Prevalence of Cardiovascular Disease in Men	Prevalence of Cardiovascular Disease in Women
Whites	30.0%	23.8%
Non-Hispanic blacks	40.5%	39.6%
Non-Hispanic whites	30.0%	23.8%
Mexican Americans	28.8%	26.6%

Estimates are age-adjusted.

2. What particular cardiovascular diseases are black Americans more at risk for as compared with other races?

The literature reveals that black Americans have a higher incidence rate of hypertension, stroke, heart failure and diabetes as compared with other races. Hypertension is a major risk factor for the development of cardiovascular disease and stroke. Black Americans have the highest incidence rate of hypertension, and development is an earlier age when compared with whites. Some researchers are calling hypertension an epidemic, with approximately 30% of the black American population having this disease known as the "silent killer."

3. **What is the incidence rate of hypertension in black Americans as compared with whites?**

Incidence rate of hypertension for ages 20 to 74 years of age		
Race	**Men**	**Women**
Black American	36.7%	36.6%
White	25.2%	20.5%

Hypertension in black Americans has an onset at an earlier age and is more severe, with a higher prevalence of blood pressures greater than or equal to 180/110 mm Hg. Studies of hypertensive pathophysiology reveal that lower levels of renin, increased salt sensitivity, and impaired salt excretions account for the higher incidence of hypertension in black Americans as compared with whites. The result is a greater incidence of end organ damage, such as left ventricular hypertrophy, renal disease, and stroke.

4. **What is the incidence rate of stroke in black Americans as compared with other races?**

Stroke rates are the highest among black Americans, followed by Asian/Pacific Islanders, whites, American Indians/Alaska Natives, and Hispanics. The risk of hemorrhagic stroke in black Americans is five times higher in men less than 45 years old and three and a half times greater in black American women than in the white population. The risk of ischemic stroke is three times greater in black American men and four times greater in black American women than in the same white population. Mortality rates from stroke in the black American population are 97% higher in men and 71% higher in women than in whites. A report from the Center for Disease Control and Prevention (CDC) reveals that 20% of black Americans have more than two risk factors associated with stroke compared with 7% of the white group. Risk factors include hypertension, diabetes, tobacco use, alcohol and illicit drug abuse, sedentary lifestyle, obesity, and family history of stroke.

5. **Is the incidence rate of heart failure higher for black Americans than for non-blacks?**

Heart failure is a leading cause of death in black Americans, accounting for a 31% higher incidence rate compared with white men and a 32% higher incidence rate in black American women compared with white women. Hypertension is the leading cause of heart failure in this population.

6. **What is the prevalence of type 2 diabetes and risk factors in black Americans?**

The incidence rate of type II diabetes in the black American population and the rate of associated complications of renal failure, blindness, and death are two times higher than in the white population. The reasoning is that the black American population has an increased number of risk factors, including diets high in fat and sugar but low in fiber, high cholesterol levels, obesity, and sedentary life styles.

7. **Does treatment for cardiovascular diseases differ in black Americans as compared with non-black Americans?**

Numerous disparities exist in the treatment of black Americans as compared with non-black Americans with respect to cardiovascular disease. Black Americans and minorities are less likely to receive:
- Appropriate cardiovascular medications. They are half as likely to take aspirin on a regular basis as compared with non-black Americans. Angiotensin-converting enzyme (ACE) inhibitors and beta-blockers are also less likely to be initiated in the black American population.
- Coronary interventions, including coronary artery bypass grafts and coronary angioplasties, compared with whites. The use of these procedures varies greatly between race and gender, with white men being most likely to receive the intervention, followed by black American men, white women, and then black American women. A striking study of Medicare patients revealed that 11% of eligible black American patients receive thrombolytic therapy compared with 68% of eligible white patients.
- Referrals for eye exams in the diabetic minority patient.
- Referrals to mental health services after hospitalization for a mental illness.

On the reverse side, black Americans and minorities are more likely to receive less desirable interventions, such as amputations of body parts as a result of complications from diabetes. These disparities in the treatment of cardio-vascular disease are recognized by leaders in health care and are currently being studied.

8. **Discuss barriers to the diagnosis and treatment of cardiovascular diseases that exist for black Americans as compared with non-black Americans?**

Barriers that may account for a lack of diagnosis of cardiovascular disease in minorities include:
- Age, ethnicity, lifestyle, socioeconomic status.
- Education, work limitations.
- Region and degree of urbanization, leading to lack of access to medical care.
- Duration of care, prior experience in the health care setting.
- Lack of appropriate monetary resources and insurance coverage.
- A lack of appropriate language access in some health care settings and clinics.
- Imprisoned populations may have delayed diagnosis and treatment.
- Attitude toward medical care and risks, functional/perceived health status.

- Delay seeking treatment and refusal of recommended treatment.
- Lack of consistent relationship with primary care provider.

9. What is salt sensitivity, and does it play a role in cardiovascular disease in the black American population?

Salt sensitivity is a direct result of the rise or fall in blood pressure when salt or sodium chloride is added or removed from the diet. As the amount of salt consumed daily increases, the blood pressure tends to rise accordingly. The reverse happens when the amount of salt consumed is reduced; the blood pressure also decreases. When less than 2 g of dietary sodium are consumed daily, hypertension is rare unless underlying pathology, such as renal stenosis, exists. Salt sensitivity is an important concept for nurses who educate and manage black Americans with high blood pressure and other minorities. Salt sensitivity has been found to be a factor in 73% of all black Americans with hypertension. Educating and counseling patients on dietary salt intake, weight reduction, and stress reduction fall within the independent role of nursing practice and are crucial in the management of hypertension and in the primary prevention of this devastating disease.

10. Do black Americans have worse outcomes for cardiovascular diseases as compared with non-black Americans?

Hypertension appears to be more severe in the black American population with a high mortality rate; 30% of the deaths of black American men and 20% of the deaths of black American women are attributed to high blood pressure. The CDC reports that the average life span for black Americans is 71.8 years compared with 77.4 years for whites.

Symptoms of heart failure present themselves earlier in the black American population and progress at a more rapid rate than in the white population. This phenomenon is possibly related to the increased incidence of hypertension, diabetes, left ventricular hypertrophy, and vascular injury seen in the black American population. This is seen in the higher incidence rate of hospitalization and repeated admissions early after diagnosis.

11. Do other minorities (Hispanics, Asians, Native Americans, or Alaska Natives) differ in regard to prevalence and death rates from cardiovascular disease?

Percentage of Deaths from Cardiovascular Disease by Race and Gender

Race	Men	Women
Black Americans	32.4%	41.6%
Asians/Pacific Islanders	35.4%	36.1%
Hispanics	25.4%	34.0%
Native Americans/Alaska Natives	26.0%	28.0%

12. What are drug polymorphisms?

A polymorphism defines a genetic variation in protein expression that alters enzymatic function. Drug polymorphisms refer to the small variations in the drug metabolizing enzymes that are present in various ethnic populations. The differences in the distribution of these polymorphic traits seem to determine the rate of metabolism of certain cardiovascular medications. The presence or lack of enzyme polymorphisms may predispose the patient to rapidly metabolizing cardiovascular medications or consideration as a slow metabolizer.

13. What are slow and fast metabolizers?

Slow metabolizers are those patients who do not inherit the essential drug-metabolizing enzyme and are more prone to development of a buildup of the medications and development of toxic drug reactions. Rapid metabolizers who clear the medications more rapidly are more prone to medication levels that may decrease too quickly, leaving the patient without coverage between doses. Their conditions may also become toxic because of the rapid uptake and high serum levels of the medication.

14. What implications do drug polymorphisms present for the treatment of cardiovascular disease?"

The polymorphisms that affect antihypertensive medications have been the most widely studied class of cardiovascular polymorphisms. Black Americans tend to have low-renin hypertension, whereas whites tend to have high-renin hypertension. Therefore black Americans tend to respond better to diuretics than to ACE inhibitors and beta-blockers. Diuretics as monotherapy are considered to be the initial treatment for hypertension in black Americans. When ACE inhibitors or beta-blockers are combined with diuretic therapy in black Americans, response tends to be as effective to this medical regimen as in the white population for the treatment of hypertension and heart failure. Alpha-blockers are also effective in black Americans for treatment of hypertension. Whites tend to respond to all antihypertensive medications, especially ACE inhibitors and beta-blockers.

Other studies have revealed that propanolol has a more dramatic effect on heart rate and blood pressure in Chinese men than in white men. The hypertensive Asian-American population tends to respond to diuretics, beta-blockers, and calcium channel blockers. Currently little scientific evidence exists that the Hispanic population should be treated any differently than the white population in management of hypertension.

15. What is the clinical significance of polymorphisms?

Polymorphisms are clinically significant with the presence of: (1) a small or narrow therapeutic range; (2) an identified enzyme pathway; and (3) medication that is known to show the effects of significant enzyme polymorphisms.

16. In the education of various culture and ethnic groups, what specific patient teaching tips should be kept in mind?

The health care provider needs to keep in mind that different cultures have diverse language patterns and beliefs and practices related to health care:

- Some black-Americans have a certain dialect that requires careful communication to prevent misunderstandings.
- Mexican-Americans believe that eye contact is important and that someone who looks and admires a child without touching the child has given the child an "evil eye."
- American Eskimos will seldom disagree with others in public to be polite; body language is extremely important.
- Jewish-Americans consider excess touching, especially from the opposite gender, offensive.
- Chinese-Americans consider excess eye contact as a sign of rudeness, and excess touching is also offensive in this culture.
- Haitian-Americans consider direct eye contact as a way to get attention and respect during communication; touch is also acceptable during conversations.
- Vietnamese-Americans consider avoidance of eye contact as a sign of respect. Also, an upturned palm is offensive during communication and the head is considered sacred and should not be patted or touched.

There are many beliefs and cultural behaviors that health care professionals should recognize and consider during the treatment and education of the patient populations they serve. It would be wise to educate oneself and develop cultural sensitivities of the variety of cultures we serve to be as effective as possible.

17. What myths regarding cardiovascular disease and race exist?

MYTH 1:
- Beta-blockers are not as effective in the black American population as in the white population for the management of heart failure.
- Fact: Carvedilol was as effective in the black American population as in the non-black American population, possibly because of its alpha-1 inhibition and antioxidant properties that are not present in other beta-blockers. The risk reduction was 54% in black Americans versus 51% in non-black Americans.

MYTH 2:
- Hypertension is as prevalent in the black American population as in the white population.
- Fact: Hypertension is more prevalent in the black American population, affecting 29 of every 100 black Americans. Hypertension is also more severe as black Americans age, causing more strokes, heart disease, and renal failure.

18. What does the future hold for study for cardiovascular diseases and ethnicity?

Healthy People 2010, the Nation's public health agenda, has made the elimination of health disparities that affect racial and ethnic minority populations a goal for this decade, according to the Department of Health and Human Services. In an attempt to reduce the racial disparities, the health objectives have proposed the same objectives for all racial and ethnic groups. The Agency for Healthcare Research and Quality began publishing an annual report on the disparities in health care delivery in 2003 in an attempt to move towards eliminating these disparities.

Another new initiative to decrease health disparities among black Americans and minorities is "Take a Loved One to the Doctor Day" supported by the Health and Human Services and ABC radio networks. This campaign was launched in November 2001 and is aimed at reducing the health care disparities between black Americans and minorities. Encouragement to seek health care screening is part of the initiative. The campaign also focuses on involving black Americans and minorities in other government programs to promote health and wellness. Information on the program, including a tool kit to assist communities to organize local health care events, can be obtained by calling 1-800-444-6472. The website address is **www.healthgap.omhrc.gov.**

Key Points

- Black men and women have a higher prevalence of cardiovascular diseases as compared with other ethnic groups.
- Disparities in the treatment of cardiovascular diseases remain an issue.
- Language patterns, beliefs, and practices need to be taken into consideration in the education of patients.

Internet Resources

Journal Article: Gender, Ethnicity and Genetics in Cardiovascular Disease:
http://www.ncbi.nlm.nih.gov/entrez/query.fcgi?cmd=Retrieve&db=PubMed&list_uids=12713680&dopt=Abstract

The Scientist Daily News: Ethnicity and CV Disease: Ethnic Variations in Cardiovascular Disease Only Partly Explained by Risk Factors:
http://www.biomedcentral.com/news/20000725/09/

U.S. Department of Health and Human Services: Race and Health: Cardiovascular Disease:
http://raceandhealth.hhs.gov/3rdpgBlue/Cardio/3pgStatCardio.htm

Bibliography

Allen JE: Landmark study tracks heart disease in blacks: cardiology researchers plan to follow 6,500 African Americans in projects aimed at ending unchecked epidemic, *Los Angeles Times,* Los Angeles, Apr 8, 2002.

American Heart Association: *2002 heart and stroke statistical update,* Dallas, 2001, The Association.

Barkauskas VH, Baumann LC, Darling-Fisher CS: Cultural considerations in health assessment. In *Health & physical assessment,* ed 3, St Louis, 2002, Mosby, pp 139-158.

Epstein AM, Ayanian JZ: Racial disparities in medical care, *N Engl J Med* 344(19):1471-1473, 2001.

Kudzman EC: Cultural competence: cardiovascular medications, *Prog Cardiovasc Nurs* 16(4):152-160, 169, 2001.

National Institutes of Health: NIH guidelines on the inclusion of women and minorities as subjects in clinical research, *Federal Register* 59:14508-14513, 1994.

Peters RM, Flack JM: Salt sensitivity and hypertension in African Americans: implications for cardiovascular disease, *Prog Cardiovasc Nurs* 15(4):138-144, 2000.

Wood AJJ: Racial difference in the response to drugs—pointers to genetic difference, *N Engl J Med* 344(18):1393-1396, 2001.

Yancy CW, Fowler MB, Colucci WS et al: Race and the response to adrenergic blockade with carvedilol in patients with chronic heart failure, *N Engl J Med* 344(18):1358-1365, 2001.

Cardiovascular Disease and Diabetes

Paul Dunn and Leslie Davis

1. What is diabetes mellitus (DM)?

Diabetes is a metabolic disease characterized by hyperglycemia that results from defects in insulin secretion, insulin action, or both. Type 1 diabetes (immunodestructive disease) is marked by relative or absolute insulin deficiency and must be managed with insulin via injection. Type 2 diabetes is marked by a combination of resistance to insulin action and an inadequate compensatory insulin secretory response. Ninety percent of people with DM have type 2. Because insulin controls the metabolism of nutrients (glucose, lipids, and protein), physiologic complications are insidious and widespread. They include macrovascular and microvascular disease, neurologic impairment, especially in the extremities, and renal/retinal degeneration.

2. What is the prevalence of diabetes in the United States?

In the United States in 2002, one in every 17 people had DM. The prevalence rate of type 2 disease in US adults increased 33% between 1990 and 1998. Because DM type 2 is so closely linked with obesity, these trends follow the increased incidence of obesity. In fact, a 30% increase in US obesity was also seen during this same period. Among adolescents, a 42% increase was seen in obesity during this period.

This incidence rate is increasing worldwide and especially in the United States. By the time one reaches age 65 years, one in every six people has diabetes. This prevalence is higher in African-Americans, Latinos, and Native Americans. No specialty area in nursing is exempt from caring for patients with this disease. Cardiovascular nurses see more diabetes in their practice than in most other health disciplines.

3. What is the impact of diabetes on cardiovascular disease (CVD)?

Many clinicians fail to appreciate this connection and its relation to CVD. Eighty-five percent of people with diabetes die of heart and cerebrovascular disease. According to the American Diabetes Association, people with diabetes should be treated as if they already have CVD. This includes preventative treatments such as aspirin and cholesterol-lowering agents.

Obesity is a primary risk for development of type 2 diabetes. In the United States today, 65% of Americans are considered overweight or obese. There is a current epidemic of teenagers with type 2 diabetes. Statistically these individuals are prime candidates for major coronary disease within 10 to 15 years.

4. What is impaired glucose tolerance (IGT), and what is its significance?

Impaired glucose tolerance is a term many people associate with what is now officially called prediabetes. The condition is a glucose level that is above normal (110 mg/dL fasting) but fails to exceed the 126-mg/dL level necessary for a diagnosis of diabetes (now called impaired fasting glucose [IFG]). The actual term IGT still exists only as a method of detecting an abnormal oral glucose tolerance when the patient is administered a 3-hour glucose tolerance test (OGTT). In this case, the term refers to a 2-hour value greater than 165 mg/dL.

Evidence remains that the presence of prediabetes still carries with it micro-vascular risk (eye, kidney, and other small vessel disease associated with heart disease) and nerve disease (especially carpal tunnel syndrome). Note that there are as many people with prediabetes as there are with diagnosed diabetes.

5. What are some of the common symptoms/sequelae of diabetes that contribute to CVD?

- Inadequate symptom identification may delay treatment. More than 50% of these cases have silent myocardial infarctions (MIs).
- Autonomic dysfunction is more common than in the general population and is manifested as episodes of postural hypotension and dizziness, paroxysmal nausea, nocturnal diarrhea, and sweating.
- Electrolyte and clotting disturbances and delayed healing are seen.
- Classic anginal symptoms are often absent. Acute dyspnea, symptoms of heart failure, indigestion, diaphoresis, and presyncope may be the presenting symptoms.

6. What are the risk factors for diabetes?

- Habitual physical inactivity.
- Overweight or obesity (body mass index [BMI], ≥ 25 kg/m^2).
- Previously identified IGT or IGT.
- Hypertension ($\geq 140/90$ mm Hg in adults).
- High-density lipoprotein–cholesterol (HDL-C) of 35 mg/dL or less (0.90 mmol/L) or a triglyceride level of 250 mg/dL or more (2.82 mmol/L).
- Family history of type 2 diabetes.
- African, Hispanic, and Native American ethnicity.
- History of gestational diabetes or delivery of a baby weighing more than 9 lb.
- Polycystic ovary syndrome.
- Preexisting peripheral arterial disease (PAD).

7. How much does diabetes affect the risk for CVD?

The annual age-adjusted risk ratios for coronary heart disease, stroke, and intermittent claudication for men and women from diabetes are as follows:
- Coronary heart disease:
  - Men = double.
  - Women = about four times.
- Stroke:
  - Men = almost four times.
  - Women = double.
- Intermittent claudication:
  - Men = almost four times.
  - Women = almost 10 times.

8. How is diabetes diagnosed in adults?

Since the 1990s, an enormous growth in the number of adolescents diagnosed with type 2 DM has been seen. Statistically speaking, by the time these teenagers reach 30 years old, a two-fold to three-fold increase will be seen in heart disease in these people. See the following table.

Diagnostic Criteria for Diabetes

Diabetes	• Acute symptoms (polyuria, polydipsia, polyphagia) with random plasma glucose value exceeding 200 mg/dL. • Two fasting plasma glucose values greater than 126 mg/dL. • Value of 200 mg/dL or greater at 2-hr period with 75-g oral glucose tolerance test.
Prediabetes	• Impaired fasting glucose (IFG) is defined as fasting plasma value between 110 and 126 mg/dL. • Impaired glucose tolerance (IGT) is defined as 2-hr plasma value between 140 and 200 mg/dL with 75-g oral glucose tolerance test.

9. What labs and control parameters are recommended?

Control Parameter	Goal in 2003
Blood pressure	130/80 mm Hg
Total cholesterol	<185 mg/dL
Low-density lipoprotein	<100 mg/dL
High-density lipoprotein	>45 mg/dL in men; >55 mg/dL in women
Triglycerides	<150 mg/dL

Continued

continued	
Control Parameter	**Goal in 2003**
Urinary microalbumin to creatinine ratio*	<30 mg/dL
A1c hemoglobin†	6.5-7.0 without significant hypoglycemia
Preprandial blood glucose	80-120 mg/dL
2-h postprandial blood glucose	<160 mg/dL

*Presence of urinary microalbumin/creatinine ratio >30 mg/dL has been found predictive of later cardiac disease with or without hypertension.
†A1c hemoglobin is not diagnostic test at this time because of lack of nationwide standardization. A1c measures glycosylated hemoglobin, which reflects ambient average glucose levels over preceding 3 months from time of test. In both type 1 and type 2 diabetes mellitus, this value is well correlated to development of complications (primarily microvascular).

10. What medications are used with diabetes and why?

Large prospective trials of both type 1 and type 2 diabetes have shown that inadequate blood pressure, lipid and glucose control, and continued smoking (in this order) are all associated with the development or worsening of microvascular and macrovascular disease.

- Blood pressure. Angiotensin-converting enzyme (ACE) inhibitors have been shown as the class of drugs preferred for hypertension in people with DM because they uniquely reduce glomerular hypertension independent of general systemic pressure. Angiotensin II blockers also show similar effects on microvascular protection in renal disease. Calcium channel blockers are not as effective as ACE inhibitors and may, in the presence of congestive heart failure (CHF), cause worsening of the disorder. The United Kingdom Prospective Diabetes Study (UKPDS) showed that controlling blood pressure by whatever means improved outcomes in microvascular disease. In recent years, the value of beta-blockers in reducing the event rate and preventing further events has been shown. The long-held belief that beta-blockers are dangerous because of the blockade of hypoglycemic symptoms has been debunked. The benefits clearly outweigh the risks.
- Lipids. People with DM can have type 4a hyperlipidemia marked by high low-density lipoprotein (LDL), low HDL, elevated triglycerides, and only a moderate elevation in total cholesterol. This condition is primarily a response to poor metabolism from inadequate insulin or insulin functioning. Cholesterol treatment goals for diabetics are as follows. The use of all lipid-lowering agents (statins, fibrates, and others) may be required. The dose of these agents should be titrated so that when combined with agents that sensitize or replace insulin the desired goal is achieved. Testing of hepatic and renal function at initiation and prescribed intervals is prudent. Note that the thiazolidinediones (glitazones) are known for worsening lipid profiles by increasing LDL, although

they do control glucose well. (See Chapter 36, Lipid-Lowering Strategies, for more details.)

- Glucose. Achievement of the goals previously listed is essential. Glucose is used as a marker for general metabolism. The function of insulin must be maximized to reduce all complications whether microvascular or macrovascular.

11. Does treatment for patients with diabetes and CVD differ from treatment for those without diabetes?

Yes. Patients with DM have two to four times more CVD than those without the disease. The advancement of disease is more rapid, and more complications are seen in vascular flow and infection. Behavioral management underpins all aspects of treatment and must be aggressive. Weight reduction and insistence on sustained cardiac rehabilitation are essential. Patients with diabetes take more medications than other people on average. Attention to cost and efficacy of these medications is important. Many patients do not readily admit to making a decision between purchasing medications and food or paying bills. Simply adding or increasing medications is not always the answer. Preventive cardiovascular nursing must be aimed at all the control parameters previously mentioned.

12. How does hyperglycemia affect the cerebrovascular system?

- Increase in neurologic ischemia from loss of endothelium-dependent vascular relaxation.
- Inducement of brain edema, leading to disruption of the blood-brain barrier and ultimately to the hemorrhagic transformation of an ischemic stroke.
- Metabolic acidosis, leading to increased lactate concentrations exaggerating ischemic damage by an increase in the formation of oxygen free radicals.
- Inhibition of vasodilation.
- Increased vascular smooth muscle proliferation.
- Thrombogenesis: impaired platelet and fibrinolytic function.
- Proatherogenic cellular processes.
- Ischemia in the microcirculation.

13. What are the common glucose-lowering drugs and their primary effects?

The following table outlines the agents used in glucose control and their function and time of action.

Secretagogues	Sensitizers	Glucose Blockers	Insulins	Length of Action
repaglinide (Prandin), nateglinide (Starlix)			Humalog, Novolog	10-90 min
		acarbose (Precose), miglitol (Glyset)	Regular	1-6 hr

Continued

continued

Secretagogues	Sensitizers	Glucose Blockers	Insulins	Length of Action
glipizide (Glucotrol), glyburide (DiaBeta, Micronase, Glynase PresTab), glimepiride (Amaryl), tolbutamide (Orinase), tolazamide (Tolinase)	metformin (Glucophage, Novo-Metformin)		NPH, Lente	4-18 hr
Chlorpropamide (Diabinese)			Ultralente, Lantus (glargine)	4-26 hr
	pioglitazone (Actos), rosiglitazone (Avandia)			3-6 wk

Clotting and endothelial function: People with DM have inadequate fibrinolysis and accelerated plaque formation on coronary vessels. Use of aspirin is standard of care for all people with DM unless absolute or relative contraindications exist (e.g., warfarin use, gastric ulceration, drug interactions).

Key Points

- Eighty-five percent of people with diabetes die of CVD.
- Atypical symptom presentation is the rule rather than the exception in diabetics. Be on the lookout for other symptoms of CVD (for example, gastrointestinal symptoms).
- Glucose control is less important than blood pressure control in type 2 DM.
- All patients with DM should be taking 81 mg acetylsalicylic acid (ASA; aspirin) and omega-3 fish oil daily unless contraindicated.

Internet Resources

American Diabetes Association:
www.diabetes.org

North Carolina Diabetes Prevention and Control Branch:
www.ncdiabetes.org

American Diabetes Association Diabetes Care Journal:
http://care.diabetesjournals.org/content/vol26/suppl_1/

Diabetes Drug Database
www.coreynahman.com/diabetesdrugsdatabase.html

MDLinx: Research updates/in the news
http://www.mdlinx.com/

Bibliography

American Diabetes Association: Standards of medical care for patients with diabetes mellitus, *Diabetes Care* 26:S33-S50, 2003.

Diabetes Control and Complications Trial Research Group: The effect of intensive insulin treatment of diabetes on the development and progression of long-term complications in insulin-dependent diabetes mellitus, *N Engl J Med* 329:977-986, 1993.

Duckworth WC, McCarren M, Abraira C: Glucose control and cardiovascular complications: the VA Diabetes Trial (VADT), *Diabetes Care* 24:942-945, 2001.

Expert Panel on Detection, Evaluation and Treatment of High Blood Cholesterol in Adults: Executive summary of the third report of the National Cholesterol Education Program (NCEP), *JAMA* 285:2486-2497, 2001.

Laight DW, Carrier MJ, Anggard EE: Antioxidants, diabetes and endothelial dysfunction, *Cardiovasc Res* 47:457-464, 2000.

UK Prospective Diabetes Study Group (UKPDS): Intensive blood glucose control with sulfonylureas or insulin compared with conventional treatment and risk of complications in patients with type 2 diabetes (UKPDS 33), *Lancet* 352:837-853, 1998.

Section VIII

Current Topics in Cardiology

Family Presence

Bonnie Taylor

1. What is family presence (FP)?

Family presence is the practice of inviting family members or significant others to remain with an individual who is undergoing a medical intervention, including certain invasive procedures and resuscitation. For most people, the primary support system consists of family and friends. During a health crisis, this support system continues to play an integral part in an individual's sense of safety and well being, thus decreasing anxiety.

2. What principle guides this practice?

Patients and their families are treated with respect by allowing their participation in experiences that provide perceptions of control, decision making, and independence.

3. What are some important needs of family members of critically ill patients?

Research indicates that the most important needs identified by family members of critically ill patients are to be:
- Physically close to the patient.
- Helpful to the patient.
- Informed of the patient's condition (including impending death).
- Comforted and supported by family and accepted, comforted, and supported by the health care staff.
- Confident that the patient receives the best possible care.

4. Who are the essential staff needed to facilitate FP?

A patient/family advocate is needed to liaise between the health care team and the family on arrival. This advocate can be a nurse, social worker, or chaplain. This individual collects vital information surrounding events and medical history for the resuscitation team to aid patient care and can then prepare family members for visiting the patient by informing them about:
- The patient's appearance/condition.
- The procedures to be performed or that are anticipated to be in progress during their visit to the bedside.
- Boundaries and restrictions: realistic expectations of acceptable behavior while in the treatment area.

This designated staff member then remains with the family to facilitate information, answer questions, and provide support as needed. Nurses, physicians, respiratory therapists, nursing assistants, and clerical staff, and any specialty consulting health care providers, must all, at a minimum, be aware of and acknowledge the presence of the family at the bedside.

5. How does a department initiate a FP program?

The first thing a department must do is survey all staff about their feelings on this topic. Some questions need to be answered by the health care team as a group. How is FP viewed by family or significant others—as a right, a privilege, or an obligation? If a general consensus appears supportive of instituting this protocol, an educational program should be developed to help staff understand what FP is and why implementing a FP program is being considered. Full multidisciplinary staff leadership support is essential for it to be successful, although anticipation is realistic that less than 100% of staff will have a favorable opinion about the decision to have this program in place. Each member of the staff has an integral role in the process and should be educated about the importance of their role and included in the development of the program.

6. How does a FP program work?

The development of fairly specific guidelines to allow for appropriate FP is important to the success of providing this family-centered approach. Precisely which actions or procedures define this activity vary and are specific to the area of practice. Having a process in place can be the basis of developing an individualized experience for each patient's circumstance.

A FP program is based primarily on the patient's wish to have the family remain at the bedside. In the event that the patient is unable to express his/her wishes, the option is explored with family members present. The reactions of the patient/family to the situation and the opinions of the health care team are considered. In many instances, FP is provided by simply never asking family to leave the bedside. If family members appear uncomfortable or have needs of their own to be met, they should be invited to a quiet room where they can temporarily remove themselves from the situation as needed. For many family and friends, the visit to the emergency department was not an expected event. They may have taken insulin and not had an opportunity to eat. They may have chronic medical problems of their own that are exacerbated by the stress of the current situation bringing them to the hospital. Also important is that in many cases, the family may have already witnessed life-saving measures, including invasive procedures and resuscitative efforts at home or an accident site before arrival in the emergency department.

7. What are the benefits and pitfalls of such a program?

Family presence during trauma or medical resuscitation and invasive procedures is controversial.

- Pitfalls:
  - Critics tout potential disruption during resuscitation/intervention efforts and fear over possible medical-legal issues. Concern for possible traumatic experiences by the family/significant other exists as well. Often the details of the events leading to the patient's arrival in the emergency department are scant. In light of such minimal information, decisions about who should be allowed to remain with the patient may be difficult to make.
  - Determining the suitability of FP must always be weighed against the potential for distraction of the staff or patient. Misunderstanding of patient care procedures by medically unsophisticated family members or significant others is a valid concern that should be addressed when developing a protocol for FP selection.
- Benefits:
  - Several studies showed that allowing family members access to the patient alleviated anxiety or anger stemming from being separated from the patient and minimized litigation. FP can show to the family that every possible measure is being taken to save their loved one's life and can emphasize the gravity of the situation. This in turn may facilitate the grieving process. In an attempt to provide compassionate care to patients and their families, the opportunity to choose FP can provide a positive experience in a difficult time.
  - Offering the option for FP can be reassuring to families and make them feel as though they do have some control and choices to be involved in the care of the patient should they choose it. Integrating a FP program can be challenging. In addition, we should be guided by the needs of patient and family in efforts to preserve dignity, confidentiality, and a holistic approach in the business of caring for humans.

8. What lies in the future for FP?

The Emergency Nurses Association strongly supports FP in the emergency department. The American College of Emergency Physicians has published a fact sheet outlining recommendations about FP and advocate that emergency departments have a policy in place addressing this issue. Far more research needs to be conducted to show measurable benefits to families, patients, staff, and hospitals. The literature suggests a favorable attitude toward FP by families and nurses.

 Key Points

- Grant the patient's wishes first and the family's wishes second.
- Do not be afraid to be transparent.
- Our responsibility as the choreographers of medical care is to support patients and families in their natural desire to be together.

Internet Resources

Emergency Nurses Association Position Statements: Family Presence at the Bedside During Invasive Procedures and Resuscitation:
http://www.ena.org/about/position/familypresence.asp

American College of Emergency Physicians: Family Presence in the Emergency Department:
http://www.acep.org/1,2082,0.html

Journal Article: Family Presence During Pediatric Resuscitation: A Focus on Staff:
http://www.critical-care nurse.org/pdfLibra.NSF/Files/McGahey_Ccn_Dec02/$file/McGaheyCEOnline.pdf

Journal Article: Family presence during cardiopulmonary resuscitation and invasive procedures: practices of critical care and emergency nurses.
http://www.ncbi.nlm.nih.gov/entrez/query.fcgi?cmd=Retrieve&db=PubMed&list_uids=12751400&dopt=Abstract

Sigma Theta Tau: Online Continuing Education Program:
http://www.nursingsociety.org/education/case_studies/cases/SC0004.html

American Medical News:
http://www.ama-assn.org/sci-pubs/amnews/pick_00/hll20918.htm

Trauma Services Operations Manual:
http://www.traumasystems.com/ostnc/Family%20Presence.htm

Nursing Spectrum: Career Fitness Online:
http://community.nursingspectrum.com/MagazineArticles/article.cfm?AID=9784

Bibliography

American Heart Association, in Collaboration with the International Liaison Committee on Resuscitation: Guidelines 2000 for cardiopulmonary resuscitation and emergency cardiovascular care, *Circulation* 102(8 suppl):I-374, 2000.

Bassler P: The impact of education on nurses' beliefs regarding family presence in a resuscitation room, *J Nurses Staff Dev* 15(3):126-131, 1999.

Bourdeaux E, Francis JL, Loyacano T: Family presence during invasive procedures and resuscitations in the emergency department: a critical review and suggestions for future research, *Ann Emerg Med* 40(2):193-205, 2002.

Eichhorn D, Meyers T, Guzzetta C et al: Family presence during invasive procedures and resuscitation: hearing the voice of the patient, *Am J Nurs* 101(5):48-55, 2001.

Emergency Nurses Association: Family presence at the bedside during invasive procedures and/or resuscitation, *Resolution* 93:2, 1993.

Haddad A: Family presence during codes, *RN* 65(11):31-34, 2002.

Mason D: Families: in the way? (editorial) *Am J Nurs* 100(2):7, 2000.

Meyers T, Eichhorn D, Guzzetta C: Do families want to be present during CPR? A retrospective survey, *J Emerg Nurs* 24(5):400-405, 1998.

Rosenczweig C: Should relatives witness resuscitation? Ethical issues and practical considerations, *Can Med Assoc J* 158(5):617-620, 1998.

Walker W: Do relatives have a right to witness resuscitation? *J Clin Nurs* 8(6):625-630, 1999.

Chapter 45

End-of-Life Care

Winnie Hennessy

1. When is "end of life" considered end of life (EOL)?

Several questions arise in the definition of EOL:
- Is EOL considered to be when a human is imminently dying, within hours of death?
- Or is EOL when a patient is expected to die within a few weeks?
- Or is EOL a phase of life, when a particular disease has reached a stage when cure is no longer feasible? For example, the phase of life and disease that represents the terminal phases of a disease, such as stage IV heart failure.

Alternatively, the Medicare benefit defines EOL as the last 6 months of life.

For the purposes of this chapter, EOL is defined as the terminal phase of any disease process, in this case end-stage heart disease.

2. What is palliative care?

Palliative medicine, a specialty practiced by doctors, was defined in 1987 in Britain as the study and management of patients with active, progressive, or far-advanced disease for whom prognosis is limited and focus of care is quality of life. In 1990, the World Health Organization (WHO) defined palliative care as "the active total care of patients whose disease is not responsive to curative treatment. Control of pain, of other symptoms, and of psychological, social and spiritual problems, is paramount. The goal of palliative care is achievement of the best quality of life for patients and their families."

Palliative care is the care offered by a team of doctors, nurses, therapists, social workers, clergy, and volunteers. The palliative care paradigm is the framework for active comprehensive therapeutic strategies for patients whose disease is not responsive to curative treatment. The WHO definition and the related paradigm were initially created for patients in the terminal stages of cancer but have been expanded to incorporate all terminal illnesses regardless of underlying disease.

3. What is establishment of goals of care?

A cornerstone of developing a meaningful palliative care plan is the establishment of goals of care with patient and family. Goals of care, in the palliative care framework, are comprehensive, collaborative, and interdisciplinary. The goals of care focus on the physical, social, psychological, spiritual, and cultural components of the disease, as experienced by a patient and family. Each of these components must be thoroughly assessed, with the findings of the assessment clearly disseminated to the health care team. From this assessment, an appropriate individual plan of care can be established. For example, one patient may have an extensive family network (minimal social needs) but have intolerable regret (extensive psychological or spiritual needs). Another patient may live alone with a limited local family network (high social and community needs) and have moderate pain and symptoms disturbances (simple medical and pharmaceutical needs) but be spiritually at peace (minimal spiritual needs).

4. What is the role of the nurse in EOL care?

The role of the nurse in EOL care is critical. The primary perspective that the discipline of nursing offers the health care system is focus on how the environment of disease and family impacts a patient's view of health and well being. The nurse not only reviews one perspective of a person's health, such as disease and physiology (medical model focus), pharmaceuticals (pharmacy focus), nutrition (dietician focus), social/community environment (social worker focus), or spiritual perspective (chaplain focus), but integrates all these perspectives when assessing, planning, implementing, and evaluating a patient's needs. This holistic perspective places nursing as a key health care provider and quality-of-life facilitator in EOL and palliative care.

5. What is hospice?

Hospice is a program of care that focuses on improving the quality of the dying experience. The National Hospice and Palliative Care Organization (NHPCO) describes the hospice philosophy as programs that provide palliative care and supportive services to individuals at the end of their lives, their families, and significant others. Hospice programs are available 24 hours a day, 7 days a week, in both home and facility-based care settings. Hospice programs address physical, social, spiritual, and emotional care. This care is provided and coordinated by a medically directed interdisciplinary team during the last phase of an illness, the dying process, and bereavement. Often, many hospices serve the same community. As with any business, services and the quality of services provided vary. Some hospices, for example, may have designated inpatient beds within a hospital system; some are free-standing (separate building with hospice beds), and some offer home care only. Therefore it is helpful to patients if nurses have an idea of the types of hospices in their local community and the services that those hospices provide.

6. What are the hospice eligibility criteria for patients with heart disease?

The following examples are guidelines to determine whether a patient with heart disease is hospice eligible:
- Symptoms of recurrent congestive heart failure (CHF) at rest classified as New York Heart Association class IV. Ejection fraction of less than 20% is helpful

objective evidence but is not required. Persistent symptoms of CHF, despite attempts with optimal treatment with diuretics and vasodilators (including angiotensin-converting enzyme [ACE] inhibitors)

Other indicators include symptomatic supraventricular or ventricular arrhythmias that are resistant to antiarrhythmic therapy, history of cardiac arrest and resuscitation in any setting, history of unexplained syncope, cardiac brain embolism (embolic cerebrovascular accident [CVA] of cardiac origin), and concomitant HIV disease.

7. Can patients receive palliative care without hospice?

Yes. Some patients may not opt for hospice care. However, palliative and supportive care strategies should still be implemented to meet the needs of the patient and family.

8. What are the most common symptoms experienced by terminally ill patients?

The most common symptoms terminally ill patients experience are:
- Asthenia (fatigue).
- Anorexia/cachexia.
- Anxiety, depression.
- Constipation.
- Delirium.
- Nausea/vomiting.
- Pain.

Additional symptoms frequently treated in palliative care include:
- Cough.
- Diarrhea.
- Dysphagia.
- Edema.
- Fever.
- Hyperacidity (reflux).
- Insomnia.
- Malodor.
- Oral candidiasis.
- "Death rattle" (noisy, moist breathing).

For patients with advanced heart failure, the most common symptoms are pain, dyspnea, abdominal fullness, depression, decrease in functional status, nausea, dry mouth, and cachexia. Pain, dyspnea, and delirium are especially prevalent and exacerbated in the last few weeks of life.

9. What are the most common medications used to treat the symptoms of patients who are terminally ill with heart failure?

Regardless of underlying disease, nursing and medical therapies to manage the symptoms of the terminally ill are driven, most often, by the individual patient's subjective experience. Pharmacological therapies to manage symptoms in terminal illness must also be compatible with medications needed to keep the heart failure stable. Most terminally ill cardiac patients are on both cardiac medical regimens to optimally manage the heart disease and drug therapies to manage the subjective experiences of terminal phase of the heart disease. These regimens are often complex as the number of medications and their interactions are complex. Therefore a patient's medication therapy may need to be reviewed from an interdisciplinary perspective. In heart failure, understanding the underlying mechanism of action is important, to not prescribe a medication that may exacerbate the heart failure, thereby complicating the unwanted symptom. Specifically, those medications with anticholinergic effects (such as Amitriptyline) may exacerbate the heart failure and further complicate the presentation of the symptom. Morphine (both sustained and normal release) is the most commonly used opioid for pain management. Morphine is also the drug of choice for management of severe dyspnea. With prescription of an opioid, a laxative with motility property (not just stool softener) must be prescribed as well for management of constipation. Constipation is an inevitable side effect of opioid therapy. Haloperidol (Haldol) is the drug of choice to treat delirium and is also commonly prescribed for the management of nausea and vomiting. Metoclopramide hydrochloride is also commonly prescribed for nausea and vomiting. Dexamethasone is commonly prescribed for asthenia and anorexia/cachexia syndromes. Death rattle, an extremely distressing symptom to family members, can be minimized with a scopolamine patches (one behind each ear). However, scopolamine patches take at least 8 hours for the desired effect; atropine ophthalmic 1% solution, two drops sublingual every 4 hours, can cover short-term needs.

10. What can be expected in the last few hours of life?

Patients who are imminently dying can range from the essentially comatose patient who simply slows respirations in a regular rhythmic slowing pattern and quietly stops breathing to the conscious patient who requires skilled management of dyspnea.

11. Are palliative care therapies limited to "low-tech" therapies?

No. Many technological advances offer unique strategies for pain and symptom control. Central venous access should not be ruled out simply because it is an invasive procedure or because the patient's condition is terminal. Central venous access may be the only access for intravenous drug therapies to manage symptoms that are out of control. One example of the need for intravenous access is the patient with heart failure who may be dependent on intravenous dobutamine. This therapy, which enhances quality of life, should not be discontinued simply because it is categorized as invasive or life promoting.

Common sense suggests, however, that the benefit of an invasive technology must outweigh the burden that the technology imposes. For example, intravenous access may not be necessary for a morphine drip because subcutaneous delivery systems are available and exceptionally well tolerated.

12. What are some of the nontraditional and low-tech therapies in palliative care?

Music therapy, as simple as allowing patients to listen to their own music with a tape or CD player, can have a profound impact on relieving suffering. Art therapy is also a powerful medium for expression of emotions and feelings. Although art supplies can be expensive, simple crayons or colored pencils and clean white paper from the computer printer at the nurses' station can serve as wonderful inexpensive supplies. Some patients benefit from writing their story, expressing their suffering or joy or life experiences in a diary. These stories can be a legacy, a connection, to the grandchildren they may not meet and can also be a great relief. Other patients may benefit from having a loved one read their favorite book to them or perhaps from listening to a book on tape. Music, art, writing, and reading are activities that the nurse can facilitate with or without family. Other therapies, such as acupuncture, massage, and aromatherapy, should also be considered. Many patients seek these therapies and do not disclose that they use them for fear of being ostracized by the traditional Western health care system.

13. How is positioning used in EOL care?

Positioning is a key element to the comfort of the patient who is within weeks of dying. Many of these patients are either bed or chair bound. Positioning a pillow underneath the head with neck support to avoid hyperextension of the neck can mean the difference between breathing at ease or with difficulty. The most common error is a pillow that is too thick and too hard. Pillows need to allow the head to remain neutral to the spine and take up the space of the natural cervical curve of the neck. Arms can be supported under the elbow and lower arm. They should be lifted onto pillows (or other support mechanism) with the elbows curved so the lower arm and hands are positioned, at a minimum, level with the patient's waist. Positioning the arms appropriately eases pain and dyspnea and conserves energy. When a patient is in bed, a slight incline of the head (5 to 10 degrees) eases breathing and eases dependent fluid from accumulating around the neck and head. This positioning also relieves intracranial pressure and improves cardiac output. Headaches may be relieved by simply raising the head of the bed by a few degrees. Placement of head and arm pillows is crucial. Gatching the knees, placing a pillow under the knees to flex the knees upward (can also be accomplished with hospital beds by raising the knees), helps relieve the strain placed on the abdominal muscles. Abdominal muscles are accessory muscles for breathing, and releasing additional strain placed on them may ease dyspnea. If the patient is positioned on his/her side, a pillow or other support under the top (upper) leg relieves the spine and supports balance. Positioning the shoulder by pulling the bottom (lower) shoulder out from underneath the patient (a few degrees) and supporting the back with a pillow is the key. This shoulder position opens the thorax and again relieves the burden of breathing and conserves energy.

14. What environmental considerations are there in the care of patients at EOL?

Patients in any setting, if possible, should be allowed to use their own pillow with their own pillowcases (if patients have excessive saliva or sweating, a towel should be used to protect the pillow; the towel should be positioned in such a way that patients see the pillow). Terminally ill patients are especially sensitive to smell and touch. Their own pillow with their own smell eases the spirit. Addition of their own afghan or blanket eases the spirit again. A display of pictures, a mobile, a drawing from a grandchild, and cards from friends all supply simple and yet deeply meaningful and comforting environmental stimuli. Music is also an environmental intervention. Music therapy is a powerful emotional trigger. Patients or families need to give input in the types of music a patient prefers and also when to play the music. Some patients prefer quiet, and others prefer the background noise of a television. Odor control is another environmental intervention that is frequently not assessed by nurses. Aromas from perfumes, hair sprays, and foods, especially when patients are nauseated, can impose a form of "silent suffering." Patients may also have malodor from lesions. It is important to ask the patient what aromas are pleasant or obtrusive and adapt the environment accordingly.

15. What considerations for hygiene and skin care should be taken with EOL care?

Nothing lifts the spirits of a patient like simple hygiene and exquisite skin care. Specific attention should be given to face, mouth, and groin areas. Many terminally ill patients do not need their arms, torso, and legs washed every day (lotion may be more appropriate); however, patients need daily attention (sometimes twice a day or more) to the face, mouth, and perineal areas. A warm, soft, moist cloth may be used to wash the face and remove old crusts from the eyes. Application of eye drops to rinse the eyes is helpful. Washing a patient's hair or shaving the legs of a woman or the face of a man (if that is the norm) can lift a patient's spirit to participate in simple social activities or promote invitations for visitors. Curling a woman's hair or applying make-up can lift a woman's spirit to encourage her engagement with the environment.

Mouth care is critical to prevent painful mouth sores. A combination of viscous liquids and topical analgesics may be helpful in keeping the oral mucosa moist. Ice chips and water may actually promote drying of the mucosa but may help with the sensation of dry mouth. Dry mouth is rarely associated with dehydration (see controversies in EOL care) but is most often a side effect of the medications the patient is taking. Dry mouth is also suspected to be the result of the disrupted physiology of the dying process.

16. How does simple hygiene impact self-worth and dignity?

Imagine if you have not washed your hair or brushed your teeth in several days. Would you want to communicate with your loved ones if you felt unclean along with the fact that you are dying? Sometimes in palliative care these simple truths are what offer our patients the best chance at quality of life while dying. In other words, reexamine the daily routines. Find out what is important to the patient when it comes to hygiene. Explore the skin type of the patient. It may be more important to provide lotion to the extremities and only use a mild soap and water to the underarms and perineal/groin areas. Many elderly persons do not wash their arms and legs every day with soap and water (much too drying for older skin).

Get to know the patient's normal hygienic routines. Families are a wonderful support here and are often relieved to be able to do something.

17. What is the difference between grieving and depression in EOL?

Distinguishing between grief (a reaction to loss) and depression (psychiatric disorder) in terminally ill patients is challenging. The challenge rests with the fact that characteristics used to assess depression (physical and psychological) are commonly present in terminally patients and families who are grieving appropriately. However, the following characteristics are a few differences shared in the literature to offer guidance:

- Temporal variation: Grief is often experienced in waves triggered in response to a specific loss, whereas a persistent flat affect that pervades all aspects of life is characteristic of depression.
- Progress with time: Grief commonly diminishes in intensity over time, whereas patients with depression stay in this state without treatment.
- Self image: Grieving patients usually have a normal self-image, whereas patients who are depressed have a sense of worthlessness and disturbed self-esteem.
- Anhedonia: Grieving patients are able to feel pleasure (upcoming anniversary, birth of a child), whereas patients who are clinically depressed cannot.
- Hopelessness: Grieving patients maintain a sense of hope (hope may shift from hope of a cure to hope for comfort), whereas pervasive hopelessness is a hallmark of depression.

Depression and grief are different conditions that require different treatments. Depression is not considered a normal part of the dying process, whereas grieving is.

18. What are the cultural implications of EOL care?

All patients live within their own cultural networks. Cultural heritage defines and informs an individual, a family, the community, and the society at large and the values and beliefs and actions that form health care decision making. These cultural perspectives are heightened and play a crucial role near EOL. The cultural perspective of the patient and the family must be clearly understood in planning and implementing the goals of care.

For example, ethnic groups have, in general, different perspectives on the withdrawal of life support. African-Americans and Mexican-Americans are less likely to withdraw life support compared with European-Americans. In some Asian groups, discussions of the prognosis and death are "protected" from the patient, with the family determining the course of decision making. However, most European-American groups use a shared family format with the patient as the primary autonomous decision maker.

19. How do patient perspectives fit into EOL care?

Interestingly, given the focus on the patient in palliative care, little research has explored what patients actually expect from the health care system in terms of EOL care. A qualitative study in Canada interviewed 126 noncancer EOL patients. Patients identified five domains of quality EOL care. These domains were: 1, receiving adequate pain and symptom management; 2, avoiding inappropriate prolongation of dying; 3, achieving a sense of control; 4, relieving burden; and 5, strengthening relationships with loved ones. This study emphasized the need to talk to the patient. Find out what is important to patients. Understand what they need from you, and then facilitate meeting the need. The needs and perspectives form the basis for establishing goals of care that are meaningful to the patient and family.

20. What considerations are important in EOL care in the acute care setting?

A nurse's role is to understand and help the family and the patient. Family dynamics are impacted by the role of the dying family member within the family. A dying matriarch, a dying child, and a dying husband and father all impact the norms of the family life and structure differently. A nurse can facilitate open visitation if permitted by the institution. If open visitation is not permitted for the dying patient, the nurse should, for the short term, advocate for the dying patient by addressing the limitations of such as policy and, for the long term, become involved in revising the visitation policy. Family presence at night can be critical for the management of the delirious or confused patient. Family members need up-to-date and current information. Families often request that the nurse explain again what the physician told them, explain procedures, and explain the "normal" course of events. Families need preparation regarding the normal dying process. Preparing family members for what "dying looks like" (agonal breathing patterns, changing skin color and texture, changing levels of consciousness) may ease the fear of the moment and is a critical supportive role of the nurse. Families need permission to feel tired, fearful, or overwhelmed and need support to promote grieving. Finally, hospice referrals, when appropriate, offer families a wealth of support. The nurse in the acute care setting can assist in facilitating a plan of care to maintain continuity and transfer of care from the acute care setting to the home.

21. Are patients enrolled in hospice ever admitted to the acute care hospital?

Yes, patients can be admitted to the hospital even if the patient is enrolled in hospice. Normally, hospice patients are admitted to the acute care setting with an exacerbation of a symptom that can no longer be managed in the home. The acute care nurse and the hospice nurse must communicate the goals of care for the patient and family on admission. As with any other patient, the ideal is that discharge planning begins with the admission of the patient. This caveat is especially important with EOL care planning and especially important if the patient (and family) desires to die at home. The acute care nurse must communicate with the hospice, relating the events of the hospital admission and how therapy may have changed, to manage the symptom.

22. What are community resources for the family?

Depending on family needs, the family may benefit from a referral to a community group that provides respite care. Other families may be ready for the help of a local support group for bereavement and grief. Social workers are wonderful resources to assist families in accessing community resources. Nurses can also offer to contact family or hospital clergy.

23. What is a current controversy in the field of EOL care?

One controversial issue in palliative care is feeding and hydration of terminally ill patients. Little evidence exists that lack of food or water impacts the suffering of patients. On the contrary, force feeding with tube feedings and promotion of hydration may increase suffering by increasing demand on waste maintenance (urination and defecation, especially when mobility becomes an issue), edema, pulmonary congestion, and pain. Thirst and dry mouth are two different sensations. Thirst is readily managed with sips of fluids at the demand of the patient. Mild to moderate dehydration in the terminally ill (not an illness-free individual) may reduce physiological burden. Terminally ill patients rarely complain of being hungry. However, if they do, hunger is easily managed by offering the patient what they desire. Families are often distressed that patients quit eating and die of starvation. In reality, it is the underlying disease that is disrupting the normal physiology of the body. The anorexia/cachexia syndrome is present in all terminal phases of diseases. Little is known about the caloric needs of the "dying physiology." Often families perceive the lack of hunger and not eating as "giving up." However, the patient is not starving to death but is dying from an underlying disease process.

Key Points

- Palliative care is not just for the dying or just for patients with cancer.
- Distinguishing between grief (a reaction to loss) and depression (a psychiatric disorder) at EOL is challenging but essential.
- Underlying disease that disrupts the normal physiology of a body is what triggers the dying process, not the lack of food or water.
- Suffering at EOL is not only physiologic but also has cultural, social, psychological, and spiritual components. The nursing holistic perspective is instrumental in reducing suffering at EOL.

Internet Resources

Center to Advance Palliative Care:
http://www.capc.org/

Hospice and Palliative Nurses Association:
http://www.hpna.org

Americans for Better Care of the Dying:
http://www.abcd-caring.com

American Academy of Hospice and Palliative Medicine:
http://www.aahpm.org/

Department of Pain Medicine and Palliative Care at Beth Israel:
http://stoppain.org

Bibliography

Albert N et al: Improving the care of patients dying of heart failure, *Cleveland Clin J Med* 69(4):321-328, 2002.

Brant JM: The art of palliative care: living with hope: dying with dignity, *Oncol Nurs Forum* 25(6):995-1003, 1998.

Braun KL et al: *Cultural issues in end-of-life decision making,* Thousand Oaks, Calif, 2000, Sage.

Ferrell BR et al: *Textbook of palliative nursing,* New York, 2001, Oxford University Press.

Hospice care: a physician's guide, 1998, National Hospice Organization.

McCaffery M et al: *Pain: clinical manual,* St Louis, 1999, Mosby.

Panke J: Difficulties in managing pain at the end of life, *Am J Nurs* 102(7):26-34, 2002.

Periyakoil VS et al: Identifying and managing preparatory grief and depression at the end of life, *Am Fam Physician* 65:883-890, 2002.

Singer P et al: Quality end-of-life care: patient perspectives, *JAMA* 281(2):163-168, 1999.

Stjernsward J et al: The World Health Organization Cancer Pain and Palliative Care Program: past, present, and future, *J Pain Symptom Management* 12(2):65-72, 1996.

The SUPPORT principle investigators: A controlled trial to improve care for seriously ill hospitalized patients: the study to understand prognoses and preferences for outcomes and risks of treatments (SUPPORT), *JAMA* 274(20):1591-1598, 1995.

Chapter 46

Genetics

Marcia Van Riper

1. What is the Human Genome Project?

The Human Genome Project is a publicly funded international effort involving more than 2000 scientists that is being coordinated by the National Institute of Health and the US Department of Energy. When the project was initiated in 1990, the ultimate goal was to map the human genome (complete set of genetic instructions in each human cell) by 2005. On February 12, 2001, the Human Genome Project's initial draft sequence and analysis of the human genome was published in *Nature*. A more polished version of the draft sequence and analysis was published. Not only does this mean that the project is being completed ahead of schedule, it is also being completed under budget. The project is also being completed right in time for the fiftieth anniversary of Watson and Crick uncovering the chemical basis of heredity with their description of DNA's double-helix structure.

2. How has the field of health care been affected by the Human Genome Project?

Recent advances in genetics made possible through the Human Genome Project have revolutionized the field of health care by providing the molecular tools needed to determine the hereditary component of most diseases. The demand for genetic services, especially genetic testing, has never been greater. In addition, the way in which these services are accessed and delivered has been dramatically changed by the convergence of genetics, electronics, and biotechnology. Genetics is rapidly becoming an integral part of routine health care. No longer is genetics something that only genetic specialists from tertiary health centers are interested in. Health care providers in all settings and roles are caring for growing numbers of individuals and families who want and deserve high-quality genetic health care.

3. What are two key findings of the Human Genome Project?

- All human beings are 99.9% identical at the DNA level.
- Approximately 30,000 to 35,000 genes exist in the human genome.

4. How will the general public benefit from the Human Genome Project?

The increased availability of genetic testing and other genetic services has given more and more individuals and families the opportunity to discover whether they are at increased risk for certain diseases or have the potential to transmit gene mutations to future generations. Awareness of genetic risk can facilitate informed health care decisions and, in some cases, promote risk reduction behaviors that help people live longer and healthier lives. Ultimately it is hoped that findings from the Human Genome Project will make diagnostic, preventative, and treatment options possible for not only genetic diseases but also common diseases, such as cancer, heart disease, and diabetes.

5. What are the minimum competencies that all health care professionals should have regarding genetics?

Members of the Core Competency and Curriculum Work Group at the National Coalition for Health Professional Education in Genetics (NCHPEG) have suggested that at a minimum each health care professional should be able to appreciate the limitations of his/her genetic expertise, understand the social and psychological implications of genetic services, and know how and when to make referrals to genetics professionals.

6. What role will nurses play in the delivery of genetic health care?

Nurses are in an ideal position to help individuals and families maximize the benefits of the genetic revolution. With their frontline position in the health care system and their longstanding history of providing holistic, family-centered care, nurses are likely to be the first health care providers to whom individuals and families turn with questions about genetic risk and susceptibility. In addition, nurses are likely to be the first health care providers from whom individuals and families seek guidance regarding the complexities of genetic testing and interpretation.

7. What are specific genetics-related activities that nurses might be involved in?

- Collaborating with genetic specialists in interdisciplinary clinical partnerships.
- Collecting, reporting, and recording genetic information.
- Offering genetic information and resources to individuals and families.
- Supporting informed choice regarding health and reproductive decisions.
- Participating in the management of individuals and families affected by genetic conditions.
- Evaluating and monitoring the impact of genetic information, testing, and treatment on individuals and families.

8. What is being done to address possible ethical, legal, and social implications of the Human Genome Project?

Individuals involved in the planning of the Human Genome Project recognized that the information gained from mapping and sequencing the human genome would have profound implications for individuals, families, and society. Although this information has the potential to dramatically improve human health, it also raises a number of complex ethical, legal, and social issues. How should this new genetic information be interpreted and used? Who should have access to it? How can people be protected from the harm that might result from its improper disclosure or use?

The Ethical, Legal, and Social Implications (ELSI) Program was established in 1990 as an integral part of the National Human Genome Research Institute (NHGRI) to address these issues. Each year, NHGRI commits more than 14 million dollars from its Human Genome Project budget to the study of ethical, legal, and social issues. The NHGRI-ELSI Program was designed to provide a new approach to scientific research by identifying, analyzing, and addressing the ethical, legal, and social implications of human genome research at the same time that the scientific issues were being studied.

9. What areas of research have been established as priorities for the NHGRI-ELSI Program?

- Privacy and fairness in the use and interpretation of genetic information.
- Responsible clinical integration of genetic technologies.
- Issues surrounding genetics research.
- Public and professional education.

10. What is genetic testing?

Genetic testing involves the analysis of human DNA (deoxyribonucleic acid), RNA (ribonucleic acid), chromosomes (threadlike packages of genes and other DNA in the nucleus of a cell), or proteins to detect abnormalities related to an inherited condition. At this time, more than 900 genetic tests are commercially available or in research development. Most of the genetic tests currently offered in clinical practice are tests for single-gene disorders in individuals with clinical symptoms or with a family history of a genetic disease.

11. What types of genetic testing are available at this time?

- Prenatal testing: testing used to determine the genetic status of a pregnancy at risk for a genetic condition (maternal serum screening, chorionic villus sampling, and amniocentesis).
- Newborn screening: testing used to screen newborn infants for abnormal or missing gene products (phenylketonuria [PKU] testing).
- Carrier testing: testing used to identify individuals who have a gene mutation for a genetic condition but do not show symptoms of the condition because the condition is inherited as autosomal recessive (e.g., cystic fibrosis, sickle cell disease, and Tay-Sachs disease).
- Predictive testing: testing used to clarify the genetic status of asymptomatic family members.

12. What are two types of predictive testing?

- Predispositional testing (testing for a BRCA1 mutation).
- Presymptomatic testing (testing for the Huntington's disease mutation).

13. What is the main difference between predispositional and presymptomatic testing?

Predispositional testing differs from presymptomatic testing in that a positive result to a predispositional test for a BRCA1 mutation (indicating that a BRCA1 mutation is present) does not indicate that the individual has a 100% risk of developing the condition (breast cancer). In contrast, a positive result to a presymptomatic test for Huntington's disease (indicating that the mutation is present) does indicate that the individual has a 100% risk of developing the condition (Huntington's disease).

14. Give examples of genetic testing for conditions that affect the heart.

- Prenatal testing for genetic disorders that are known to be associated with congenital heart disease (Down syndrome, Turner's syndrome, trisomy 13 syndrome, trisomy 18 syndrome, and velocardiofacial syndrome).
- Newborn screening for hyperlipidemia, familial hypercholesterolemia, and hemochromatosis.
- Genetic screening for cardiovascular disorders, such as hypertrophic cardiomyopathy, as part of the preparticipation sports physical examinations.
- Targeted screening of relatives of individuals already diagnosed with inherited cardiac conditions, such as familial hypercholesterolemia.

15. What are the rights of the individual in regards to genetic testing?

The decision to undergo genetic testing should be the decision of the individual being tested. There should be no coercion. Sometimes the suggestion to undergo testing does not originate from the individual who is considering testing. The suggestion may have come from an insurance company, a family member, an adoption agency, a potential mate, or an employer. Before any testing is done, the individual being tested must give consent and it must be informed consent. Strictly speaking, an individual can give informed consent for genetic testing only after full disclosure of pertinent information concerning the genetic test and full understanding of the risks, benefits, and limitations of the test. Individuals who choose to undergo genetic testing have a right to know who will have access to the test results before they undergo the test. They also have a right to know how and when they will be informed of the results.

16. What is pharmacogenomics?

Pharmacogenomics is the use of genetic information to individualize drug therapy. Dr Francis Collins, director of NHGRI, has speculated that pharmacogenomics may become part of standard practice for a large number of disorders and drugs by 2020. The expectation is that with identification of common variants in genes that are associated with the likelihood of a good or bad response to a specific drug, drug prescriptions can be individualized based on the individual's unique genetic make-up. A primary benefit of pharmacogenomics is the potential to reduce adverse drug reactions.

17. What are some of the major challenges involved in bringing pharmacogenomics from the research bench to the bedside?

- Most health care professionals receive little, if any, instruction about pharmacogenomics as part of formal training.
- The economic impact of introducing genotyping as a guide for developing individual therapy has not been addressed. Who will provide the genotyping? How much will it cost? Who will pay for it? Will it be covered by insurance?

18. Give an example of how pharmacogenomics information could be used in cardiovascular nursing.

Pharmacogenomic information could be helpful in the care of patients receiving warfarin to prevent or treat thromboembolisms. Warfarin is metabolized primarily by the CYP2C9 enzyme. Individuals who are deficient in CYP2C9 enzyme activity may require a lower warfarin dose or more frequent monitoring and may be at higher risk for bleeding episodes. CYP2CP enzyme genotype assays are readily performed in research labs and are currently being developed for commercial use. It is likely that clinicians would be able to interpret the results and use them as they care for patients taking warfarin. To date, a definitive study has not linked CYP2C9 to adverse drug reactions and warfarin use, but several studies have found an association between the CYP2CP genotype and adverse drug reactions. Other genetic polymorphisms that may affect individual responses to cardiovascular drugs are reviewed and discussed in an article by Humma and Terra (2002).

19. How is genetics applicable to nursing care for the cardiovascular patient?

Recent discoveries in molecular biology and genetics have made it clear that cardiovascular disease may result from a variety of genetics-related causes: single-gene mutations, chromosomal defects, the interactions of multiple genes and environmental factors, and environmental factors operating in a susceptible genetic background. High-throughput genomic technology, also known as microarray or "DNA chip," is increasingly used to identify genetic predictors of cardiovascular disease. Unfortunately, genetic risk assessment for cardiovascular disease is less advanced and less widely performed than it is for cancer and other diseases. In addition, much more must be learned about associations between genetic polymorphisms and responses to cardiovascular drugs before pharmacogenomics information can be routinely incorporated into therapeutic decisions.

20. **What are some of the genetics-related activities that advanced practice nurses in cardiovascular nursing might provide?**
    - Identifying individuals with cardiovascular conditions that have a significant genetic component.
    - Performing genetic health assessments.
    - Identifying elements of a family history suggestive of increased risk for cardiovascular conditions with a significant genetic component.
    - Facilitating the informed consent process.
    - Offering genetic information and assessing comprehension.
    - Providing genetic counseling.
    - Identifying individual, family, and community resources.
    - Making a referral to genetic specialists.
    - Providing psychosocial interventions for families who are adjusting to a recent genetic diagnosis.
    - Providing care for individuals and families affected by or at risk for cardiovascular conditions that have a significant genetic component.
    - Serving as a consultant to other health care professionals.
    - Collaborating with experts in genetics.
    - Recognizing risks for stigma and discrimination.
    - Serving as an advocate for individuals with genetic conditions and their family members.
    - Developing, conducting, and evaluating genetic research.
    - Coordinating and participating in multidisciplinary genetic studies.
    - Participating in the development of recommendations to address the ethical, legal, and social implications of existing and future genetic services.
    - Applying findings from genetic research.
    - Participating in public and private educational efforts in genetics.

21. **Identify two of the current controversies concerning genetics and cardiovascular disease.**
    - Testing of individuals with a family history of cardiac disease for specific variants of the ApoE gene.
    - The use of gene therapy/gene transfer for the treatment of vascular disease.

 Key Points

- Genetics is rapidly becoming an integral part of routine health care.
- Recent discoveries have made it clear that cardiovascular disease may result from a variety of genetics-related causes.
- The decision to undergo genetic testing should be the decision of the individual being tested.
- Pharmacogenomics is the use of genetic information to individualize drug therapy.

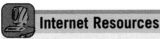 **Internet Resources**

AACN: Clinical Issues- Foundations of Genetics:
http://www.aacn.org/AACN/jrnlci.nsf/GetArticle/ArticleThree94?OpenDocument

Centers for Disease Control and Prevention: Office of Genetics and Disease Prevention:
http://www.cdc.gov/genomics/default.htm

Genetics Program for Nursing Faculty at the Cincinnati Children's Hospital Medical Center:
http://www.cincinnatichildrens.org/education/gpnf/

Genetic Science Learning Center:
http://gslc.genetics.utah.edu/

Life a Study of Genetics and Molecular Biology:
http://library.thinkquest.org/20465/games.html

Online Talking Glossary of Genetics:
http://www.genome.gov/glossary

Human Genome Project of the U.S. Department of Energy:
http://www.ornl.gov/hgmis/

National Human Genome Research Institute:
http://www.nhgri.nih.gov/ and http://www.nhgri.nih.gov/educationkit/

Online Mendelian Inheritance in Man (OMIM):
http://www3.ncbi.nlm.nih.gov/omim/

Online Talking Glossary of Genetics:
http://www.genome.gov/glossary.cfm

Bibliography

Cheek DJ, Cesan A: Genetic predictors of cardiovascular disease: the use of chip technology, *J Cardiovasc Nurs* 18:50-56, 2003.

Collins F, Guttmacher A: Genetics moves into the medical mainstream, *JAMA* 286:2322-2324, 2001.

Collins F, McKusick VA: Implications of the human genome project for medical science, *JAMA* 285:540-544, 2001.

Guttmacher AE, Collins FS: Genomic medicine—a primer, *N Engl J Med* 347:1512-1520, 2002.

Humma L, Terra S: Pharmacogenetics and cardiovascular disease: impact on drug response and applications to disease management, *Am J Health Syst Pharm* 59:1241-1252, 2002.

International Human Genome Sequencing Consortium: Initial sequencing and analysis of the human genome, *Nature* 409:860-921, 2001.

Lea DH: What nurses need to know about genetics, *Dimens Crit Care Nurs* 21:50-60, 2002.

Lea DH, Jenkins JF, Francomano C: *Genetics in clinical practice: new directions for nursing and health care*, Sudbury, Mass, 1998, Jones and Bartlett.

Lea DH, Williams JK: Are you ready for the genetics revolution? *Am J Nurs* 101:11, 2001.

Mahowald MB, McKusick VA, Scheuerle AS et al: *Genetics in the clinics: clinical, ethical, and social implications for primary care*, St Louis, 2001, Mosby.

Merkle C, Montgomery D: Gene therapy with vascular endothelial growth factor reduces angina, *J Cardiovasc Nurs* 18:38-43, 2003.

Phillips KA, Veenstra DL, Oren E et al: Potential role of pharmacogenomics in reducing adverse drug reactions, *JAMA* 14:2270-2279, 2001.

Roses AD: Pharmacogenetics and the practice of medicine, *Nature* 405:857-865, 2000.

Sparks EA, Frazier L: Heritable cardiovascular disease in women, *J Obstet Gynecol Neonatal Nurs* 31:217-228, 2002.

Special Issue: *J Cardiovasc Nurs* 13:4, 1999.

Tinkle MB, Cheek DJ: Human genomics: challenges and opportunities, *J Obstet Gynecol Neonatal Nurs* 31:30-38, 2002.

Wung S: Genetic advances in coronary artery disease, *MEDSURG Nurs J* 11:296-300, 2002.

Index

C

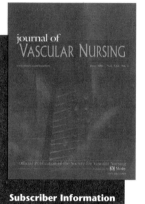